Breast and Axilla Localisation Techniques

Raghavan Vidya • Nisha Sharma
Editors

Breast and Axilla Localisation Techniques

Current Trends, Techniques and Tips

Springer

Editors
Raghavan Vidya
Department of Breast Surgery
The Royal Wolverhampton NHS Trust
Wolverhampton, UK

Nisha Sharma
Department of Breast Radiology
St James's University Hospital
Leeds, UK

ISBN 978-3-032-17994-4 ISBN 978-3-032-17995-1 (eBook)
https://doi.org/10.1007/978-3-032-17995-1

This Springer imprint is published by the registered company Springer Nature Switzerland AG
The registered company address is: Gewerbestrasse 11, 6330 Cham, Switzerland

This book is dedicated to all our patients, the clinicians and industry who have supported and allowed us to embrace precision surgery to advance and shape the future of breast cancer care.

Preface

Breast cancer remains one of the most common cancers worldwide, and despite significant advances in systemic therapies and diagnostics, surgery continues to be a cornerstone of its management. With improvements in imaging, a growing proportion of breast cancers are now impalpable at diagnosis, underscoring the increasing importance of precise preoperative localisation. For decades, wire-guided localisation served as the gold standard. Yet, with evolving technology, logistical challenges associated with wire placement and the pursuit of improved patient experience and surgical precision, non-wire localisation techniques have emerged and rapidly progressed to the forefront of modern breast surgery. Simultaneously, axillary management has undergone a profound transformation. The paradigm has shifted away from radical clearance towards more tailored, minimally invasive strategies such as targeted axillary dissection. These advances reflect a broader movement in breast cancer care—towards precision, individualisation and preservation without compromising oncological outcomes. This book was conceived to capture these significant developments.

As the first text devoted exclusively to the localisation of breast lesions and the contemporary management of the axilla, it brings together the experience and insights of leading global experts. The intention is not only to summarise current trends but also to deepen understanding, refine technique and provide clear, practical guidance for clinicians navigating this rapidly evolving field.

The journey of this book began 18 months ago. Like many clinical endeavours, its progress was influenced by service pressures, competing demands and the ever-changing landscape of breast care. Yet, through the commitment of our contributors and the support of our publishers and editors, the project has finally come to fruition. We are deeply grateful to all the authors who generously shared their expertise and to everyone who helped bring this work into the light of day.

This is a practical, user-friendly text designed to support breast surgeons, radiologists, radiographers, trainees and multidisciplinary teams in contemporary practice. Our aim is to provide clear, accessible, experience-based guidance that enhances patient care and supports clinicians as they adapt to advancing technologies and evolving standards.

It is with great enthusiasm that we present this work, and we trust that the knowledge shared within these pages will contribute meaningfully to clinical practice and to the advancement of breast cancer care worldwide.

Wolverhampton, UK Raghavan Vidya
Leeds, UK Nisha Sharma

Acknowledgements

Reflecting on the evolution of wire localisation, it is remarkable to observe how successive technological innovations have continually reshaped the management of breast lesions. The transition from traditional wire-guided techniques to contemporary wireless localisation systems represents a pivotal advance in surgical precision, patient experience and overall outcome optimisation. Inspired by this progression, I organised the first meeting on breast and axilla localisation in Wolverhampton in 2018, establishing a multidisciplinary forum that fostered collaboration and the exchange of emerging evidence and best practices.

My fascination with the art and science of plastic and reconstructive surgery began in India and deepened during my formative years at Stanley Medical College—an institution with a distinguished legacy spanning over three centuries. I am deeply grateful to my teachers at Holy Angels Convent and Adarsh Vidyalaya, whose early guidance laid the foundation for my education and values. I also extend my sincere thanks to my mentors and colleagues at Stanley Medical College and Coimbatore Medical College, as well as to the Edinburgh Breast Unit, and my colleagues in the Wessex and West Midlands regions, for the invaluable training and support I received.

No journey is complete without the steadfast support of family, and I am profoundly grateful to mine. My father, the late Mr. Raghavan; my mother, Annapoorani; my sister, Chitra, and brother-in-law, Vaidyanthan; my husband, Dr. S. Venkatachalam; and my son, Abhinav, have been my anchors. Their patience, encouragement and sacrifices have made every achievement possible. I also wish to honour the late Mr. Raja Krishnan of Quilon and Mrs. Kumari Rajakrishnan for their enduring support. A special tribute goes to my late brother, Mahesh Vishnu, to whom I offer heartfelt and respectful remembrance.

Finally, I extend my heartfelt gratitude to all the authors who contributed to this book, generously sharing their expertise and detailing their surgical techniques. I am deeply thankful to my patients, whose trust and collaboration form the very foundation of meaningful clinical progress. I also wish to express my sincere appreciation to Springer Verlag for their invaluable support in bringing this work to publication.

Raghavan Vidya, UK

As a breast radiologist, it is amazing to see how technology has advanced in the last decade to support oncoplastic techniques allowing women the choice of breast surgery.

When I started as a consultant in 2007, wire localisations were the only means of supporting breast conservation in women with impalpable breast cancers. The way we localised and performed surgery had not changed for three decades. Then there was a shift from mastectomy to support breast conserving oncoplastic surgery for women with multifocal or multicentric disease. This was a significant shift in the landscape, which was important for women, but led to a significant silent increase in workload for breast imaging. This meant more biopsies, requirement for contrast-based imaging and the need to be able to localise the biopsy proven cancers to support the surgeons to deliver successful single stage operations. The advent of non-wire localisers has transformed the patient pathway and raised the expectation of both patients and surgeons.

I feel privileged to have witnessed such a positive transformation.

I was born in Glasgow and completed my medical training at University of Glasgow. After my MRCP, I decided to pursue a career in Radiology and late in my training chose to specialise in breast. I started my radiology training in Glasgow but completed it at Leeds. I am grateful to my parents for their unwavering support and belief in me. My husband for all his support—personally and professionally. All my friends and colleagues that I have met through my journey, who have helped shape me, provided me with opportunities and kept me going when the path has been difficult or obscured.

My driver and passion is to improve the pathway for all women and men affected by breast cancer by utilising innovations and technologies that support earlier and accurate diagnoses.

Nisha Sharma, UK

Contents

Chapter 1
Current Update in the Management of Screen-Detected Breast Cancers

Aiswarya Sukumar, Ngee-Ming Goh, Thomas Hubbard, and Nisha Sharma

Contents

A. Sukumar · N.-M. Goh
Department of Breast Surgery, Royal Devon University Hospital NHS Trust, Exeter, UK
e-mail: aiswarya.sukumar@nhs.net; ngee-ming.goh@nhs.net

T. Hubbard (✉)
Department of Breast Surgery, Royal Devon University Hospital NHS Trust, Exeter, UK

Faculty of Health and Life Science, University of Exeter, Exeter, UK
e-mail: thubbard1@nhs.net

N. Sharma
Department of Breast Radiology, St. James's Hospital, Leeds, UK
e-mail: nisha.sharma2@nhs.net

R. Vidya, N. Sharma (eds.), *Breast and Axilla Localisation Techniques*,
https://doi.org/10.1007/978-3-032-17995-1_1

1.1 Introduction

Breast cancer is the most common cancer in women in the UK. There are approximately 56,822 new cases of breast cancer each year [1], of which at least 23% could have improved outcomes if detected early. Early detection is therefore crucial in improving outcomes with population-based screening serving as the bedrock for screening programmes across the world. Breast screening became prevalent in the mid-1980s, although global interest began earlier, with the American Cancer Society recommending mammography as early as 1976 [2]. Screening mammograms employ low dose X-rays to detect early tumours before they become symptomatic. This is pivotal in reducing breast cancer mortality. Although breast screening uptake increased to 64.6% in 2022–2023 from 62% in the previous year, it remains below the recommended acceptable threshold of 70% [3]. Newer imaging modalities such as digital breast tomosynthesis (DBT) [4], multiparametric breast MRI [5] and recently even artificial intelligence [6] has been used to improve breast imaging accuracy and efficiency. Screen-detected breast cancers are often small and pre-invasive in nature making them amenable to curative treatment as opposed to larger tumours. However, there are debates surrounding overdiagnosis during routine screening mammography especially in older women, prompting discussion around the need for personalised screening approaches. It is therefore more important than ever to examine the current trends and challenges in breast cancer screening. Through this chapter, we aim to look at the National Health Service (NHS) Breast Screening programme, the characteristics of cancers detected through the screening and the treatment approaches tailored to screen-detected cancers.

1.2 NHS Breast Screening Programme

NHS Breast Screening Programme was introduced in 1988 based on the recommendations by Sir Patrick Forrest in his report in 1986 [7].The working group chaired by Sir Forrest was appointed by the UK Ministers of Health to examine whether UK policy should be revised to include mammographic screening for asymptomatic women. This was based on the mounting evidence from international trials such as the Malmo trial [8]and the Swedish Two-County trials [9] which advocated for the introduction of screening. The group advised four stages in the screening which began with screening to detect an abnormality, followed by clinical examination, biopsy, and treatment for the screen-detected cancer. The report recommended mammographic screening for women aged 50–64, every 3 years. It also emphasised the importance of continued research and quality assurance to ensure that this remains cost-effective and efficient [7]. This was crucial in the formation of the NHS breast screening programme.

In 2012, Cancer Research UK and the Department of Health, commissioned another working group chaired by Sir Michael Marmot to study the efficiency and harm of breast screening programmes. This group concluded that breast screening extends lives, probably preventing up to 1300 breast cancer deaths annually. However, it also emphasised overdiagnosis—cancers detected by screening, proven pathologically as cancers but would not have been detected in the absence of screening. These cancers would be treated with surgery, chemotherapy, or radiotherapy but it is unsure if these cancers would have become apparent without screening leading to progression of symptoms or remained indolent throughout the woman's lifetime. The panel recommended further trials examining the need for treatment, and tailor treatment options for DCIS, continued support for the Sloane project [10], which has an extensive database of screen-detected DCIS which might further our understanding in the management of these cases in the long run [11].

The screening programmes delivered by UKHSA (UK Health Security Agency), formerly Public Health England in partnership with NHS Trusts currently invites women aged 50–70 for a routine mammogram every 3 years. Invitations are sent based on GP registrations, and the women invited undergo a two-view digital mammography at a static unit or a mobile breast screening unit. There are ongoing discussions to expand the ages to include women from ages 47–73. AgeX trial thus was implemented to look at the benefits and harm of screening programmes in women aged 47–49 and women aged 71–73 in two separate trials and the final report is expected in 2031 [12].

Recent developments include trials such as PROCAS lifestyle study (Predicting Risk of Breast Cancer at Screening) which ran from 2009 to 2015. It aimed to accurately predict the breast cancer risk by incorporating risk factors such as family history and lifestyle as standard in the breast screening programme [13]. Another such study is the ATHENA–M project which created a large high-quality and representative dataset of individual women's screening trajectories and outcomes in England from 1997 to 2018. This aided in the evaluation and optimisation of screening processes [14].

With the increasing availability of new imaging technologies such as Digital Breast Tomosynthesis and Contrast-Enhanced Mammography, and the explosion in the understanding of genetic risk factors for breast cancer, more adaptive and tailored screening is being investigated. Risk-adapted screening approaches will aim to personalise breast cancer management with the aim of reducing overdiagnosis while refining prognostic precision [15, 16].

1.3 Higher Risk Screening

Although screen-detected cancer is overwhelmingly from the mammographic programme, another arm of the NHS Breast Screening Programme is those women at high risk of breast cancer which defines high risk as women with a strong family history of breast cancer or ovarian cancer, and Women are considered as high-risk if the 10-year risk of developing breast cancer is more than 8%, or lifetime risk is greater than 30% [17]. This 10 year risk estimate can be assessed by software programmes such as BOADICEA (CanRisk) or Tyrer Cuzick. Those at very high risk are those with previous chest wall irradiation or genetic mutations including BRCA1, BRCA 2 and TP53 [18].

Women at higher risk are offered earlier and more frequent surveillance screening compared to the general population. Surveillance screening typically includes two imaging modalities—MRI and mammogram. The UK's National Institute for Health and Care Excellence (NICE) guidelines recommend that high risk women can be offered an annual MRI concurrently with mammograms from the age of 30 except in TP53 mutation carriers, due to their increased sensitivity to radiation induced damage. In the NHS BSP high-risk programme, women are offered breast MRI from age of 25 and mammography and breast MRI from 40 years of age. Annual MRI should be offered to women with TP53 mutation from the age of 20. Studies have shown that MRI (71–94%) has an increased sensitivity compared to mammography (36–59%) albeit with a lower specificity [17]. The Magnetic Resonance Imaging for Breast Screening (MARIBS) trial examined the cost-effectiveness of MRI screening in high-risk women in the UK. It confirmed the higher sensitivity of contrast-enhanced MRI in detecting breast cancers, and acceptable specificity in comparison with mammograms [19].

The high-risk screening population is more often associated with aggressive tumour biology including higher grade cancers and rapid progression, triple negative or HER-2 positive subtypes at a younger age, reinforcing the need for an annual MRI and/or mammogram [20]. Therefore, the treatment of these high-risk cancers in younger patients is generally much more aggressive than for standard screen-detected cancers.

1.4 DCIS (Ductal Carcinoma In Situ)

Ductal Carcinoma In Situ (DCIS) is a precursor to invasive breast carcinoma characterised by the proliferation of neoplastic epithelial cells of the mammary ducts, confined within the basement membrane. The aetiology behind DCIS is largely unknown but some cases of DCIS are linked to genetic predispositions such as BRACA1 and BRACA2 [21]. Advances in screening techniques have led to a marked increase in the detection of DCIS. Prior to the introduction of screening, DCIS was typically an incidental finding. It now accounts for approximately 25% of breast cancers detected through screening.

DCIS is commonly identified on mammograms by the presence of microcalcifications [21]. Low-grade DCIS is characterised by low mitotic counts, monomorphic nuclei proliferation and evenly spaced luminal epithelial cells with uniform chromatin distribution whereas high-grade DCIS is characterised by high mitotic counts, pleomorphic nuclei and randomly spaced luminal epithelial cells with coarse chromatin. Biomarkers such as oestrogen and progesterone receptors are expressed in

70–80% of DCIS and has prognostic implications and predicts response to endocrine therapy. Other biomarkers include HER-2 receptor, p-53, Ki-67 seen in high-grade DCIS [22]. DCIS, although a precursor of invasive disease, a substantial proportion of cases do not progress to invasive cancer.

There are several trials currently underway to risk stratify DCIS, determine its natural history and optimise management to reduce over treatment. These studies are limited by the difficulty in accurately identifying which cases are DCIS are truly low-risk. The LORD (Low-risk DCIS Observation or Radiotherapy) trial is one such randomised trial, later modified to patient preference trial, that aims to compare standard treatment with active surveillance with regular mammograms for low-grade DCIS [23]. The COMET (Comparing an Operation to Monitoring, With or Without Endocrine Therapy) trial is another randomised trial, whose findings support the short-term safety of active surveillance to standard treatment for ER, PR positive, HER2 negative low-risk DCIS [24]. The LORIS (Low Risk DCIS) trial is a multicentre, phase three, randomised study for women aged 46 or higher with low-risk DCIS which examines if active surveillance is non-inferior to surgery in terms of ipsilateral invasive breast cancer-free survival time [25].

1.5 Invasive Breast Cancer

1.5.1 Prognostic Variable in Screen Detected Breast Cancer Outcomes

Survival rates for breast cancer are approximately 95%, 85% and 75% at 1, 5 and 10 years, respectively. There are several prognostic factors that influence outcomes and overall survival in breast cancer. Tumour size, lymph node involvement, hormone receptor status, margins, lymphovascular invasion, and tumour biology are some of these factors. Large tumour size, positive lymph nodes or lymphovascular involvement, negative hormone receptors and positive surgical resection margins are associated with poorer prognosis [26]. As previously noted, screen-detected cancers are often smaller in size and therefore associated with a more favourable prognosis. Survival statistics may also be inflated by including indolent cancers which may not have become clinically apparent during the patient's lifetime. Due to advances in mammographic screening, any population studies examining disease-free survival time and time to metastasis may be skewed by overdiagnosis, lead time and length time bias [27].

A West Midlands study of over 1900 patients compared screen-detected with symptomatic detected cancers in prognostic variable comparable groups. This found the survival differences were small, suggesting the survival advantage seen in the screen-detected group is primarily due to the difference in tumour size and nodal status [28].

1.5.2 Size of Cancers Detected in Screening

Tumour size is an important prognostic factor in breast cancer as it influences the probability of lymphatic spread, and subsequently, overall survival. Screening plays a key role in identifying cancers before they reach a larger size. Screen-detected cancers have a median size of 8 mm compared to 15 mm in symptomatically detected cancers [29]. Of all cancers detected through the NHS Breast Screening Programme, 79.3% were invasive. Small, invasive tumours (<15 mm) comprised 47.2% of all invasive cancers and 37.5% of all cancers [30].

Tumour size plays a crucial role in determining the treatment modalities particularly in smaller cancers. A large proportion of smaller cancers are now diagnosed due to the breast screening programme. Even a small variation in size can alter the staging of the tumour and consequently its management—making it eligible or ineligible for breast-conserving surgery, radiotherapy or systemic therapy. However, tumour size alone is not adequate to determine the prognosis of breast cancer. Other factors such as nodal status, molecular subtype and hormonal receptor status determine prognosis and survival and direct the treatment pathway [31].

1.5.3 Genetic Signatures

Genomic expression profiling is increasingly recognised as providing improved prognostic and decision-making information than traditional clinicopathological risk factors. These advances in genomic assays play a role in enhancing tailored decision-making and identifying those suitable for de-escalation of systemic therapies. The utility of the 21 gene panel Oncotype dx prognostic ‘recurrence score’ in guiding treatment plans was quickly realised through the TailorRx [32] and Rxponder trials [33]. This has allowed for a significant reduction in the volume of chemotherapy administered for patients in a non-high-risk recurrence score group [34].

Another example of genetic scoring is the Oncotype DX Breast DCIS Score test which generates a score thereby predicting the risk of recurrence or progression to invasive disease and response to radiotherapy after DCIS [35]. MammaPrint (70 GS) is a 70-gene signature assay which analyses the expression of 70 genes in the tumour sample and predicts the risk of recurrence in women with early-stage, HR positive, HER2 negative breast cancer [36]. Prosigna is a PAM-50 assay which identifies the intrinsic subtype of the tumour and predicts the risk of distant recurrence [37].

1.6 Other Lesions Detected at Screening

Other lesions detected in screening are pathological abnormalities such as breast lesions of uncertain malignant potential (B3 lesions). B3 lesions can co-exist with in situ and invasive cancers, and their rate of upgrade to DCIS and invasive cancer is highly unpredictable and variable, making their management challenging [38]. They are identified on screening, confirmed via core-needle biopsy, and if surgery is required, it is often performed as an excisional biopsy following lesion localisation [38, 39]; The NHS BSP provide comprehensive guidelines on the management of these lesions, and subsequent surveillance is recommended [40]. The NHS BSP now recommend vacuum-assisted excision (VAE) as an alternative to surgery for many B3 lesions.

1.7 Treatment

Screen-detected cancers are treated like any other breast cancer, but they tend to be smaller, less advanced with a high proportion of DCIS. Therefore, we will focus on treatment of pre-invasive and small breast cancers.

Breast cancer treatment can largely be categorised as surgery, chemotherapy, radiotherapy and immunotherapy. Treatment decisions are guided by the stage, hormone receptor status and tumour biology. As screen-detected cancers are caught often early, and are small, treatment approaches are usually less aggressive [41].

1.7.1 Breast Surgery

Surgical treatment in screen-detected breast cancer consists of breast-conserving surgery (BCS) and mastectomy, with axillary surgery (sentinel node biopsy or axillary node clearance (ANC)) for invasive disease and no axillary surgery for DCIS.

Surgery involves either BCS in the form of wide local excision, or mastectomy depending on the tumour location, size, genetic factors and patient preference. Breast-conserving surgery in combination with radiotherapy has become the standard of care for breast cancers when technically feasible and there is no contraindication to radiotherapy. It involves removing the affected breast tissue with a margin while maintaining the cosmetic appearance of the breast. The NSABP 06 trial demonstrated its oncological equivalence to mastectomy in 1976 in invasive breast cancer, and new data suggests there may even be some oncological benefit to performing BCS—though the mechanism of this is unknown [43, 44]. Advanced oncoplastic techniques, such as volume replacement and volume displacement, allow for larger volume tissue resection and maintenance of a satisfactory cosmetic result, and the indications for BCS continue to grow [45]. Although there has never been a formal

RCT to compare BCS to mastectomy in DCIS, it has been adopted from extrapolation of the oncological safety demonstrated in invasive disease trials (e.g. NSABP B06). Due to the size of the tumours detected, BCS is commonly utilised in the management of DCIS.

Studies have shown that the rate of mastectomy is lower in the screened population (25.3%) when compared to the symptomatic group (31.1%) [46].

Overall, for both invasive cancer and DCIS, lesions that are multicentric, locally widespread, containing diffuse microcalcifications, or in patients with a previously irradiated thoracic wall, typically require mastectomy [47].

Margins have been a contentious issue over the years, with recommended safe widths changing and there being differing guidance around the world. Balancing advancements in oncoplastic techniques and improved cosmetic outcomes against the cost of re-excisions and most essentially oncological outcomes is important, and hence large teams (Houssami 2014 [48]/Bundred 2022 [49]) undertook meta-analyses. Methodology, findings and recommendations differed resulting in the Association of Breast Surgery (ABS) commissioning the Sheffield Centre for Health and Related Research (ScHARR) to independently review the two meta-analyses. In 2024, NICE guidelines [50] were updated and concordant ABS Guidelines [51] were published, confirming the importance of accurate preoperative imaging assessment and ratifying a 'clear' margin to be one with no invasive disease or DCIS within 1 mm of the inked radial margin. Notable mention was made of need for multidisciplinary team (MDT) discussion when disease was within 1 mm, citing varying patient factors such as low or high risk of recurrence, age and fitness of patient and patient wishes. Prospective audit internally by individual breast units was recommended.

With DCIS, whilst dispute still exists, the diffuse nature of the disease and differing adjuvant regimens is well recognised, thus necessitating slightly differing guidance—NICE [50] and ABS [52] currently recommends a 2 mm margin [52]. Some of the studies informing this is a meta-analysis by Ezzat et al. [53], and a data registry study by Robertson et al. [54] that both reached the same conclusion that 2 mm was the optimal margin for reducing local recurrence rate. It is clear that representative tissue sampling, good preoperative imaging and localisation are vital, and the importance of intraoperative specimen imaging is highlighted within the ABS guidelines as strongly recommended and as representing best practice for all screen-detected non-palpable lesions. It plays a vital part in confirming complete excision and in guiding when and which margins need re-excision.

1.7.2 Localisation

As lesions are predominantly impalpable, localisation is often required prior to wide local excision. Wire-guided localisation is a conventional method a thin wire is inserted into the lesion. However, it needs to be done either on the day of the surgery and is often dependent on the availability of the breast imaging team. Additionally, it carries a risk of being displaced. This technique is now being replaced by a myriad of different localisation approaches which allow localisation to be decoupled from the day of surgery, offering departments greater logistical flexibility, though their cost-effectiveness, safety and efficacy are still to be completely validated, and carry other disadvantages including interference with MRI and questionable suitability for patients with pacemakers and defibrillators. Other localisation techniques that are in use include radioactive seed localisation, radio-occult lesion localisation and radiofrequency identification tags [55]. One group investigating this is the iBRA-NET (implant Breast Reconstruction evaluation-NETwork)—a UK-based group prospectively auditing these techniques with some published data showing non-inferiority in terms of safety and efficacy comparing Magseed® [56], SCOUT® Radar, Hologic LOCalizer™ and Sirius Pintuition®. The merits of the different localisation systems are discussed in more detail in subsequent chapters.

1.7.3 Nodal Surgery

For the screening patient, axillary surgery follows standard guidelines with preoperative staging via ultrasound and lymph node biopsy when indicated. Those with invasive disease and a preoperative negative axilla proceed to sentinel lymph node biopsy (SLNB) alongside their primary surgery. Those with DCIS and having BCS should have SLNB omitted, unless there is a high risk of invasive disease. Due to the difficulties post-mastectomy, SLNB was perceived to be a necessary option for those undergoing mastectomy—the advent of MagTrace® has however shifted the ground further, allowing SLNB omission in even more patients by enabling surgeons to perform a delayed SLNB if required [57].

There is also the continuing trend of de-escalation to consider for the axilla. Updated American Society of Clinical Oncology [58] (ASCO) guidelines following the SOUND [59] and INSEMA [60] trials now ask clinicians to consider omission of SLNB in post-menopausal patients, over the age of 50, with negative preoperative axillary staging, and T1, grade 1–2, ER-positive, Her2-negative invasive breast cancer. Given the characteristics of screen-detected invasive cancers, these guidelines are pertinent with UK guidelines updated awaited.

For those patients with biopsy-proven axillary lymph node metastasis, axillary node clearance remains the standard recommendation, though this too is being challenged. Whilst the ATNEC [61] trial may be applicable for those screening cases requiring neoadjuvant chemotherapy, of greater relevance for the screening cohort is likely to be the TADPOLE study [62]. This UK-based trial is aiming to compare targeted axillary dissection (TAD) to ANC in patients with low volume nodal disease having upfront surgery, with primary end points being lymphoedema rates and locoregional recurrence. Recruitment is due to start in 2025. The European TAXIS study plans to randomise 1500 to either TAD followed by axillary clearance and regional nodal irradiation, or receive TAD followed by regional nodal irradiation and has been recruiting for many years and has published its feasibility sub-study [63].

1.7.4 Adjuvant Therapies

Radiotherapy

The offer of adjuvant radiotherapy then follows BCS once clear margins are confirmed with invasive cancer. Following the IMPORT–LOW [64] trial this can be as partial breast irradiation in patients with a low risk of recurrence (aged over 50, tumour 3 cm or less, N0, ER-positive, Her2-negative, grade 1–2) and for whom endocrine therapy is recommended. The regime length has also substantially changed since the FAST-FORWARD [65] trial, with a 26 Gy, 1-week routine proven to be non-inferior to the 40 Gy, 3-week routine. The obvious logistical benefits, particularly advantageous during the Covid-19 pandemic, accelerated the uptake and introduction of the hypofractionated and newer method.

When in relation to DCIS, once clear margins are achieved, *consideration* of adjuvant radiotherapy is recommended following BCS. It is generally accepted that there is a lack of up-to-date evidence in this domain, with older studies not reflecting current practice, newer proposed studies struggling to recruit, and scepticism about tools such as the Van Nuys Prognostic Index [66] (VNPI) given its first iteration was released in 1996. It is no surprise that NICE thus notes the importance of shared decision-making.

Following mastectomy, radiotherapy should still be offered to those with positive nodes (macrometastases) or involved margins, with T3 and T4 tumours to be considered as well. Results from the SUPREMO trial [67], which will soon be available to guide adjuvant radiotherapy post-mastectomy in patients with 'intermediate risk', such as, lymphovascular invasion and positive lymph nodes are no longer an absolute indication for chest wall radiotherapy.

There is less of a role for radiotherapy post-mastectomy in the DCIS patient. A prospective large-scale audit run by the Sloane group via the NHS Breast Screening Programme [68] (NHSBSP) has demonstrated that in UK practice, between 2003 and 2012, only 1.1% of DCIS patients were given radiotherapy post-mastectomy. This was associated with close margins (<1 mm), DCIS size and the presence of microinvasion—characteristics the authors pose may warrant radiotherapy to reduce ipsilateral recurrence—whilst conceding the lack of trials to clarify this.

Continuing the trend of de-escalation onto radiotherapy, after the Early Breast Cancer Trialists's Cooperative Group's meta-analysis demonstrated only modest survival benefit [69], albeit reducing recurrence in node-negative patients, further trials have emerged to promote the potential omission of radiotherapy. PRIME2 [70] completed recruitment in 2009 and recently published 10-year outcomes. In patients over 65 years of age with ER-positive, N0 disease, tumours <3 cm and receiving BCS with clear margins and having endocrine treatment, they demonstrated omission or radiotherapy to have higher incidence of local recurrence. However, there was no significant difference in distant recurrence or overall survival.

Subsequently PRIMETIME [71] was designed and is currently in follow-up. The lower age limit was lower at 60, with tighter tumour characteristics (<2 cm, grade 1–2, ER-positive, Her2-negative, N0) and with usage of the Ki67 tumour marker to calculate a IHC4+C score to risk-stratify patients. Whilst all patients should have 5 years of endocrine therapy, the 'very low risk' group would also be offered omission of radiotherapy.

Endocrine Therapy

NICE guidance for endocrine therapy is broadly established with a well evidenced update in 2018. In ER-positive disease, men and pre- and peri-menopausal women, and post-menopausal patients of low risk, are recommended 5 years of adjuvant Tamoxifen, with post-menopausal patients of medium or high risk to be offered an aromatase inhibitor (AI) instead. Given the likely tumour profile of patients in the screening programme, neoadjuvant endocrine therapy (NET) would be relatively uncommon, though still to be considered in the post-menopausal patient with an aim towards tumour size reduction when BCS is not feasible but desired. EndoNET [72] is a trial currently recruiting in the UK to better evaluate the effectiveness of NET, given the scarcity of evidence.

For the patient with ER-positive DCIS, following BCS endocrine therapy should be offered if radiotherapy has been recommended but not given.

Of note, specific applications such as ovarian function suppression (OFS) and extended adjuvant endocrine treatment would again be uncommon given the characteristics of the screening cohort, as well as primary endocrine therapy or bridging therapy for patients either indefinitely or temporarily unfit for surgery.

Guidance also exists to help manage the side effects of endocrine therapy, with a particular reminder to offer a dual energy X-ray absorptiometry (DEXA) scan to women either starting an AI, experiencing treatment-induced menopause or starting OFS, and in turn commencing bisphosphonate therapy when appropriate. Notably bisphosphonates themselves are increasingly used in higher risk patients to reduce bone metastasis.

Chemotherapy

Chemotherapy plays an important role in improving outcomes and prolonging survival in early-stage breast cancer. Anthracycline-based chemotherapy regime is often advised for women with node-positive cancers or high-risk node negative cancers. Trials such as TRYPHAENA [73] illustrated improved outcomes by incorporating docetaxel–carboplatin-based neoadjuvant chemotherapy to dual HER2 blockade regimen. NATT [74] trial demonstrated that anthracycline-based chemotherapy was more beneficial in patients with early breast cancer than anthracycline-free chemotherapy. Chemotherapy remains the mainstay of treatment for triple negative breast cancer, with immunotherapy being increasingly used in the neoadjuvant setting [75]. Chemotherapy in combination with endocrine therapy remains a viable option for both early and metastatic ER positive cancers [76].

Greater options are now also available for ER-positive, node positive and high-risk patients with the advent of cyclin-dependent kinase (CDK) 4/6 inhibitors. Abemaciclib is a recommended option for such patients provided they have at least four positive axillary lymph nodes, or one to three nodes alongside grade 3 disease or a tumour size of at least 5 cm [77]. Palbociclib and Ribociclib are options for those with locally advanced or metastatic disease, though a consultation period has closed and a further NICE committee meeting has taken place to consider extending Ribociclib's role.

1.8 Non-Invasive Management

Lastly, ongoing interest into the non-invasive management of early breast cancer has resulted in trials such as SMALL [78] and ICE3 [79]. SMALL is a UK based study comparing standard surgery to vacuum-assisting excision (VAE). With radiological advancements allowing increasingly accurate and larger volume excisions, the study is specifically recruiting patients with screen-detected (age > 47 years) small (<15 mm), low grade (1), unifocal and strongly ER and PR positive (Allred score 7–8), Her2-negative, normal axillary ultrasound and without any previous ipsilateral disease. The VAE arm would have no axillary surgery but by default be offered adjuvant radiotherapy and endocrine treatment. The ambitions are thus to evaluate the local recurrence risks of the two arms, but also the relative adequacy of the VAE technique compared to standard surgery in terms of margins and additional surgery or re-excisions.

ICE3 is a US trial that has evaluated the non-operative option of cryoablation. Similarly, it chose low-risk cases (grade 1–2, unifocal, <15 mm, ER/PR-positive, Her2-negative, lymph node negative) but in older patients (age > 60 years). Published results showed a 5-year ipsilateral breast tumour recurrence of 4.3% and breast cancer survival of 96.7%. As a small study of 194 patients, with only a single arm and no standardisation of adjuvant treatment, the authors noted the limitations whilst proposing further studies to confirm whether cryoablation is a safe alternative.

In the fullness of time, it therefore seems likely that there will be a group of low-risk patients with early screen-detected breast cancer that will be having non-operative management—a true continuation of the de-escalation trend.

1.9 Summary

- Breast cancer screening detects breast cancers early and reduces breast cancer-related mortality.
- Screen-detected cancers are commonly pre-invasive or small invasive cancers with good prognostic clinicopathological features.
- Treatment of screen-detected breast cancers is the same as for symptomatic breast cancer; but due to tumour characteristics, management is predominantly surgical, where breast-conserving surgery predominates.
- As screen-detected cancers reduce in size at diagnosis, there is increasing interest in the non-operative management of these tumours.

References

1. https://www.cancerresearchuk.org/health-professional/cancer-statistics/statistics-by-cancer-type/breast-cancer.
2. Nicosia L, Gnocchi G, Gorini I, et al. History of mammography: analysis of breast imaging diagnostic achievements over the last century. Healthcare (Basel). 2023;11(11):1596. https://doi.org/10.3390/healthcare11111596.
3. https://www.gov.uk/government/publications/breast-screening-consolidated-programme-standards/nhs-breast-screening-programme-screening-standards-valid-for-data-collected-from-1-april-2021.
4. Kleinknecht JH, Ciurea AI, Ciortea CA. Pros and cons for breast cancer screening with tomosynthesis – a review of the literature. Med Pharm Rep. 2020;93(4):335–41. https://doi.org/10.15386/mpr-1698.
5. Marino MA, Helbich T, Baltzer P, Pinker-Domenig K. Multiparametric MRI of the breast: a review. J Magn Reson Imaging. 2018;47(2):301–15. https://doi.org/10.1002/jmri.25790.
6. Ng AY, Glocker B, Oberije C, et al. Artificial intelligence as supporting reader in breast screening: a novel workflow to preserve quality and reduce workload. J Breast Imaging. 2023;5(3):267–76. https://doi.org/10.1093/jbi/wbad010.
7. Forrest APM. Breast cancer: the decision to screen. J Public Health Med. 1991;13(1):2–12. https://doi.org/10.1093/oxfordjournals.pubmed.a042572.
8. Andersson I, Aspegren K, Janzon L, et al. Mammographic screening and mortality from breast cancer: the Malmö mammographic screening trial. BMJ. 1988;297(6654):943–8. https://doi.org/10.1136/bmj.297.6654.943.
9. Tabár L, Vitak B, Chen TH, et al. Swedish two-county trial: impact of mammographic screening on breast cancer mortality during 3 decades. Radiology. 2011;260(3):658–63. https://doi.org/10.1148/radiol.11110469.
10. Clements K, Kearins O, Lawrence G, Bishop H. The Sloane Project: a UK prospective audit of screen-detected non-invasive carcinoma of the breast. Breast Cancer Res. 2006;8(Suppl 1):P50. https://doi.org/10.1186/bcr1465.
11. Marmot MG, Altman DG, Cameron DA, Dewar JA, Thompson SG, Wilcox M. The benefits and harms of breast cancer screening: an independent review. Br J Cancer. 2013;108(11):2205–40. https://doi.org/10.1038/bjc.2013.177.
12. https://www.ceu.ox.ac.uk/research/agex-trial/agex-trial.
13. https://www.cancerresearchuk.org/about-cancer/find-a-clinical-trial/a-study-looking-breast-cancer-risk-screening-procas.

14. Brettschneider J, Morrison B, Jenkinson D, et al. Development and quality appraisal of a new English breast screening linked data set as part of the age, test threshold, and frequency of mammography screening (ATHENA-M) study. Br J Radiol. 2024;97(1153):98–112. https://doi.org/10.1093/bjr/tqad023.
15. Tsarouchi MI, Hoxhaj A, Mann RM. New approaches and recommendations for risk-adapted breast cancer screening. J Magn Reson Imaging. 2023;58(4):987–1010. https://doi.org/10.1002/jmri.28731.
16. Trapani D, Sandoval J, Aliaga PT, et al. Screening programs for breast cancer: toward individualized, risk-adapted strategies of early detection. Cancer Treat Res. 2023;188:63–88. https://doi.org/10.1007/978-3-031-33602-7_3.
17. Gilbert FJ. Breast cancer screening in high risk women. Cancer Imaging. 2008;8 Spec No A(Spec Iss A):S6–9. https://doi.org/10.1102/1470-7330.2008.9002.
18. https://www.gov.uk/government/publications/breast-screening-higher-risk-women-surveillance-protocols/protocols-for-surveillance-of-women-at-higher-risk-of-developing-breast-cancer#:~:text=women%20with%20a%20lifetime%20risk,including%20the%20age%20of%2050.
19. Leach MO, Boggis CR, Dixon AK, et al. Screening with magnetic resonance imaging and mammography of a UK population at high familial risk of breast cancer: a prospective multicentre cohort study (MARIBS) [published correction appears in Lancet. 2005;365(9474):1848]. Lancet. 2005;365(9473):1769–78. https://doi.org/10.1016/S0140-6736(05)66481-1.
20. Sokolova A, Johnstone KJ, McCart Reed AE, Simpson PT, Lakhani SR. Hereditary breast cancer: syndromes, tumour pathology and molecular testing. Histopathology. 2023;82(1):70–82. https://doi.org/10.1111/his.14808.
21. Tomlinson-Hansen SE, Khan M, Cassaro S. Breast ductal carcinoma in situ. [Updated 2023 Feb 27]. In: StatPearls [Internet]. Treasure Island: StatPearls Publishing; 2025. Available from: https://www.ncbi.nlm.nih.gov/books/NBK567766/.
22. Sanati S. Morphologic and molecular features of breast ductal carcinoma in situ. Am J Pathol. 2019;189(5):946–55, ISSN 0002-9440. https://doi.org/10.1016/j.ajpath.2018.07.031.
23. https://www.dcisprecision.org/clinical-trials/lord/.
24. Hwang ES, Hyslop T, Lynch T, et al. Active monitoring with or without endocrine therapy for low-risk ductal carcinoma in situ: the COMET randomized clinical trial. JAMA. 2025;333(11):972–80. https://doi.org/10.1001/jama.2024.26698.
25. https://associationofbreastsurgery.org.uk/professionals/research/trials/closed-in-follow-up/loris#:~:text=Overview,diagnosed%20with%20low%20risk%20DCIS.
26. Allison KH. Prognostic and predictive parameters in breast pathology: a pathologist's primer. Mod Pathol. 2021;34(Supplement 1):94–106, ISSN 0893-3952. https://doi.org/10.1038/s41379-020-00704-7.
27. Cox B, Sneyd MJ. Bias in breast cancer research in the screening era. Breast. 2013;22(6):1041–5, ISSN 0960-9776. https://doi.org/10.1016/j.breast.2013.07.046.
28. Allgood PC, Duffy SW, Kearins O, et al. Explaining the difference in prognosis between screen-detected and symptomatic breast cancers. Br J Cancer. 2011;104(11):1680–5. https://doi.org/10.1038/bjc.2011.144.
29. Starikov A, Askin G, Blackburn A, et al. Mode of detection matters: differences in screen-detected versus symptomatic breast cancers. Clin Imaging. 2021;80:11–5. https://doi.org/10.1016/j.clinimag.2021.06.032.
30. https://digital.nhs.uk/data-and-information/publications/statistical/breast-screening-programme/england%2D%2D-2022-23/mainreport2223#section-6-cancers-detected.
31. Provencher L, Diorio C, Hogue JC, Doyle C, Jacob S. Does breast cancer tumor size really matter that much? Breast. 2012;21(5):682–5. https://doi.org/10.1016/j.breast.2012.07.003.
32. Sparano JA, Gray RJ, Makower DF, Pritchard KI, Albain KS, Hayes DF, Geyer CE, Dees EC, Goetz MP, Olson JA, et al. Adjuvant chemotherapy guided by a 21-gene expression assay in breast cancer. N Engl J Med. 2018;379:111–21.

33. Kalinksy K, et al. 21 Gene assay to inform chemotherapy benefit in node-positive breast cancer. N Engl J Med. 2021;385(25):2336–47.
34. Loncaster J, Armstrong A, Howell S, et al. Impact of Oncotype DX breast recurrence score testing on adjuvant chemotherapy use in early breast cancer: real world experience in Greater Manchester, UK [published correction appears in Eur J Surg Oncol. 2018;44(1):194. doi: 10.1016/j.ejso.2017.06.002]. Eur J Surg Oncol. 2017;43(5):931–7. https://doi.org/10.1016/j.ejso.2016.12.010.
35. https://www.breastcancer.org/screening-testing/oncotype-dx.
36. Cardoso F, van't Veer LJ, Bogaerts J, Slaets L, Viale G, Delaloge S, et al. 70-Gene signature as an aid to treatment decisions in early-stage breast cancer. N Engl J Med. 2016;375:717–29.
37. Jensen MB, Nielsen TO, Bartlett J, et al. Prosigna Risk of Recurrence score and intrinsic subtypes are associated with adjuvant anthracycline chemotherapy benefit in high-risk breast cancer. NPJ Breast Cancer. 2025;11:26. https://doi.org/10.1038/s41523-025-00738-7.
38. Pinder SE, Shaaban A, Deb R, et al. NHS Breast Screening multidisciplinary working group guidelines for the diagnosis and management of breast lesions of uncertain malignant potential on core biopsy (B3 lesions). Clin Radiol. 2018;73(8):682–92. https://doi.org/10.1016/j.crad.2018.04.004.
39. Rubio IT, Wyld L, Marotti L, et al. European guidelines for the diagnosis, treatment and follow-up of breast lesions with uncertain malignant potential (B3 lesions) developed jointly by EUSOMA, EUSOBI, ESP (BWG) and ESSO [published correction appears in Eur J Surg Oncol. 2024;50(3):107943. doi: 10.1016/j.ejso.2023.107943]. Eur J Surg Oncol. 2024;50(1):107292. https://doi.org/10.1016/j.ejso.2023.107292.
40. https://assets.publishing.service.gov.uk/media/5a808356e5274a2e8ab50931/Clinical_guidance_for_breast__cancer_screening__assessment_Nov_2016.pdf.
41. Sharma A, Ives C. Management of breast cancer: basic principles. Surgery. 2022;40:113–20.
42. Dillon MF, Hill AD, Quinn CM, et al. Surgical intervention in screen-detected patients versus symptomatic patients with breast cancer [published correction appears in J Med Screen. 2004;11(4):211]. J Med Screen. 2004;11(3):130–4. https://doi.org/10.1258/0969141041732238.
43. Fisher B, Anderson S. Conservative surgery for the management of invasive and noninvasive carcinoma of the breast: NSABP trials. National Surgical Adjuvant Breast and Bowel Project. World J Surg. 1994;18(1):63–9. https://doi.org/10.1007/BF00348193.
44. Rajan KK, Fairhurst K, Birkbeck B, et al. Overall survival after mastectomy versus breast-conserving surgery with adjuvant radiotherapy for early-stage breast cancer: meta-analysis. BJS Open. 2024;8(3):zrae040. https://doi.org/10.1093/bjsopen/zrae040.
45. de Boniface J, Szulkin R, Johansson ALV. Survival after breast conservation vs mastectomy adjusted for comorbidity and socioeconomic status: a Swedish national 6-year follow-up of 48 986 women. JAMA Surg. 2021;156(7):628–37. https://doi.org/10.1001/jamasurg.2021.1438.
46. James TA, Wade JE, Sprague BL. The impact of mammographic screening on the surgical management of breast cancer. J Surg Oncol. 2016;113(5):496–500. https://doi.org/10.1002/jso.24184.
47. Fajdic J, Djurovic D, Gotovac N, Hrgovic Z. Criteria and procedures for breast conserving surgery. Acta Inform Med. 2013;21(1):16–9. https://doi.org/10.5455/AIM.2013.21.16-19.
48. Houssami N, Macaskill P, Marinovich ML, Morrow M. The association of surgical margins and local recurrence in women with early-stage invasive breast cancer treated with breast-conserving therapy: a meta-analysis. Ann Surg Oncol. 2014;21(3):717–30. https://doi.org/10.1245/s10434-014-3480-5.
49. Bundred JR, Michael S, Stuart B, Cutress RI, Beckmann K, Holleczek B, et al. Margin status and survival outcomes after breast cancer conservation surgery: prospectively registered systematic review and meta-analysis. BMJ. 2022;378:e070346. https://doi.org/10.1136/bmj-2022-070346.
50. National Institute for Health and Care Excellence. Early and locally advanced breast cancer: diagnosis and management. NICE guideline. NG101. 2025. https://www.nice.org.uk/guidance/ng101. Published 18 July 2018. Accessed 8 June 2025.

51. Chagla L, Rigby K, Wyld L, et al. The management of radial surgical margins in relation to breast conservation surgery for invasive breast cancer. The Association of Breast Surgery. https://associationofbreastsurgery.org.uk/media/so1frd0u/invasive-radial-surgical-margins-v1ii.pdf. Accessed 8 June 2025.
52. Gandhi A, Cunnick G, Gibson E, et al. Association of Breast Surgery recommendations for the management of radial surgical margins in patients undergoing breast conserving surgery for ductal carcinoma in situ (DCIS). The Association of Breast Surgery. https://associationofbreastsurgery.org.uk/media/3z5bk0nj/dcis-margins-guidance-2024-v2.pdf. Accessed 8 June 2025.
53. Ezzat A, Shanthakumar D, Laskar N, Cutress R, et al. Impact of resection margin width on local recurrence following breast-conserving surgery and whole breast radiotherapy for pure ductal carcinoma in situ: a systematic review and meta-analysis. BMJ Oncol. 2025;4:e000633.
54. Robertson J, Sibbering M, Ndebele-Mahati S, et al. Surgical margins in breast conserving surgery (BCS) for ductal carcinoma in-situ (DCIS) and clinical outcomes: significant associations with increased recurrence and overall survival. Cancer Res. 2024;84(9_Supplement):PS01–10.
55. Banys-Paluchowski M, Kühn T, Masannat Y, et al. Localization techniques for non-palpable breast lesions: current status, knowledge gaps, and rationale for the MELODY study (EUBREAST-4/iBRA-NET, NCT 05559411). Cancers (Basel). 2023;15(4):1173. https://doi.org/10.3390/cancers15041173.
56. Dave R, Barrett E, Morgan J, Harvey J, iBRA-NET Localisation Study Collaborative. Wire- and magnetic-seed-guided localization of impalpable breast lesions: iBRA-NET localisation study. Br J Surg. 2022;109(3):274–82. https://doi.org/10.1093/bjs/znab443.
57. Karakatsanis A, Eriksson S, Pistiolis L, et al. Delayed sentinel lymph node dissection in patients with a preoperative diagnosis of ductal cancer in situ by preoperative injection with superparamagnetic iron oxide (SPIO) nanoparticles: the SentiNot study. Ann Surg Oncol. 2023;30:4064–72. https://doi.org/10.1245/s10434-022-13064-0.
58. Park KU, et al. Sentinel lymph node biopsy in early-stage breast cancer: ASCO guideline update. J Clin Oncol. 2025;43:1720–41. https://doi.org/10.1200/JCO-25-00099.
59. Gentilini OD, Botteri E, Sangalli C, et al. Sentinel lymph node biopsy vs no axillary surgery in patients with small breast cancer and negative results on ultrasonography of axillary lymph nodes: the SOUND randomized clinical trial. JAMA Oncol. 2023;9(11):1557–64. https://doi.org/10.1001/jamaoncol.2023.3759.
60. Reimer T, Stachs A, Veselinovic K, Kühn T, Heil J, Polata S, et al. Axillary surgery in breast cancer – primary results of the INSEMA trial. N Engl J Med. 2025;392:1051–64. https://doi.org/10.1056/NEJMoa2412063.
61. The ATNEC Study. 2025. https://sites.google.com/nihr.ac.uk/atnec/ATNEC. Accessed 8 June 2025.
62. NIHR. Targeted Axillary Dissection versus axillary node clearance in patients with POsitive axillary Lymph nodes in Early breast cancer: a multicentre, pragmatic, phase III randomised controlled trial. 2025. https://fundingawards.nihr.ac.uk/award/NIHR158400. Accessed 8 June 2025.
63. Weber W, Matrai Z, Hayoz S, et al. Tailored axillary surgery in patients with clinically node-positive breast cancer: pre-planned feasibility substudy of TAXIS (OPBC-03, SAKK 23/16, IBCSG 57–18, ABCSG-53, GBG 101). Breast. 2021;60:98–110.
64. Coles C, Griffin C, Kirby A, et al. Partial-breast radiotherapy after breast conservation surgery for patients with early breast cancer (UK IMPORT LOW trial): 5-year results from a multicentre, randomised, controlled, phase 3, non-inferiority trial. Lancet. 2017;390(10099):1048–60.
65. Brunt A, Haviland J, Wheatley D, et al. Hypofractionated breast radiotherapy for 1 week versus 3 weeks (FAST-Forward): 5-year efficacy and late normal tissue effects results from a multicentre, non-inferiority, randomised, phase 3 trial. Lancet. 2020;395(10237):1613–26.
66. Silverstein M, Lagios M, Craig P, et al. A prognostic index for ductal carcinoma in situ of the breast. Cancer. 1996;77:2267–74. https://doi.org/10.1002/(SICI)1097-0142(19960601)77:11<2267::AID-CNCR13>3.0.CO;2-V.

67. SUPREMO. 2025. https://www.supremo-trial.com/. Last accessed 8 June 2025.
68. Clements K, Dodwell D, Lawrence G, et al. Radiotherapy after mastectomy for screen-detected ductal carcinoma in situ. Eur J Surg Oncol. 2015;41(10):1406–10. https://doi.org/10.1016/j.ejso.2015.07.021.
69. Early Breast Cancer Trialists' Collaborative Group (EBCTCG), Darby S, McGale P, et al. Effect of radiotherapy after breast-conserving surgery on 10-year recurrence and 15-year breast cancer death: meta-analysis of individual patient data for 10,801 women in 17 randomised trials. Lancet. 2011;378(9804):1707–16. https://doi.org/10.1016/S0140-6736(11)61629-2.
70. Kunkler IH, Williams LJ, Jack WJL, Cameron DA, Dixon JM. Breast-conserving surgery with or without irradiation in early breast cancer. N Engl J Med. 2023;388(7):585–94. https://doi.org/10.1056/NEJMoa2207586.
71. PRIMETIME. 2025. https://www.hra.nhs.uk/planning-and-improving-research/application-summaries/research-summaries/primetime/. Accessed 8 June 2025.
72. EndoNET Study. 2025. https://www.nds.ox.ac.uk/research/surgical-intervention-trials-unit/endonet. Accessed 8 June 2025.
73. Schneeweiss A, Chia S, Hickish T, et al. Pertuzumab plus trastuzumab in combination with standard neoadjuvant anthracycline-containing and anthracycline-free chemotherapy regimens in patients with HER2-positive early breast cancer: a randomized phase II cardiac safety study (TRYPHAENA). Ann Oncol. 2013;24(9):2278–84. https://doi.org/10.1093/annonc/mdt182.
74. Chen X, Ye G, Zhang C, et al. Superior outcome after neoadjuvant chemotherapy with docetaxel, anthracycline, and cyclophosphamide versus docetaxel plus cyclophosphamide: results from the NATT trial in triple negative or HER2 positive breast cancer. Breast Cancer Res Treat. 2013;142(3):549–58. https://doi.org/10.1007/s10549-013-2761-1.
75. Schmid P, Cortes J, Pusztai L, et al. Pembrolizumab for early triple-negative breast cancer. N Engl J Med. 2020;382(9):810–21. https://doi.org/10.1056/NEJMoa1910549.
76. Hu W, Xu D, Li N. Research status of systemic adjuvant therapy for early breast cancer. Cancer Control. 2023;30:10732748231209193. https://doi.org/10.1177/10732748231209193.
77. National Institute for Health and Care Excellence. Abemaciclib with endocrine therapy for adjuvant treatment of hormone receptor-positive, HER2-negative, node-positive early breast cancer at high risk of recurrence. NICE Technology appraisal guidance TA810. 2025. https://wwwniceorguk/guidance/ta810/chapter/1-Recommendations. Published 20 July 2022. Accessed 8 June 2025.
78. SMALL Trial. 2025. https://www.birmingham.ac.uk/research/crctu/trials/small/small-trial. Accessed 8 June 2025.
79. Fine RE, Gilmore RC, Tomkovich KR, et al. Cryoablation without excision for early-stage breast cancer: ICE3 trial 5-year follow-up on ipsilateral breast tumor recurrence. Ann Surg Oncol. 2024;31(11):7273–83. https://doi.org/10.1245/s10434-024-16181-0.

Chapter 2
Surgical Management of Non-Palpable Breast Lesions

Salvatore M. Nardello, Abhishek Chatterjee, and Raghavan Vidya

Contents

S. M. Nardello (✉) · A. Chatterjee
Division of Surgical Oncology, Tufts Medical Centre, Boston, MA, USA
e-mail: Salvatore.Nardello@TuftsMedicine.org; Abhishek.Chatterjee1@TuftsMedicine.org

R. Vidya
Department of Breast Surgery, The Royal Wolverhampton NHS Trust, Wolverhampton, UK
e-mail: Raghavan.Vidya@nhs.net

R. Vidya, N. Sharma (eds.), *Breast and Axilla Localisation Techniques*,
https://doi.org/10.1007/978-3-032-17995-1_2

2.1 Introduction

Increased screening of breast cancer has markedly increased the detection of non-palpable breast lesions, including early-stage cancers and high-risk lesions which typically warrant surgical excision to rule out underlying carcinoma. These lesions, often identified through advancements in mammography, ultrasound, and/or magnetic resonance imaging (MRI), require precise localization for surgical excision due to their non-palpable nature. Precise localization techniques and surgical excision results in successful excision of the targeted non-palpable lesion with limited excision of adjacent healthy tissue.

Historically, wire-guided localization has been the gold standard, but with limitations such as wire displacement, patient discomfort, and logistical constraints, wireless technologies have evolved. Among these techniques, radioactive, magnetic, RFID, and radar reflective technologies have emerged to improve the limitations experienced with standard wire localization.

Concurrently, oncoplastic surgery has transformed breast conservation by integrating oncologic resection with aesthetic reconstruction, enhancing outcomes for patients with non-palpable lesions. Oncoplastic surgery also allows more patients to undergo breast conservation increasing the need for localization. Oncoplastic surgery enables more favourable cosmetic outcomes and reduces positive margin rates [1]. Numerous wireless localization technologies have emerged to respond to limitations with wires, thus enabling surgeons to offer effective solutions for non-palpable breast lesions, such as radioactive seeds, magnetic localization, radar reflectors, and radiofrequency tags. This chapter centres on wireless technologies due to the authors' extensive experience with wireless technology. Our focus on wireless technology reflects its practical application in our practice, aiming to improve not only oncologic outcomes, but improve workflow efficiency, and the overall patient experience. Wireless localization techniques allow us to provide detailed insights into its integration with surgical techniques, particularly oncoplastic approaches, axillary management, while recognizing that it is one of many innovative tools shaping modern breast surgery. Over time, wireless technologies have employed an innovative, wire-free technique leveraging a tiny marker to assist surgeons in overcoming numerous obstacles associated with conventional localization methods.

2.2 A Timeline of Localization: From Wires to Wireless Techniques

Preoperative needle-wire localization techniques first began in the 1970s following mammographic detection of breast abnormalities [2]. Since the 1970s, image-guided wire placement has been the mainstay for pinpointing lesions identified by breast imaging (Fig. 2.1). Over the years, technology has emerged improving some

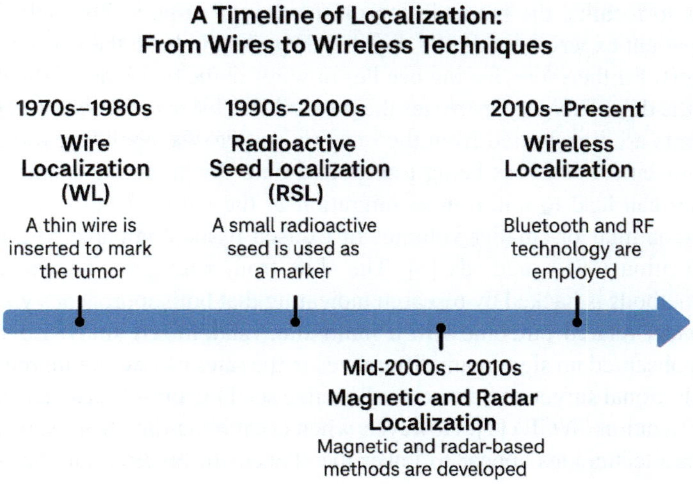

Fig. 2.1 A timeline of progression of technology

of the disadvantages of wire placement such as workflow inefficiencies, pain associated with protruding wires, potential displacement leading to the inability to remove the targeted lesion and/or clip and limiting incision options. These downfalls have led to the emergence of newer techniques such as radioactive seed localization with I-125; however, its general use is limited by strict nuclear regulations. Non-radioactive, wire-free alternatives have emerged as favourable alternatives such as SAVI SCOUT™, which uses infrared and radar, Magseed™, which uses a magnetic seed, MOLLI™, which uses a magnetic marker [3], LOCalizer™ which uses miniature radiofrequency identification (RFID) tag [4] and EnVisio™, which uses an electromagnetic localization system [5].

Localizing non-palpable breast lesions began in the early 1970s, when mammography revealed cancers too subtle to feel. Using a hooked wire inserted under mammographic guidance to mark lesions for excision [6], wire-guided localization emerged as a pioneering solution [2]. This technique, refined over the 1980s, became the gold standard, offering a 93–98% success rate in lesion retrieval [7]. Wire displacement, patient discomfort, and the logistical issues between radiology and surgery spurred innovation over the next several decades to improve patient experience and surgical precision.

2.3 Advancements and Impact on Patient Care

Each leap in localization technology has brought distinct advantages. Wire-guided localization, despite being the gold standard for decades, was associated with higher rates of wire displacement, patient discomfort, and larger excisions. Regarding patient comfort and logistics, wire-free methods avoid the need for needle and wire placements to localize the breast lesion on the day of surgery. This subsequently improves patient experiences on the day that they already have the stress of undergoing surgery. Furthermore, having needles or wires in the breast as a form of localization on the day of surgery increases the possibilities for wire migration especially when patients are transported from the imaging suite to the operating room where common movements such as being transported onto the operating room bed from the stretcher can lead to unfortunate migration of the wires. Additionally, studies demonstrate similar or smaller volumes of excised tissue compared to traditional wire localization (WL) methods [8]. The shift from wire-guided localization to wire-free methods is backed by research indicating that both approaches yield comparable cancer-related outcomes. In a multi-site, randomized study, Lovrics and colleagues observed no significant differences in the rates of positive margins or the need for additional surgeries between radioactive seed localization (RSL) and wire-guided localization (WGL) [9]. However, when combining data from various studies, wire-free techniques appear to lower the chances of positive surgical margins and the necessity for follow-up excisions compared to WGL. For example, pooled data showed that the SAVI SCOUT ™ system led to fewer re-excisions (8.6% versus 18.8%) and positive margins (10.6% versus 15.0%) than WGL. Together, these findings indicate that wire-free methods are just as effective and safe as WNL, while possibly improving surgical results [10]. In addition to cancer outcomes, wire-free technologies provide a clear improvement in patient comfort and overall experience [11]. By removing the external wire, patients have responded positively to wire-free systems as the protruding wire and placement lead to significant anxiety [12].

2.3.1 Cost-Effectiveness of Wireless Technology

Overall, wire-free breast localization techniques have demonstrated cost-effectiveness and operational advantages over traditional WL methods in various studies [13–15]. These techniques offer potential benefits in terms of reduced surgery delays, lower costs, and improved patient and surgeon experiences. Wire-free breast localization techniques, including radar localization (RL) and radiofrequency identification (RFID) tags, have been assessed for their cost-effectiveness relative to traditional wire localization (WL) methods.

A study conducted by Nguyen et al. demonstrated that RL utilizing the SCOUT ™ Surgical Guidance System proved more cost-effective than WL for wide local excision of non-palpable breast cancer. RL minimized surgery delays, resulting in cost savings and presenting an incremental cost–utility ratio of AUD$493 per quality-adjusted life-year (QALY) gained [13]. Heindl et al. evaluated the feasibility and cost-effectiveness of RFID tags for breast lesion localization in routine clinical practice. Benefits included reduced preoperative radiography, decreased patient discomfort, and enhanced scheduling flexibility [14]. According to Zhang et al., radioactive seed localization (RSL) showed lower costs and improved operating room efficiency compared to WL. The average cost per patient for RSL was significantly lower, and RSL optimized the utilization of radiology resources, leading to shorter patient wait times [15].

Wire-free breast localization techniques have demonstrated their cost-effectiveness and operational advantages over traditional WL methods across multiple studies, offering potential benefits in terms of reduced surgery delays, lower costs, and improved experiences for both patients and surgeons. This underscores the need to evaluate factors beyond initial device expenses, including the potential for fewer re-excisions, minimized surgical delays, enhanced operating room productivity, and increased patient experience to determine the true financial benefit of these technologies [16].

2.3.2 *Excisional Biopsy: Diagnosing the Uncertain*

For non-palpable high-risk or discordant lesions where imaging or percutaneous biopsy yields inconclusive results, excisional breast biopsy remains an indispensable diagnostic modality. Precise localization is paramount to ensure accurate targeting with minimal tissue disruption. Following preoperative marking, utilizing either traditional wire-guided techniques or contemporary wireless systems, a strategically planned incision is executed, prioritizing both complete lesion resection and optimal cosmesis. The lesion is excised en bloc to facilitate definitive histopathological diagnosis. Specimen orientation is essential for accurate pathologic correlation, while placement of a biopsy cavity marker (e.g. titanium clip) serves dual purposes: it delineates the site for potential adjuvant therapy and provides a reference for longitudinal surveillance imaging. Incision design demands foresight, as placement must account for possible subsequent oncologic or reconstructive procedures, ensuring compatibility with future surgical approaches and avoiding compromise of therapeutic outcomes. This technique underscores the balance between diagnostic precision, patient-centred aesthetics, and multidisciplinary treatment planning.

2.3.3 *Standard Breast Conservation and Partial Mastectomy*

Breast-conserving surgery (BCS), or partial mastectomy, reigns as the cornerstone for early-stage (Stage I–II) non-palpable breast cancers. The goal is clear: achieve negative margins—defined as $\geq$1 mm for invasive cancer and $\geq$2 mm for ductal carcinoma in situ (DCIS) per NICE guidelines—while preserving cosmesis [17]. It is worth noting that in the United States, per the American Society of Breast Surgeons guidelines, negative margins for invasive breast cancer are defined as no tumour on ink, and $\geq$2 mm for DCIS [18]. In Europe, BCS dominates, accounting for approximately 80% of eligible cases, a testament to screening advancements and patient preference for breast preservation [19]. Localization is critical for the success of BCS. Surgeons measure outcomes by excised tissue volume (ideally minimized), localization reliability, and positive margin rates. Improvements in technology reflect a shift toward precision, ensuring cancer control without sacrificing the form of the breast, a foundation oncoplastic surgery builds upon.

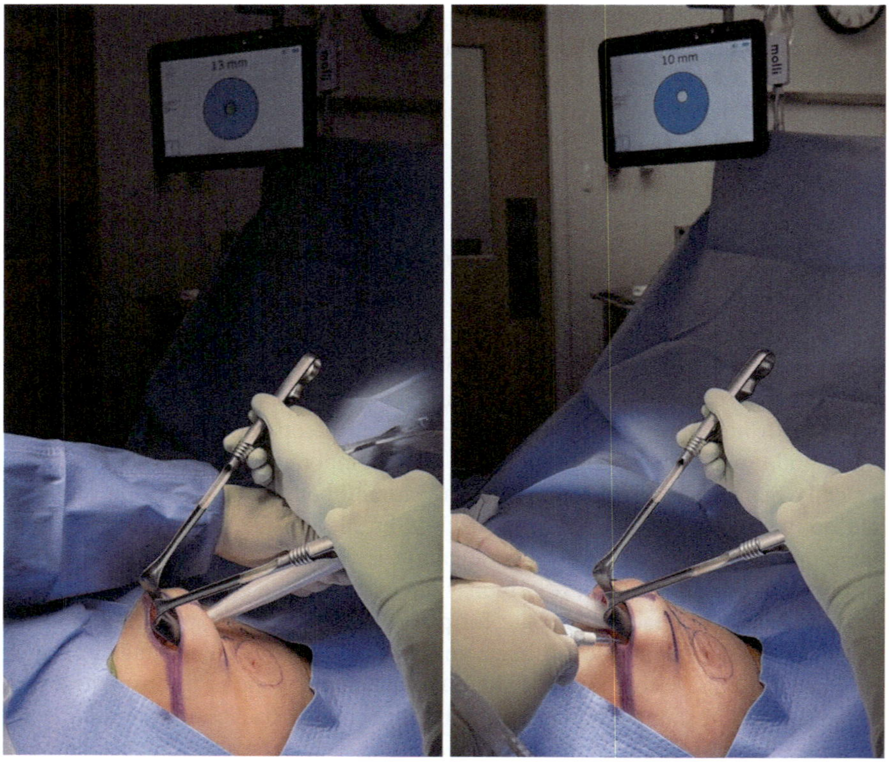

Oncoplastic techniques allow the surgeon to access the impalpable breast lesion through a hidden scar technique

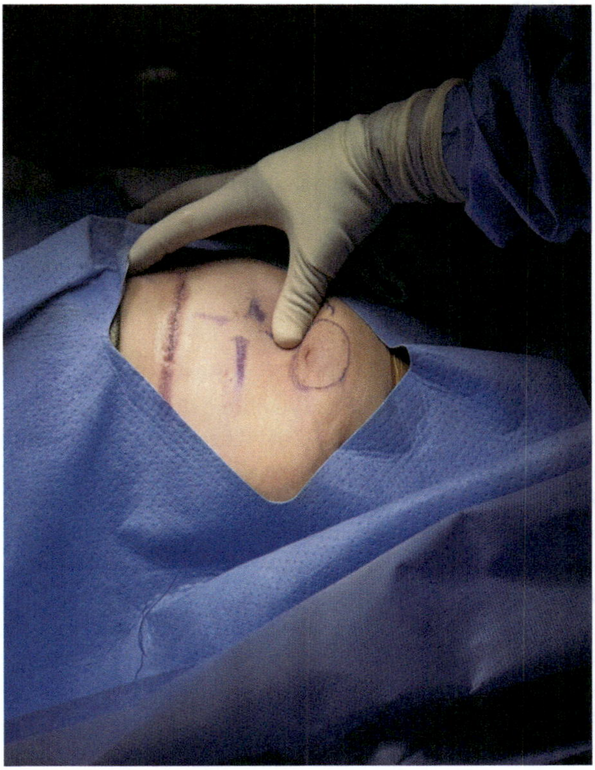

Well-hidden inframammary incision following successful wireless localized excisional biopsy

2.4 Oncoplastic Surgery: The Fusion of Function and Form

Oncoplastic surgery is defined as breast conservation combining strict oncologic and aesthetic principles during cancer resection [20]. Oncoplastic surgery utilizes volume displacement (Level 1 and Level 2) when up to 50% of the breast tissue is removed as well as volume replacement techniques such as implant-based reconstruction, local/regional flap reconstruction when >50% of the breast is removed [20]. Oncoplastic surgery has many benefits. Oncoplastic surgery offers lower re-excision rates, wider margins, and superior patient satisfaction, all while matching standard BCS in survival [21].

2.4.1 Level 1 Oncoplastic Surgery

For defects under 20% of breast volume, Level 1 techniques—like local tissue rearrangement, crescent mastopexy or donut mastopexy offer effective ways of reducing the contour deformity and offer more cosmetically appropriate incisions and better access to lesions not typically amenable to a hidden scar technique [20].

2.4.2 Level 2 Oncoplastic Surgery

In cases where defects encompass 20–50% of breast volume, Level 2 oncoplastic techniques are recommended, specifically volume displacement mammoplasty and circumvertical mammoplasty designs [20]. These approaches utilize the breast reduction framework, often the Wise pattern skin incision, affording the breast surgeon optimal exposure for the resection of non-palpable lesions. This method ensures the potential for wide, oncologically recommended margins while effectively addressing the defect. Utilizing techniques similar to a breast reduction, these techniques are particularly advantageous for patients presenting with a higher tumour-to-breast volume ratio or those facing complex cosmetic challenges affecting both the ipsilateral and contralateral breasts. In such instances, a contralateral reduction mammoplasty may be indicated to achieve symmetry and enhance overall aesthetic outcomes.

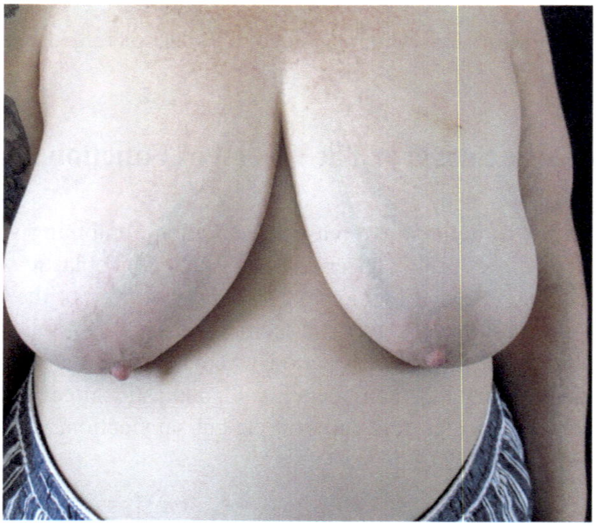

A 60-year female presenting with left-sided breast cancer at the 12:00 radian, breast asymmetry and symptomatic macromastia

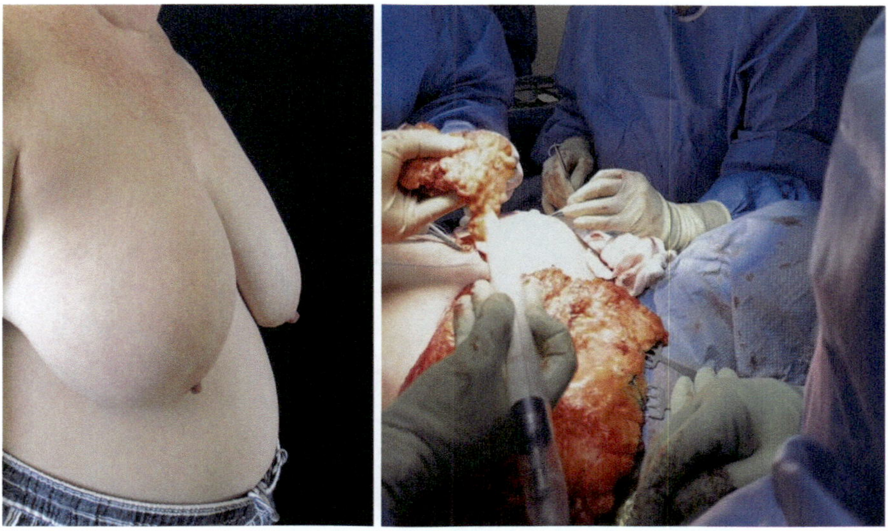

Level 2 Volume displacement design. A large partial mastectomy was performed and a probe was used to confirm successful inclusion of the targeted clip

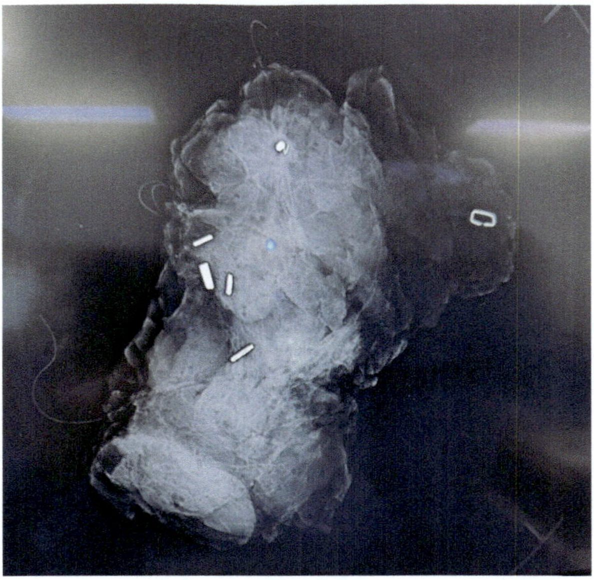

Intraoperative specimen radiograph confirming successful inclusion of the biopsy clip, wireless localization device, and mass

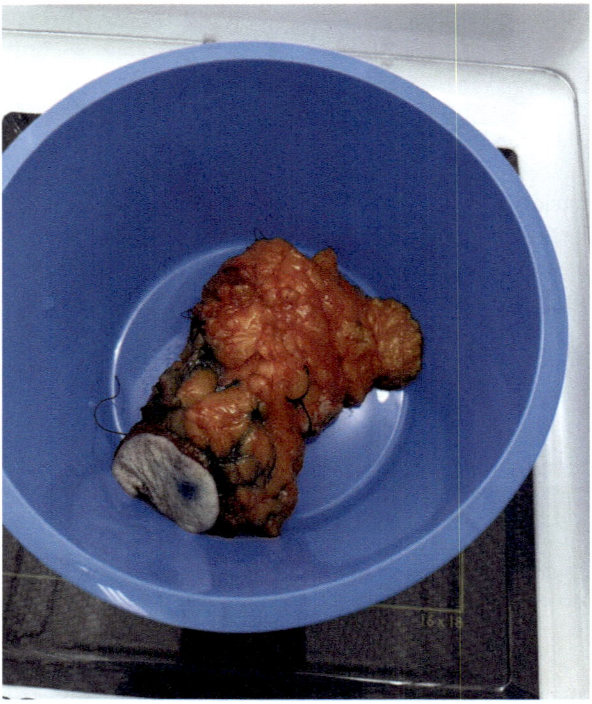

Gross specimen of large oncoplastic partial mastectomy including the superior keyhole and positional sutures designating the margins

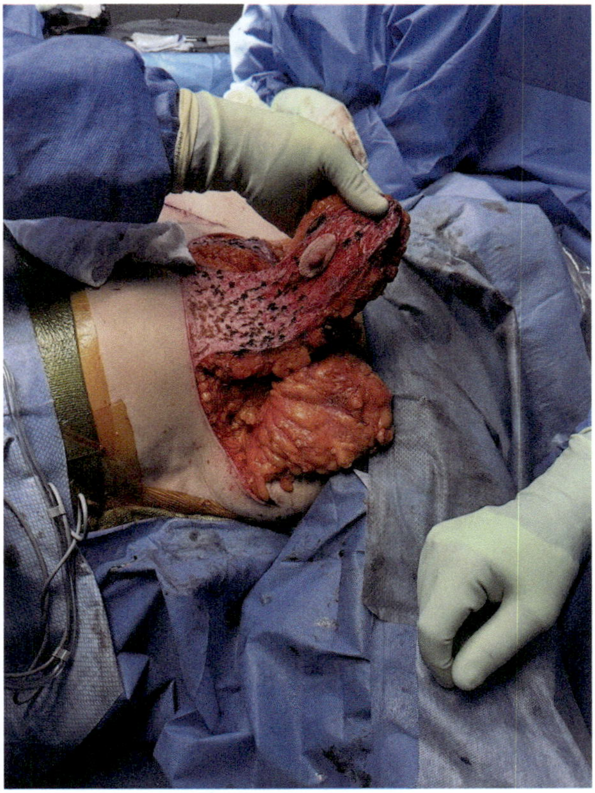

Inferior pedicle demonstrating a well-vascularized pedicle and nipple areolar complex. The inferior pedicle will be used to autoaugment the defect at the 12:00 position. The large resection maximizes negative margin rates and alleviates ptosis and symptomatic macromastia

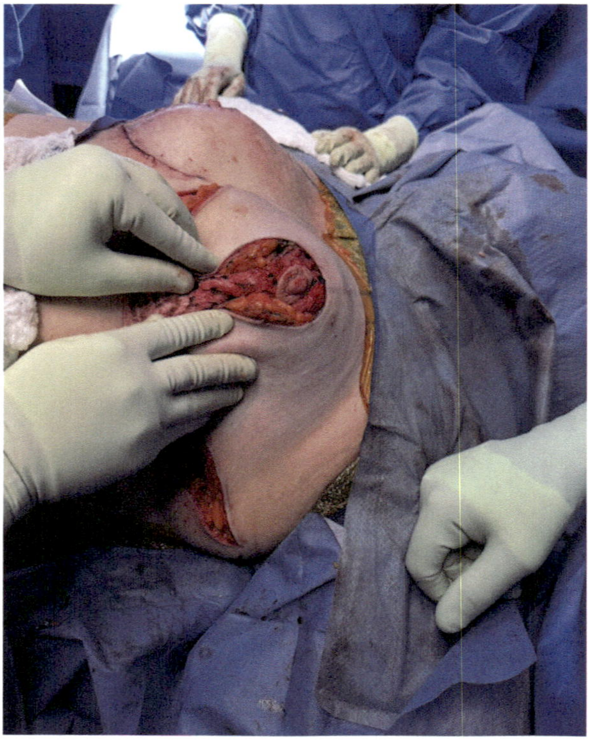

The inferior pedicle is autoaugmented into the superior keyhole

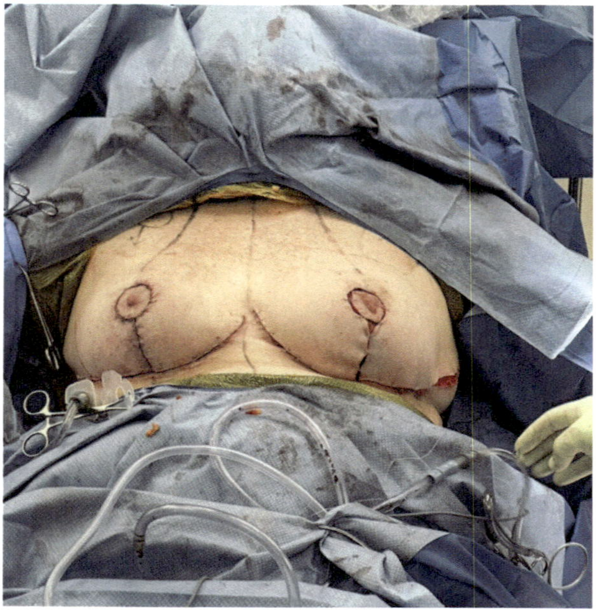

The incisions are stapled and the patient is sat up to assess for breast symmetry

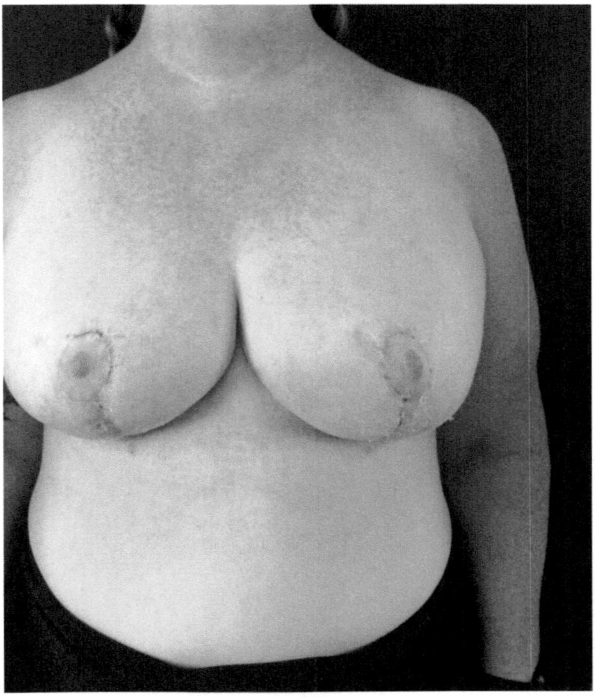

8 weeks post-operatively. The cancer was resected to negative margins

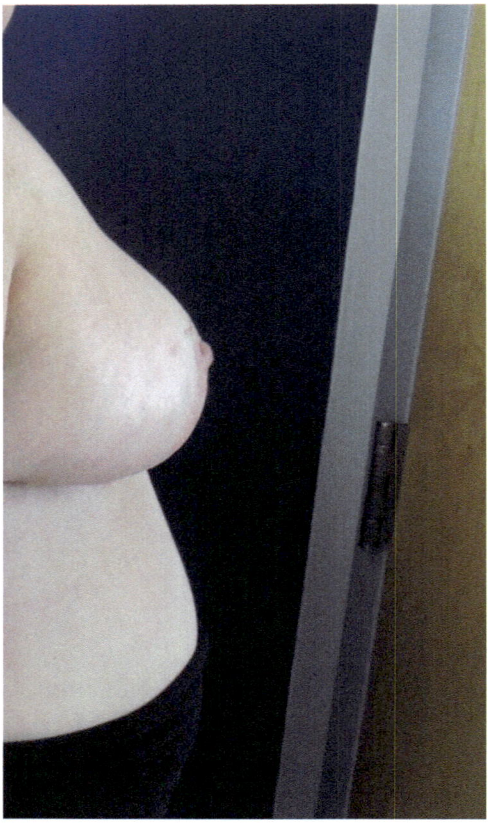

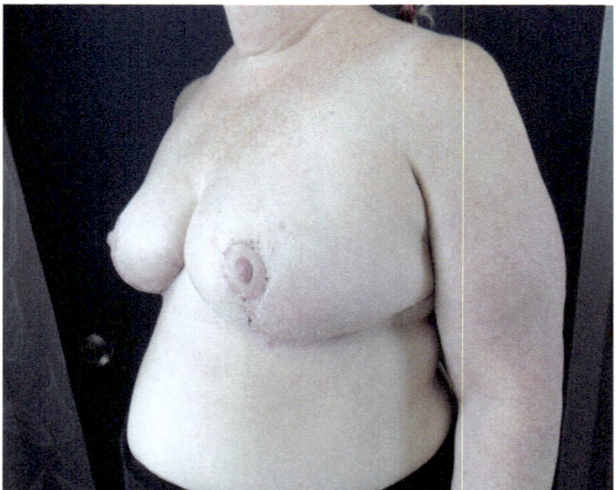

2.4.3 Volume Replacement Surgery

Volume replacement breast surgery utilizes pedicled flaps and flaps like the lateral intercostal artery perforator (LICAP), thoracodorsal artery perforator (TDAP), or anterior intercostal artery perforator flap (AICAP). These flaps harvest tissue from the adjacent chest wall and offer the surgeon the ability to excise lesions in cosmetically challenging areas such the lower pole to prevent a bird's beak deformity. With minimal donor site morbidity and the ability to offer partial breast reconstruction simultaneously as the cancer resection, volume replacement surgery is particularly advantageous for maintaining symmetry while performing unilateral surgery.

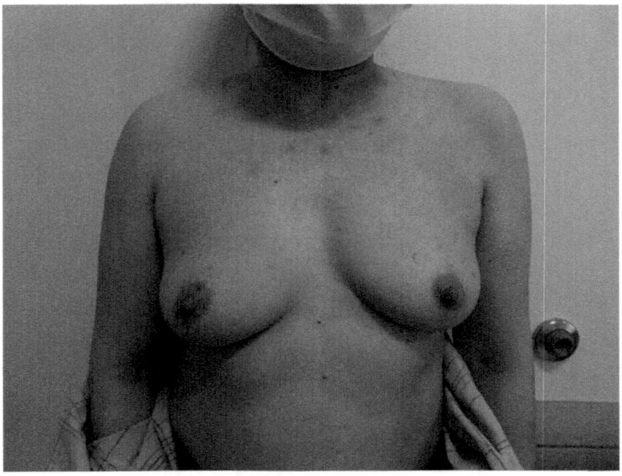

Preoperative Photo. Given lack of ptosis and breast size, a volume replacement technique was chosen to minimize asymmetry and deformity

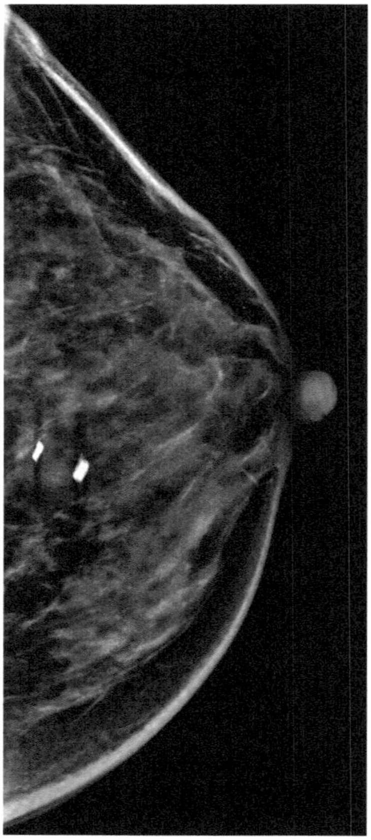

Left LMO mammogram demonstrating the post-biopsy clip and the wireless localization marker 'goal posting' the cancer

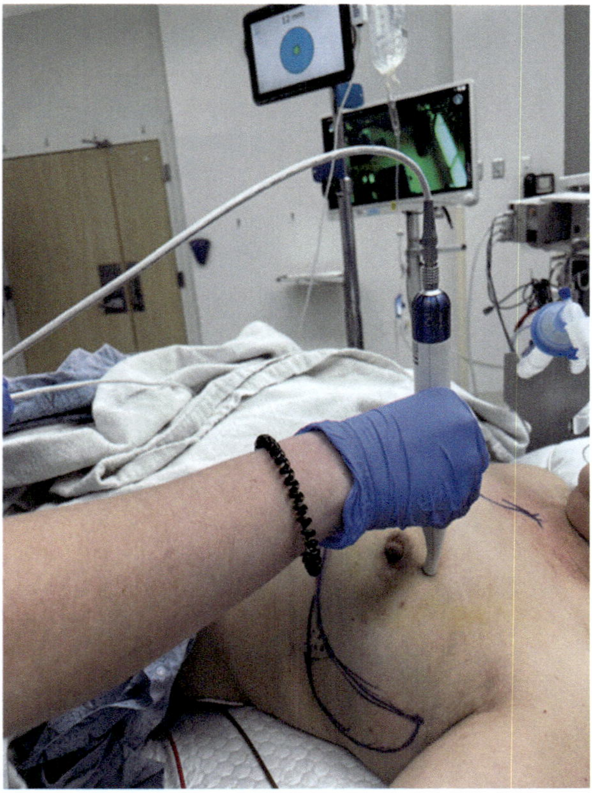

The patient is marked for a left lateral intercostal artery perforator flap (LICAP), and utilizing the wireless localization device, the cancer is identified at the 12:00 position. Due to the patient's breast size, she elected to undergo unilateral surgery and volume replacement to autoaugment the defect created from the partial mastectomy

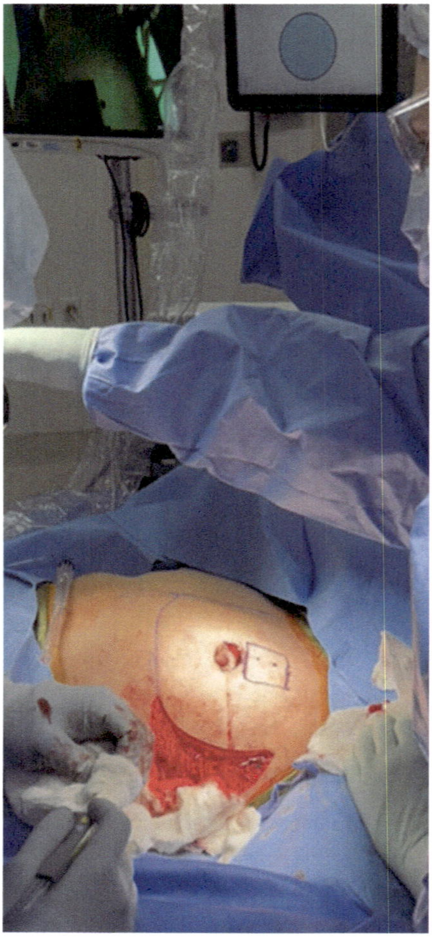

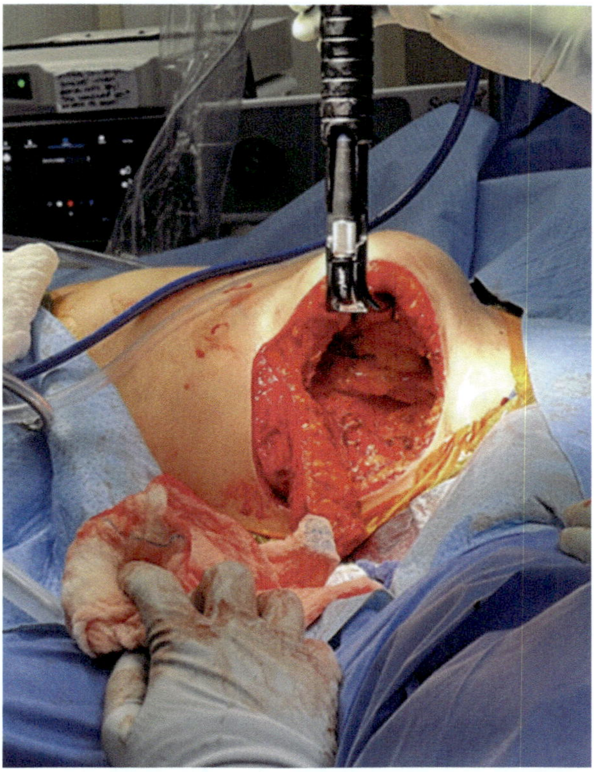

The cancer was excised through the lateral left breast and a separate periareolar incision was made to mobilize the tissue medially

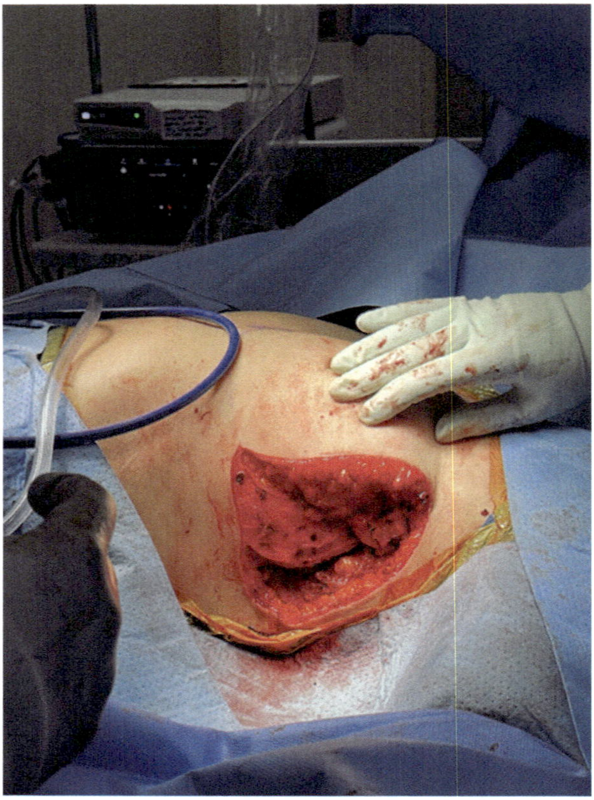

The lateral intercostal artery perforator (LICAP) was used to autoaugment the defect created from the partial mastectomy

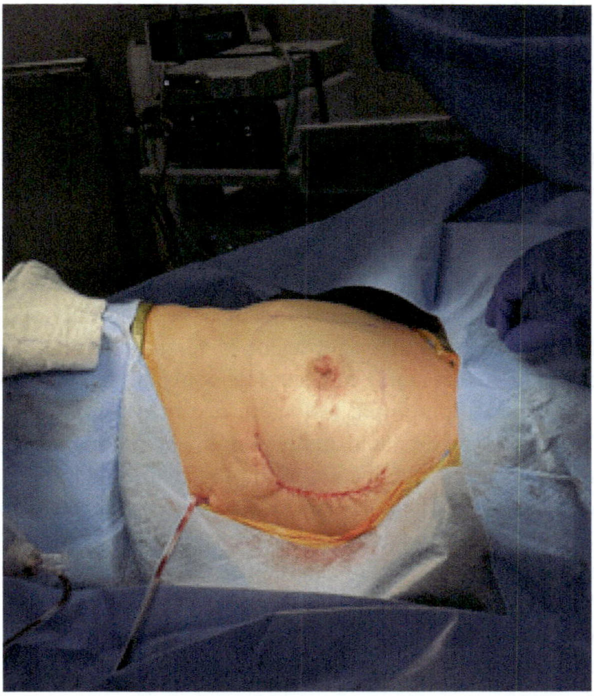

The periareolar incision is closed along with the lateral intercostal artery perforator (LICAP) donor site and a drain is fashioned into place

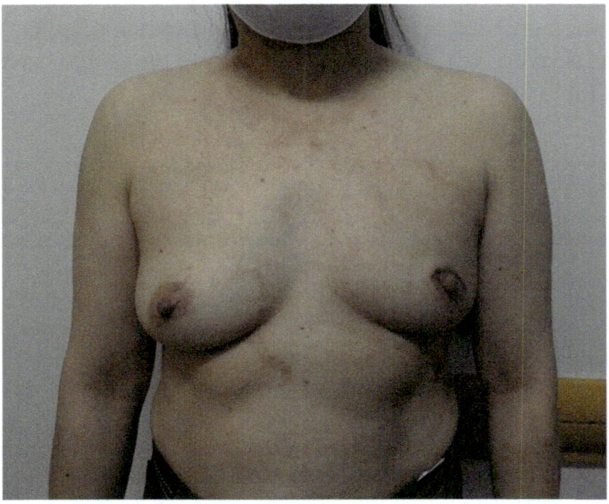

8 weeks after her left partial mastectomy and lateral intercostal artery perforator (LICAP) breast

2.4.4 *Wireless Localization During Oncoplastic Surgery: Tips and Tricks*

Wireless localization has revolutionized the preoperative preparation for oncoplastic breast surgery (Table 2.1). This approach enhances patient comfort, improves precision in lesion targeting, especially in the large breast, and provides surgeons with greater flexibility during complex procedures. In larger breasts, the depth and volume of tissue can complicate the localization. Traditional wires require longer needles, increasing the chance for greater pain and migration, while some wireless technologies falter when lesions lie beyond their detection threshold. Therefore, selecting the appropriate technology for lesion localization is crucial and should be tailored to breast size, lesion depth, and surgical goals. Some wireless technologies stand out when identifying multiple lesions in one breast or when lesions require bracketing. The authors recommend multidisciplinary preoperative planning with Radiology to ensure optimal localization. Radiologists should have a general understanding of what surgery is being performed to avoid compromising the pedicle with an overzealous localization approach.

Oncoplastic surgery employs pedicles such as the superomedial or inferior pedicle for partial breast reconstruction. Knowing the exact location preoperatively by utilizing the hand-held localization device and tablet allows the surgeon to map the incision pattern and pedicle orientation. For example, a lesion identified at the 6:00 radian would favour a superomedial pedicle approach preserving upper breast fullness while ensuring lesion excision. Drawing this location during the preoperative marking is essential to achieve our oncologic and aesthetic goals.

Oncoplastic surgery requires multidisciplinary planning. By utilizing wireless technologies, surgeons can achieve precise lesion excision, adapt to anatomical challenges, and leverage real-time tools to maximize oncologic outcomes and aesthetic results (Table 2.1).

Table 2.1 Key aspects of wireless localization during oncoplastic surgery

Aspect	Details
Technology selection	Choose the appropriate wireless technology based on breast size, lesion depth, and surgical goals
Challenges in large breasts	Localization can be difficult in large breasts due to depth and tissue volume. Traditional wire methods may cause more pain and migration
Pedicle consideration	Selection of pedicles such as superomedial or inferior is crucial for planning the incision and preserving breast fullness while excising the lesion
Wireless localization	Improves precision and patient comfort. Helps map lesions and determine incision location for effective surgery
Multidisciplinary planning	Collaboration between surgeons and radiologists ensures optimal localization and surgical planning, minimizing errors
Preoperative marking	Essential for accurately mapping the lesion location and the planned incision to meet oncologic and aesthetic goals
Localization devices	Hand-held localization devices with tablets allow real-time mapping of lesion location, pedicle orientation, and incision plan

2.4.5 Axillary Management Using Wireless Localization

Axillary management in breast cancer has evolved significantly. Given the morbidity associated with axillary dissection, neoadjuvant treatments are used to downstage a clinically positive axilla making patients candidates for sentinel lymph node biopsy. Studies such as ACOSOG Z1071 highlight the challenge of accurately assessing residual nodal disease after neoadjuvant chemotherapy [22]. Additional studies demonstrate the use of clipping the biopsy-proven lymph node to reduce the false negative rate of sentinel lymph node biopsy after neoadjuvant chemotherapy. The authors concluded that clip placement and resection of the clipped biopsy-proven node at diagnosis should be considered to reduce the false negative rate [23].

Wireless technologies, such as MOLLI™, radiofrequency identification (RFID) tags, and radioactive seed localization (RSL), offer precise preoperative targeting of axillary lymph nodes, enhancing surgical accuracy and potentially reducing the need for extensive axillary dissection. For instance, McGugin et al. demonstrated that RFID tag localization is comparable to traditional wire-guided methods for non-palpable breast lesions, suggesting similar efficacy in axillary applications [8]. Zhang et al. further highlight RSL's advantages, noting improved operating room efficiency and cost-effectiveness compared to wire localization, which could extend to axillary procedures [15]. This precision is especially vital in the neoadjuvant setting, where accurate identification of previously positive nodes post-chemotherapy can influence de-escalation strategies, as supported by findings from the BrighTNess trial [19]. Thus, wireless localization represents a transformative approach in axillary management, optimizing outcomes for patients with node-positive breast cancer.

Beyond trial data, practical advantages of wireless systems amplify their value in axillary management. Unlike wire localization, which can protrude externally and complicate scheduling, wireless methods allow placement days or weeks in advance, as noted in historical reflections on wire techniques by Hall et al. [2]. This flexibility is particularly beneficial for axillary nodes, which may be deeper and harder to access than breast lesions, ensuring surgeons can operate with optimal timing and precision. Chatterjee et al. discuss oncoplastic surgery principles that, while focused on breast conservation, parallel is the need for meticulous axillary planning to balance oncologic efficacy with reduced morbidity [20]. Removing the targeted node minimizes the risk of leaving residual disease, a concern heightened in node-positive cases where systemic therapy response varies.

In conclusion, wireless localization represents a transformative leap in axillary management for breast cancer, particularly for biopsy-proven node-positive disease. By ensuring the accurate removal of targeted lymph nodes, these technologies enhance staging accuracy, reduce false-negative rates, and support tailored surgical approaches. The shift from wire-based to wireless systems not only improves clinical outcomes but also streamlines operative workflows, underscoring their growing importance in modern breast cancer care.

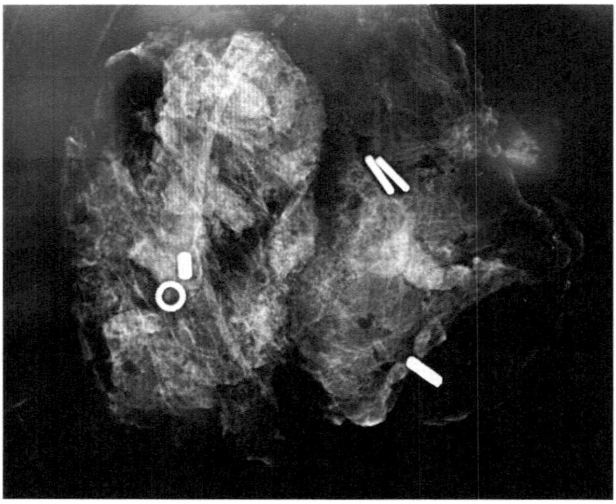

Targeted axillary dissection specimen demonstrates the biopsy twirl-shaped marker and the wireless marker which was utilized to ensure successful excision of the biopsy-proven metastatic lymph node

2.5 Summary

The toolbox for breast lesion localization is varied, with each method tailored to the patient and treating team. Successful lesion localization should focus on precise lesion identification, offer effective and reproducible localization techniques, have high patient satisfaction, achieve negative margins, minimize the volume of adjacent healthy tissue excision, preserve cosmetic outcomes, maintain reliable coordination with Radiology and Pathology, be safe, cost-effective, and efficient.

References

1. Losken A, et al. Oncoplastic surgery versus standard breast conservation: a meta-analysis. Plast Reconstr Surg. 2022;149(4):567–79.
2. Hall FM, Kopans DB, Sadowsky NL, Homer MJ. Development of wire localization for occult breast lesions: Boston remembrances. Radiology. 2013;268(3):622–7. https://doi.org/10.1148/radiol.13121943.
3. Jeffries DO, Dossett LA, Jorns JM. Localization for breast surgery: the next generation. Arch Pathol Lab Med. 2017;141(10):1324–9. https://doi.org/10.5858/arpa.2017-0214-RA.
4. LOCalizer™ Wire-free Guidance System | Hologic® Breast Surgery.
5. Technology—Elucent Medical. https://elucent.com/technology/.
6. Frank HA, Hall FM, Steer ML. Preoperative localization of nonpalpable breast lesions demonstrated by mammography. N Engl J Med. 1976;295(5):259–60. https://doi.org/10.1056/NEJM197607292950505.

7. Corsi F, et al. Wire-guided localization for non-palpable breast lesions: a review of 500 cases. Breast Care. 2013;8(5):359–63.
8. McGugin C, Spivey T, Coopey S, Smith B, Kelly B, Gadd M, Hughes K, Dontchos B, Specht M. Radiofrequency identification tag localization is comparable to wire localization for non-palpable breast lesions. Breast Cancer Res Treat. 2019;177(3):735–9. https://doi.org/10.1007/s10549-019-05355-0.
9. Lovrics PJ, Goldsmith CH, Hodgson N, et al. A multicentered, randomized, controlled trial comparing radioguided seed localization to standard wire localization for nonpalpable, invasive and in situ breast carcinomas. Ann Surg Oncol. 2011;18(12):3407–14. https://doi.org/10.1245/s10434-011-1699-y, https://pubmed.ncbi.nlm.nih.gov/21533657/.
10. Shirazi S, Hajiesmaeili H, Khosla M, Taj S, Sircar T, Vidya R. Comparison of wire and non-wire localisation techniques in breast cancer surgery: a review of the literature with pooled analysis. Medicina (Kaunas). 2023;59(7):1297. https://doi.org/10.3390/medicina59071297, https://pmc.ncbi.nlm.nih.gov/articles/PMC10383802/.
11. Banys-Paluchowski M, Kühn T, Masannat Y, et al. Localization techniques for non-palpable breast lesions: current status, knowledge gaps, and rationale for the MELODY study (EUBREAST-4/iBRA-NET, NCT 05559411). Cancers (Basel). 2023;15(4):1173. https://doi.org/10.3390/cancers15041173, https://pmc.ncbi.nlm.nih.gov/articles/PMC9954476/.
12. Wazir U, Tayeh S, Perry N, Michell M, Malhotra A, Mokbel K. Wireless breast localization using radio-frequency identification tags: the first reported European experience in breast cancer. In Vivo. 2020;34(1):233–8. https://doi.org/10.21873/invivo.11765, https://pmc.ncbi.nlm.nih.gov/articles/PMC6984090/.
13. Nguyen CL, Cui R, Zhou M, et al. Cost-effectiveness of radar localisation versus wire localisation for wide local excision of non-palpable breast cancer. Ann Surg Oncol. 2024;31(6):3916–25. https://doi.org/10.1245/s10434-024-15142-x, https://pubmed.ncbi.nlm.nih.gov/38472677/.
14. Heindl F, Schulz-Wendtland R, Jud S, Erber R, Hack CC, Preuss C, Behrens A, Pöschke P, Emons J. Evaluation of a wireless localization system for nonpalpable breast lesions—feasibility and cost-effectiveness in everyday clinical routine. In Vivo. 2022;36(5):2291–7. https://doi.org/10.21873/invivo.12965.
15. Zhang Y, Seely J, Cordeiro E, Hefler J, Thavorn K, Mahajan M, Domina S, Aro J, Ibrahim AM, Arnaout A, Gravel D, Nessim C. Radioactive seed localization versus wire-guided localization for nonpalpable breast cancer: a cost and operating room efficiency analysis. Ann Surg Oncol. 2017;24(12):3567–73. https://doi.org/10.1245/s10434-017-6084-z.
16. Cheung BHH, Co M, Lui TTN, Kwong A. Evolution of localization methods for non-palpable breast lesions: a literature review from a translational medicine perspective. Transl Breast Cancer Res. 2024;5:12. https://doi.org/10.21037/tbcr-23-49, https://pmc.ncbi.nlm.nih.gov/articles/PMC11093046/.
17. National Institute for Health & Care Excellence (NICE). Early and locally advanced breast cancer: diagnosis and management. 2025. https://www.nice.org.uk/guidance/ng101. Accessed 12 Mar 2025.
18. The American Society of Breast Surgeons. Resource guide on breast cancer breast conservation surgery margins. 2024. https://www.breastsurgeons.org/docs/statements/asbrs-rg-margins.pdf.
19. Golshan M, Loibl S, Wong SM, Huober JB, O'Shaughnessy J, Rugo HS, Wolmark N, McKee MD, Maag D, Sullivan DM, Metzger-Filho O, Von Minckwitz G, Geyer CE Jr, Sikov WM, Untch M. Breast conservation after neoadjuvant chemotherapy for triple-negative breast cancer: surgical results from the BrighTNess randomized clinical trial. JAMA Surg. 2020;155(3):e195410. https://doi.org/10.1001/jamasurg.2019.5410.
20. Chatterjee A, Gass J, Patel K, Holmes D, Kopkash K, Peiris L, Peled A, Ryan J, El-Tamer M, Reiland J. A consensus definition and classification system of oncoplastic surgery developed by the American Society of Breast Surgeons. Ann Surg Oncol. 2019;26(10):3156–63. https://doi.org/10.1245/s10434-019-07345-4.

21. Clough KB, Kaufman GJ, Nos C, et al. Improving breast cancer surgery: a classification and quadrant per quadrant atlas for oncoplastic surgery. Ann Surg Oncol. 2010;17:1375–91. https://doi.org/10.1245/s10434-009-0792-y.
22. Boughey JC, Suman VJ, Mittendorf EA, Ahrendt GM, Wilke LG, Taback B, Leitch AM, Kuerer HM, Bowling M, Flippo-Morton TS, Byrd DR, Ollila DW, Julian TB, McLaughlin SA, McCall L, Symmans WF, Le-Petross HT, Haffty BG, Buchholz TA, Nelson H, Hunt KK, Alliance for Clinical Trials in Oncology. Sentinel lymph node surgery after neoadjuvant chemotherapy in patients with node-positive breast cancer: the ACOSOG Z1071 (Alliance) clinical trial. JAMA. 2013;310(14):1455–61. https://doi.org/10.1001/jama.2013.278932.
23. Boughey JC, Ballman KV, Le-Petross HT, McCall LM, Mittendorf EA, Ahrendt GM, Wilke LG, Taback B, Feliberti EC, Hunt KK. Identification and resection of clipped node decreases the false-negative rate of sentinel lymph node surgery in patients presenting with node-positive breast cancer (T0-T4, N1-N2) who receive neoadjuvant chemotherapy: results from ACOSOG Z1071 (Alliance). Ann Surg. 2016;263(4):802–7. https://doi.org/10.1097/SLA.0000000000001375.

Chapter 3
The Challenges in Management of Positive Surgical Margin Following Localisation of Non-Palpable Breast Cancers

Billy Ho Hung Cheung and Ava Kwong

Contents

B. H. H. Cheung
Division of Breast Surgery, Department of Surgery, School of Clinical Medicine, LKS Faculty of Medicine, The University of Hong Kong, Hong Kong, China
e-mail: billychh@hku.hk

A. Kwong (✉)
Breast Surgery Centre (Island East), Hong Kong Sanatorium and Hospital, Hong Kong, China
e-mail: avakwong@hku.hk

R. Vidya, N. Sharma (eds.), *Breast and Axilla Localisation Techniques*,
https://doi.org/10.1007/978-3-032-17995-1_3

3.1 Introduction

The increasing implementation of population-based breast cancer screening programmes, coupled with improved imaging technologies, has led to a significant rise in the detection of early breast cancers [1, 2]. Throughout the years, various techniques have evolved, from the traditional wire-guided localization (WGL) to newer methods including radioactive seed localization (RSL), magnetic seed localization (MSL), and radar-based technologies [3]. Each method presents its unique advantages and challenges, but all share the common goal of achieving complete tumour excision with appropriate surgical margins.

Clear surgical margins remain one of the most critical determinants of successful breast cancer surgery [4]. The presence of positive margins is associated with an increased risk of local recurrence. It often necessitates reoperation, leading to additional psychological stress, potential cosmetic compromise, and increased healthcare costs [5]. Compared to palpable tumours, non-palpable breast cancers carry a higher likelihood of positive surgical margins (Odds ratio (OR) 1.51) [6], with incomplete excisions observed in as many as 38.5% of cases [7].

Hence, it is essential to improve our understanding of margins and non-palpable breast cancers. This chapter focuses on the specific challenges associated with positive surgical margins of non-palpable breast cancers, including risk factors, preventive measures, treatment options, and future perspectives. Despite scientific advances, managing positive margins remains complex and requires careful consideration from various perspectives.

3.2 Clinical Importance of Surgical Margins and Current Standard of Practice

Clear surgical margins remain one of the most critical aspects in breast-conserving surgery (BCS) with significant implications for both oncological outcomes and patient quality of life.

3.2.1 Oncological Outcomes

The relationship between margin status and local recurrence has been extensively studied. A 2014 meta-analysis including 33 studies with 28,162 patients showed that positive margins doubled the risk of local recurrence (odds ratio (OR) 1.96 for positive/close vs. negative; OR 1.74 for close vs. negative, and 2.44 for positive vs. negative) [4]. Another more recent meta-analysis, published in 2022, involving 68 studies evaluated the relationship between margins and recurrence [8]. They reviewed the tumour on ink margins (involved) and found that they were associated not only with local recurrence (hazard ratio (HR) 1.98), but also with distant recurrence (HR 2.10). Moreover, close margins were also associated with increased distant recurrence (HR 1.38) and local recurrence (HR 2.09) compared with negative margins, after adjusting for receipt of adjuvant chemotherapy and radiotherapy.

To further highlight the importance of clear margins for survival, another meta-analysis involving more than 40,000 patients demonstrated that for every four local recurrences avoided at 5 years, one breast cancer death is prevented at 15 years (rate ratio 1.23), underlining the critical importance of achieving adequate margins [9].

3.2.2 Cosmetic and Quality of Life Considerations

Beyond oncological outcomes, re-excision surgery, which is required most of the time when there is a positive margin, can significantly impact cosmetic outcomes and patient satisfaction [10]. This is evident in a prospective study examining 80 patients with re-excisions vs. 359 without. The study showed a significant worsening in aesthetic status in the re-excision group after adjustment for confounders [11]. This is coupled with the fact that a relatively high percentage (8.5% in a trial involving 2200 patients [12]) of women may eventually require a completion mastectomy. Thus, a positive margin can significantly alter patients' initial expectations.

Quality of life can also be affected before and after re-excision. When re-excision is required, the patient is subjected to another waiting time for another elective procedure, which can create an extra burden to the patient's psychological health and social life [13]. Specific to re-excision following BCS, a prospective study involving more than 2000 patients with BCS showed that there is a lower breast satisfaction (as demonstrated by well-validated BREAST-Q [14]) and sexual well-being 2 years post-operatively [15]. However, this difference did not persist in the long term.

Hence, the surgeon needs to minimize positive margins and the need for re-excision.

3.2.3 Definition of Margin Safety with Current Guidelines

Most current guidelines shared similar recommendations based on current evidence (Summary in Table 3.1).

Invasive Ductal Carcinoma

For invasive ductal carcinoma, the most typical cell type, consistency was shown across US guidelines, with all major organizations adopting the 'no ink on tumor' standard. This consensus emerged from the 2014 Society of Surgical Oncology (SSO) and the American Society for Radiation Oncology (ASTRO) (SSO/ASTRO) guidelines, supported by Level 1A evidence showing no benefit from wider margins when combined with contemporary multimodal therapy [16]. This is based on a meta-analysis involving 33 studies with 28,162 patients with a median follow-up of 6.6 years [4]. The same criteria were also adopted by the National Comprehensive Cancer Network (NCCN) guideline [17].

However, a 2022 meta-analysis confirmed that involved or close pathological margins after breast-conserving surgery for early stage, invasive breast cancer are associated with increased distant and local recurrences [8]. Based on this, in 2024, the NICE guidelines issued an update, recommending consideration of further surgery if the invasive component was within 1 mm (0–1 mm) of the radial margin [18]. The guidelines suggested the decision process should include the benefits and risks to the patient's circumstances, comorbidities, tumour characteristics, and potential treatments.

Table 3.1 Summary of recommendations of margins from current guidelines

	No ink on tumour	2-mm margin	No margin necessary	Uncertain
Invasive breast cancer	X			
Invasive breast cancer + DCIS	X			
Invasive breast cancer with neoadjuvant chemotherapy	X			
Invasive lobular carcinoma	X			
Pure DCIS		X		
DCIS with microinvasion		X		
Pure nonclassic LCIS				X
Pure LCIS at the surgical margin			X	
Atypia at the surgical margin			X	

Adopted from NCCN guideline 2024 [17]

In cases of invasive breast carcinoma with concurrent ductal carcinoma in situ (DCIS), the established negative margin criterion of 'no ink on tumor' should be applied to the invasive margin, irrespective of the DCIS extent [17], as these mixed lesions demonstrate biological behaviour, therapeutic requirements, and prognostic outcomes more closely aligned with invasive carcinoma rather than pure DCIS. For cases presenting specific technical or anatomical challenges, a multidisciplinary approach with careful consideration of clinical parameters and comprehensive patient consultation should be undertaken.

Ductal Carcinoma In Situ

For DCIS, a meta-analysis with a total of 4660 patients from trials examining BCS and RT for DCIS found that a negative margin significantly reduced the risk of ipsilateral breast tumour recurrence (IBTR) [19]. Specifically, a 2-mm margin was superior to a margin less than 2 mm (OR 0.53), and there was no significant difference in the rate of IBTR between margins of 2 mm and greater than 5 mm. Based on this comprehensive meta-analysis, the SSO/ASTRO and NCCN maintain a ≥2 mm standard [17, 20]. On the other hand, while another meta-analysis published in 2025 reconfirmed the benefit of lower local recurrence risk with a margin width up to 2 mm, there is a lack of data comparing 1.1–2 mm with >2 mm [21]. The association between recurrence and close margins is not significant after the application of boost radiotherapy, suggesting boost radiotherapy could be a possible alternative to re-excision in patients with close margins <2 mm.

In cases of ductal carcinoma in situ (DCIS) with microinvasion (defined as invasive tumour ≤1 mm), the management, including margin widths, should align with DCIS guidelines (e.g. ≥2 mm) rather than invasive carcinoma guidelines, given the lesion's predominantly DCIS composition and treatment approach [17].

Lobular Pathology

For invasive lobular carcinoma, SSO/ASTRO guidelines continued to support 'no ink on margin' as the standard, and there is no need for a wider margin [16]. The risk of ipsilateral breast tumour recurrence (IBTR) for ILC is similar to that of invasive ductal carcinoma (IDC), and studies have shown that wider margins in ILC do not yield lower IBTR rates [22, 23]. For classic lobular carcinoma in situ (LCIS) at the margin, re-excision is not indicated.

For nonclassic lobular carcinoma in situ, the optimal margin is uncertain [17]. On the other hand, an extensive single-institute study suggested that nonclassic LCIS at or near the margin with concurrent invasive carcinoma will not affect local recurrence [24].

3.3 Risk Factors for Positive Margins

Achieving negative surgical margins in breast-conserving surgery for non-palpable cancers is crucial for minimizing local recurrence and optimizing patient outcomes. Several factors influence the likelihood of achieving positive margins, and understanding these factors is vital for effective surgical planning and decision-making. These factors can be broadly categorized into tumour characteristics and patient-specific factors.

3.3.1 Tumour Characteristics

The tumour's inherent biology and morphology play a significant role in margin status. Ductal carcinoma in situ (DCIS) generally carries a higher risk of positive margins compared to invasive ductal carcinoma, likely due to its diffuse nature and the potential for microscopic extension beyond the clinically or radiologically apparent lesion [25]. A population-based study involving over 4000 patients compared IDC and DCIS and suggested a threefold increased risk of positive margins in DCIS [25]. In comparison, a more recent study suggested approximately a ninefold increased risk of a positive margin when DCIS is concurrently present with IDC [26].

On the other hand, invasive lobular carcinoma (ILC) has a significantly higher risk of positive margins compared to invasive ductal carcinoma, attributed to its diffuse growth pattern, lack of desmoplastic reaction, and difficulty in clinical and radiological assessment [27, 28]. A large single-institute study revealed that the rate of re-excision after BCS for ILC was significantly higher at 35.1% compared to 17.7% for IDC, and 20.0% for DCIS [29]. Of note, in the setting of ILC, discordance between imaging results and pathology is well documented; hence, careful case selection is essential [30]. Pleomorphic lobular carcinoma in situ (LCIS), a more aggressive variant of classical LCIS, presents similar challenges [31].

Furthermore, biological subtypes affect local recurrence rates, which in turn could impact margin status. HER2-positive and triple-negative tumour subtypes tend to exhibit more aggressive biological behaviour, including higher rates of proliferation and invasion [32]. This aggressive growth pattern can make complete surgical excision more challenging, leading to a higher likelihood of residual tumour cells at the margin [26]. Similarly, other features of a more aggressive tumour upon histology examination, including extensive intraductal component, necrosis, and higher grade, were shown to increase the risk of positive margins [33–35].

Large tumours may also contribute to a higher rate of positive margins, as supported by recent studies [36, 37]. Similarly, elevated risk for a larger tumour was also shown in the post-neoadjuvant setting [38].

On the other hand, a non-palpable tumour, with difficulty in accurately localizing the cancer and the margins despite current techniques, still increases the risk of involved margins. Compared to palpable tumours, non-palpable breast cancers posted an elevated positive surgical margin risk (Odds ratio (OR) 1.51) [6].

Multifocal/multicentric disease presents a particular challenge, with significantly higher positive margin rates compared to unifocal disease [26]. This can be reflected by the risk of involvement due to satellite tumour foci, and additional imaging-invisible lesions [39]. Hence, careful preoperative planning with MDT involving a radiologist for optimal preoperative localization will be necessary [40].

In the modern era, when neoadjuvant treatments (NATs) are more commonly used, they may also increase the risk of positive margins, partly due to non-uniform tumour regression after systemic treatment [41]. The risk increased further in patients where a complete pathological response cannot be achieved, and, contrary to high-grade tumours in the upfront setting, slower-growing tumours, such as those with oestrogen receptor positive, may be exposed to an increased risk due to their response to NAT [38, 42].

3.3.2 *Patient-Specific Factors*

Several patient-specific characteristics significantly influence the risk of positive margins in breast-conserving surgery. Breast density emerges as a crucial factor, with extremely dense breasts showing higher positive margin rates, as the tumour extent may be underestimated, and increases the risk of re-excision [43].

Aligned with breast density, younger women often present with denser breast tissue and also more aggressive tumour behaviour. Hence, it is also considered a risk factor for residual disease at the margin [28, 33, 44] (Table 3.2).

Table 3.2 Summary table for risk factors for positive margins

Tumour factor	Patient factor
DCIS, including concomitant lesion	Dense breast
Lobular type	Young patient
Aggressive subtype and features	
Multifocal tumours	
Large tumour	
Non-palpable tumour	
Neoadjuvant treatment	

3.4 Prevention Strategies

3.4.1 Preoperative Planning Optimization

Preoperative planning is critical for minimizing positive margins in breast-conserving surgery (BCS). Optimal imaging, careful patient selection, and precise tumour localization are key components to reducing re-excision rates. First, multimodal imaging should be carefully reviewed and discussed in MDT whenever appropriate. MRI, in particular, can more accurately assess lesion boundaries, especially in patients with dense breasts or multifocal disease, thereby enabling more detailed surgical planning and decreased re-excision risk [45, 46].

Accurate tumour localization is equally essential. Discussion with a radiologist may be required to identify the optimal imaging modality and localization technique that is both familiar to the surgeon and the radiologist [3].

In addition, patient selection is crucial for successful BCS, which is informed by tumour size, breast-to-tumour ratio, and the presence of multifocal or multicentric disease. Given the presence of high-risk features, intraoperative margin assessment may be selectively performed to ensure margins and successful breast conservation.

3.4.2 Improved Surgical Techniques

Localization Methods

Various methods of localization have been developed and utilized for non-palpable breast cancer [3]. However, no single modality is consistently superior to others. Hence, it is crucial for the surgeon to have close communication with the radiologist to choose the most familiar methods.

Oncoplastic Surgery (OPS) and Locoregional Flap

Oncoplastic surgery (OPS) can reduce the need for reoperation in anatomically suitable patients [47]. Commonly, OPS allows excision of a larger volume than simple excision, providing a wider margin and thereby reducing the risk of positive margin [48]. In a population-based study, OPS is associated with a modest but significant decrease in re-excision rate [49]. Moreover, in cases with involved margins, the conversion rate to mastectomy was also reduced with OPS. Similarly, the use of a locoregional flap may allow a relatively large defect to be adequately replaced, enabling a larger resection volume and hence improving margin clearance.

Cavity Shaving

Cavity shaving involves the systematic excision of additional tissue from the walls of the surgical cavity following a standard lumpectomy. By removing thin rims of tissue from each margin, the surgeon reduces the likelihood of leaving behind positive margins. A landmark randomized controlled trial revealed that the addition of cavity shaving halved the rates of positive margins (19% vs. 34%) and re-excision in patients with BCS (10% vs. 21%) [50]. The addition of cavity shaving did not lead to excessive excised tissue volume according to a 2017 meta-analysis [51].

3.4.3 Intraoperative Assessment Strategies

Several intraoperative margin assessment (IOMA) techniques have been developed to address the limitations of traditional methods, which often involve a delay in results and can lead to additional surgeries. These techniques can be broadly categorized into pathological, imaging, spectroscopic, optical, electrical, and molecular imaging approaches.

Pathological Techniques

Pathological techniques such as cytology and frozen section analysis are among the most established methods. Imprint cytology (IC) has demonstrated high diagnostic accuracy [52]. The technique involves pressing the lumpectomy specimen onto glass slides, which are then stained and analysed, offering a rapid assessment of the entire surface area while preserving tissue for permanent sectioning. However, it is less sensitive for ductal carcinoma in situ, invasive lobular carcinoma, and lobular carcinoma in situ, and less specific for the presence of atypical cells.

On the other hand, frozen section is another commonly used technique for intraoperative analysis. The tissue is rapidly frozen to −20 °C, cut at low temperature, mounted on slides, and stained for examination [53]. However, it can be time-consuming and labour-intensive. It also causes tissue loss during processing and may not accurately represent the entire specimen due to sampling limitations [54–56]. Additionally, the abundant adipose tissue in the breast produces significant artefacts in Frozen Section (FS), limiting its accuracy. A recent meta-analysis showed that the pooled specificity is around 97%, but the pooled sensitivity is lower at 81% [53].

Imaging Techniques

Imaging techniques, including specimen radiography and intraoperative ultrasound (IOUS), are also used for margin assessment [57]. Specimen radiography confirms the presence of a targeted lesion in the excised specimen, but has limitations in identifying diffuse microscopic processes. As with all breast radiography, the density of breast tissue could affect assessment, making it more challenging to evaluate dense breast tissue [58]. Compression is required for better mammographic views; however, it may alter tissue planes and affect accuracy. Digital specimen mammography is preferred over conventional specimen mammography because it eliminates the need for specimen compression and can be acquired with a small electronic device in or near the operating room, allowing for a more timely assessment [59]. The predictive value might be further enhanced with artificial intelligence assistance [60].

Intraoperative ultrasound (IOUS) is another established technique. Even though IOUS is operator dependent, studies have shown that the learning curve is relatively short [61]. It can be used to guide excision and to assess specimen completeness of removal and margin status. According to a recent systematic review, negative margin rates in the IOUS arm are significantly lower than those with wire-guided localization when data from three randomized controlled trials were included [62]. This was also confirmed by 41 cohort studies, with over 3000 patients analysed [62].

Automated three-dimensional breast ultrasound (ABUS) systems have been developed in recent years to overcome the shortcomings of hand-held ultrasound (HHUS) [63]. ABUS reconstructs the 3D images of the specimen from automatically acquired B-mode images. However, a specially trained medical assistant will be required for image acquisition, and it can only be used for ultrasound-visible lesions.

Novel Intraoperative Margin Assessment Technologies

Micro-Computed Tomography (MCT)

More advanced imaging methods, such as micro-computed tomography (MCT), are being explored. MCT uses a rotating sample and X-ray beams to create multiplanar, cross-sectional images [64]. Micro-CT provides rapid, volumetric scanning of an entire BCS resection with high reconstruction resolutions [64]. A large series involving 200 cases demonstrated that the receiver operating characteristic (ROC) curve of the Volumetric Specimen Imaging (VSI) was higher than those of the other specimen imaging methods [65]. The full-3D specimen imaging can improve the correlation between the main lumpectomy specimen margin status and surgical pathology. However, some studies showed no significant improvement when compared to standard specimen radiography [66, 67]. With ongoing technological advances, it has the potential to improve margin assessment.

Spectroscopic Techniques

Spectroscopic techniques analyse biochemical differences between malignant and benign tissue.

Optical spectroscopy has shown good diagnostic accuracy with a pooled sensitivity of 0.86 and specificity of 0.92 [68]. Raman spectroscopy (RS), which uses a laser to measure scattered light and identify unique vibrational spectra, is being investigated for real-time margin assessment [69].

Several commercially available devices are already on the market. The MarginProbe system (Dilon Technologies) [73], which operates on the principle of electrical impedance, has received FDA approval. Evidence from a systematic review indicates that its use significantly lowers re-excision rates in breast-conserving surgery, with no associated negative impact on cosmetic outcomes or the volume of tissue resected [70]. A separate device, ClearEdge (LsBiopath, Fig. 3.1a–c) [71], utilizes bioimpedance spectroscopy to analyse tissue resistance with alternating current. Data from a phase II cohort study have shown good diagnostic accuracy.

Optical Tissue Imaging Techniques

Optical tissue imaging techniques, such as optical coherence tomography (OCT), provide high-resolution, real-time images. OCT can image up to 2 mm beneath the tissue surface, allowing for microscopic assessment of tumour margins [72]. The pooled sensitivity was high at 0.91 and specificity at 88 for margin assessment in BCS, and its ability to image subsurface tissue is an advantage.

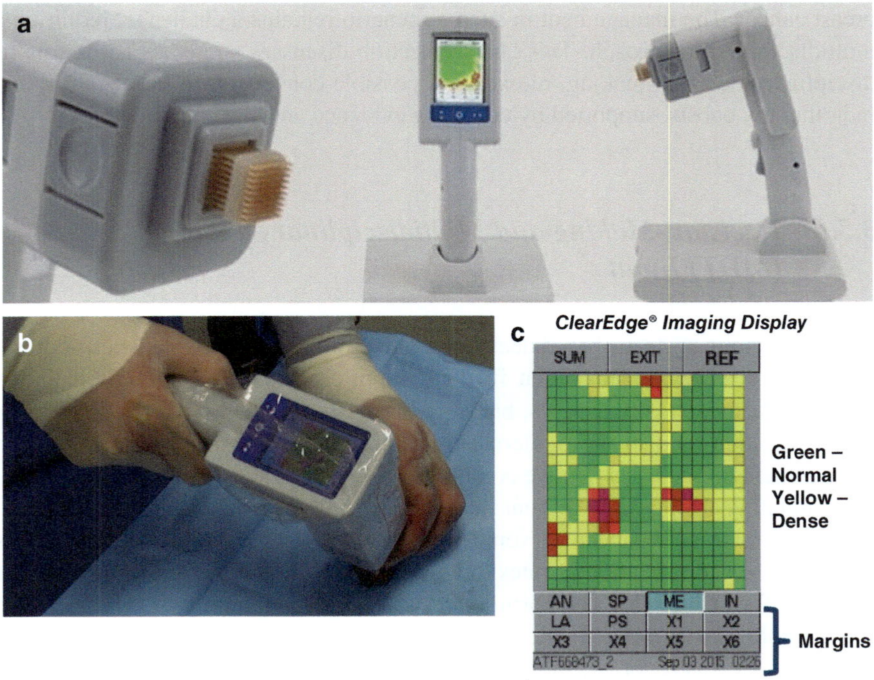

Fig. 3.1 (**a**–**c**) ClearEdge intraoperative imaging for breast cancer surgery [74]

Molecular Imaging
Finally, molecular imaging, such as fluorescence imaging, can detect residual cancer cells using molecular markers. The Lumicell Imaging System (LUM) system uses a fluorescent agent to image the tumour cavity to identify residual tumour, making it a direct visualization method for residual tumour compared to the indirect method of specimen assessment [75]. A feasibility study involving 45 patients was enrolled with the use of the LUM system, showing a sensitivity of 0.84 and specificity of 0.73 [75].

These technologies demonstrate the ongoing effort to improve the accuracy and efficiency of intraoperative margin assessment, ultimately aiming to reduce re-excision rates, improve patient outcomes, and make breast-conserving surgery more effective.

3.5 Management of Positive Margins in Non-Palpable Breast Cancer

Despite the advances in preoperative workup, surgical techniques, and intraoperative assessment, positive margins cannot be avoided entirely, especially in non-palpable breast cancer. The management in such a scenario remains a challenge, requiring a multidisciplinary approach. This chapter section discusses strategies across multidisciplinary decision-making, re-excision, possible conversion to mastectomy, and radiotherapy boosts, supported by emerging evidence and current guidelines.

3.5.1 Decision-Making and Multidisciplinary Team (MDT) Input

A multidisciplinary team-based decision-making process is valuable when addressing positive margins. This often involves input from breast surgeons, radiation oncologists, medical oncologists, breast radiologists, and pathologists [76]. This is especially important in the modern era, with complex treatment algorithms and management options, as effective communication among these specialists is crucial to formulating an optimal treatment strategy, especially when the margin is involved.

From a disease perspective, some researchers have sought to identify factors predicting re-excision success rates to guide surgical decisions. A normogram was proposed for DCIS [35]. The normogram was developed mainly based on clinical and pathological factors. In their external validation, an estimated concordance index of 0.71 was reported, suggesting the potential for this valuable tool to guide treatment recommendations, particularly for re-excision vs. completion mastectomy.

In deciding how to proceed, clinicians must consider factors such as the extent and location of the positive margin, tumour biology and molecular subtype, patient-specific preferences (e.g. desire for breast symmetry or aversion to multiple surgeries), and the feasibility of alternative treatments. For example, a study showed that older women were less likely to undergo reoperations after positive margins, but there was no difference in survival [77]. This was postulated Based on differences in tumour biology, such as lower-grade and less lymphovascular invasive tumours among older people. Shared decision-making has been emphasized as a patient-centred approach.

3.5.2 Re-Excision Surgery

When margins are deemed positive, re-excision is frequently the first recommended next step to ensure adequate oncologic control. Factors known to impact IBTR rates should be considered in determining the need for re-excision, especially when the margin is clear but close in DCIS, or when the positive margin is anterior, which has been shown to have a lower risk of residual tumour [20, 78, 79].

A frequent concern regarding re-excision is the risk of further positive margin, particularly in higher-risk tumours such as DCIS or ILC. A large cohort study has shown that, even though the margin-positive rate of ILC after the first lumpectomy is relatively high (37.6%), the re-excision success rate is 74.2% in patients who chose to undergo re-excision, giving an overall BCS success rate of 78.3% [80].

There have been concerns raised about the risk of increased recurrence in re-excision. Studies showed that multiple re-excisions do not affect local recurrence and provide a safe oncological outcome if negative margins can eventually be achieved [81, 82]. Hence, numerous re-excisions are still safe in carefully selected patients, and the need for mastectomy solely due to multiple re-excisions may not be necessary. Nonetheless, the patient must understand the risk of further involved margin and the need for further surgery. And there is a subgroup of patients who will still eventually need to resort to complete mastectomy due to extensive, multicentric disease.

With the use of oncoplastic surgery, BCS was made possible despite a larger resection volume compared to the breast. Despite the potentially higher tumour-to-breast ratio from the first operation, oncoplastic surgery, including level II procedures, is not contraindicated for re-excision, and it was found to be possible and appropriate as long as the remaining volume allows [28, 83]. However, some studies have suggested that at least in the short term, the aesthetic outcome could be impaired after re-excision [11], which could impact patients' quality of life, especially in the short-term [15]. Therefore, careful patient selection and well-planned surgery remain paramount, with the potential use of Oncoplastic surgery (OPS) when a high total excision volume is involved. In some scenarios, a locoregional flap can be utilized to fill the resected cavity [84].

In selected patients, the intraoperative frozen-section assessment can be used. Especially when a target margin is aimed at, the procedure for frozen section and the resources required might become more reasonable. Although intraoperative frozen section for BCS showed a decrease in margin involvement, there are only a handful of retrospective studies about its use in re-excision scenarios, and its efficacy remains unproven [85, 86]. One study concluded that underlying tumour characteristics should be more important in predicting clearance after re-excision [85]. Hence, the use in re-excision should be considered on a case-by-case basis, and this also highlights the importance of MDT input.

3.5.3 Conversion to Mastectomy

In some instances, re-excision may not be feasible or sufficient to achieve oncologically clear margins. Conversion to mastectomy represents a definitive option, particularly when tumour biology or breast size–tumour size ratios undermine the success of further breast conservation. Several factors may make completion mastectomy a more favourable option, including a larger tumour, a tumour with high-risk features, ILC, limited residual breast volume, high risk of gross deformity, and a higher number of margin involvement [49, 80, 87]. In addition, patients may prefer completion mastectomy to minimize the risk of further margin involvement and the need for a third surgery, which could create a psychological burden [13].

In patients where an optimal cosmetic outcome is preferred, immediate reconstruction at the time of completion of mastectomy can be offered. It remains a reasonable choice despite a potentially slight increase in risk of revision compared to primary mastectomy with immediate reconstruction [88].

Of note, according to the literature, up to 54% of mastectomies performed after Breast-Conserving Therapy (BCT) contained no residual tumour [89]. Hence, it is essential during counselling that there is always a chance of no further residual tumour in the residual breast, and the implication of mastectomy has to be clearly explained, especially in patients whose original wish was for breast conservation.

3.5.4 Radiotherapy Boost

Finally, a targeted radiotherapy (RT) boost can be a safe option in carefully selected patients. It is also considered when reoperation is contraindicated or not preferred. According to the long-term follow-up results from a Randomized Controlled Trial (RCT) compared between patients with additional RT boost vs. whole-breast irradiation only, there is an improved local control in the patients receiving RT boost, with the 20-year cumulative incidence of ipsilateral breast tumour recurrence at 16.4% in the no boost group vs. 12.0% in the boost group [90].

In more recent years, an increasing body of evidence supports the role of high-dose radiotherapy in carefully selected scenarios, particularly for ductal carcinoma in situ (DCIS). Dose escalation to the tumour bed (≥66 Gy total) was shown to achieve excellent local control in patients with DCIS who have close (<2 mm) or focally/minimally involved margins [91]. In this study, 61 patients (29%) underwent re-excision before irradiation, and 147 patients (71%) received breast irradiation with boost, without re-excision. Seven-year IBTR rates were 9.3% without and 9.6% with re-excision. No differences were observed when adjusting for margin status.

The margin needed for DCIS also creates a subgroup of patients with 'close' margins, where the margin was clear from the DCIS tumour cells but more than 2 mm. The need for another excision in this group of patients was being challenged frequently, as the chance of further presence of tumour cells in the remaining breast is low. Tailored radiation doses based on the margin width may be an option for this patient group. According to a recent study, local recurrence-free survival remained similar between those with close margins and those with negative margins when a tailored radiation dose was prescribed [92].

When considering invasive disease, a radiotherapy boost can also be an option in older or medically frail patients with positive margins, as suggested by a study involving 550 invasive ductal carcinoma (IDC) patients followed for a median of 58 months [93]. In that cohort, a modest increase in the total equivalent dose in 2 Gy fractions (EQD2) delivered to the tumour bed—ranging from 65.81 to 66.25 Gy for positive margins—was not associated with a significant difference in local control for older patients compared with re-excision. However, in younger patients, re-excision plus standard RT remained significantly superior (local recurrence-free survival 89.2% vs. 97.6%). These findings underscore the importance of patient selection: a radiotherapy boost may offer a safe alternative to surgery in well-defined subsets of the population (e.g. older patients with comorbidities), but it is less likely to replace re-excision in younger, higher-risk patients.

However, although a boost provides a degree of reduction in ipsilateral breast tumour recurrence (IBTR), the absolute benefit is not sufficient to reduce the rate of IBTR to that seen with negative margins and the use of a boost [94]. Moreover, a radiotherapy boost can lead to increased long-term side effects, especially fibrosis. Hence, in general, re-excision is still more advisable in most patients with positive margins [20].

3.5.5 Section Summary

As our understanding of multifaceted risk factors grows, individualized treatment strategies will continue to evolve. For now, the focus remains a multidisciplinary team-based approach that incorporates patient preferences, tumour biology, and best-practice guidelines. Although re-excision remains the safest choice, completion mastectomy might help avoid further surgery, while radiation boost could be preferred in selected patients (Flowchart 3.1).

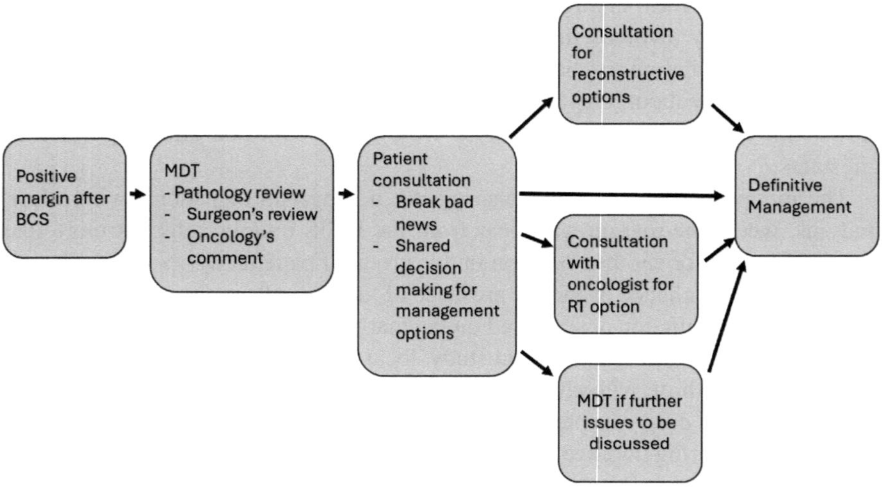

Flowchart 3.1 Workflow after positive margin

3.6 Special Scenarios

3.6.1 Multifocal/Multicentric Tumour

Multifocal and multicentric breast cancers present distinct challenges, particularly when attempting breast-conserving surgery (BCS). While re-excision is a possible option with careful planning, patients must be counselled about the possibility of multiple surgeries and the increased likelihood of ultimately converting to mastectomy if repeated re-excisions fail to secure clear margins. MDT with radiologists' and pathologists' valuable input may also help to better localize the involved area for re-excision and the extent of potential residual disease. With careful planning, it can remain oncologically safe if a clear margin can ultimately be achieved by re-excision [95].

3.6.2 Elderly Patient

Management strategies differ substantially in older adults due to comorbidities, frailty, and life expectancy. Some elderly patients may face a higher operative risk from repeat procedures, making re-excision for a positive margin less desirable. Furthermore, limited functional reserves and potential delays in adjuvant therapies (e.g. radiation or endocrine therapy) influence the clinical decision. Shared decision-making and comprehensive geriatric assessments are crucial at this juncture. In select older patients with small-volume residual disease and hormone receptor–positive tumours, an alternative might be to omit a second surgery and/or radiation boost. However, there is no universal consensus, and recommendations should be tailored to tumour biology, patient performance status, and patient preference.

3.6.3 Use of Oncoplastic Surgical Technique

If positive margins are found after oncoplastic breast surgery (OBS), surgeons may face complex reconstructive challenges because a significant volume of tissue has already been rearranged or partially removed. A second oncoplastic revision is possible—particularly if the remaining breast volume can tolerate another resection. A detailed review with the first operating surgeon is crucial to locate the corresponding margin that requires re-excision, and collaboration with plastic surgery might be needed to plan further tissue rearrangement [83].

On the other hand, in a patient with prior simple BCS, oncoplastic breast surgery (OBS) during re-excision can offer a valuable solution by allowing more generous excision while maintaining a favourable cosmetic result. As oncoplastic techniques integrate plastic surgery principles—such as tissue rearrangement, glandular flaps, or local tissue advancement—to resect additional breast tissue and keep the breast aesthetically acceptable, the need for conversion to mastectomy might be less [96].

3.6.4 Locoregional Flap

In some instances, locoregional flaps—such as a latissimus dorsi mini-flap—are used initially to fill a large defect and maintain cosmetic integrity. When a margin is positive, the flap itself may obscure the tumour bed, especially when the operated site has already healed, making re-excision more technically challenging. Further imaging, especially doppler, might be required, and surgeons must confirm the flap's vascular supply and viability, as revisions can compromise blood flow and healing. If the flap can be partially mobilized and repositioned, a more localized procedure could still be safe without long-term oncological compromise [97]. However, if re-excision risks flap necrosis or yields suboptimal clearance, mastectomy may be necessary.

In some scenarios, a locoregional flap can be utilized to fill the resected cavity when a larger volume of tissue must be removed to ensure clear margins [84]. Incorporating a local rotation flap or a latissimus dorsi mini-flap can preserve breast shape and symmetry, particularly if the excision is located in an area where simple closure would cause significant deformity. Locoregional flaps can be especially advantageous in smaller-breasted individuals or when the tumour is in a cosmetically sensitive area (e.g. the lower pole of the breast). Though it may require longer surgery time and requires technical expertise, a locoregional flap is a valuable option to avoid mastectomy while achieving negative margins.

3.6.5 Second Margin Positive

A particularly challenging scenario emerges when a second margin is found to be positive after re-excision. This outcome raises concerns about multifocal or extensive disease that may not be adequately controlled with further partial breast resections. In these recurrently positive margin cases, many clinicians consider mastectomy—possibly with immediate reconstruction—to definitively secure local control [82]. For patients strongly desiring breast conservation, a thorough re-evaluation is required, including detailed imaging (MRI if not already performed), potential use of oncoplastic surgery, or consultation with radiation oncology regarding an intensified boost. Nevertheless, with every additional resection, the risk of adverse cosmetic outcomes and potential delays in adjuvant therapy increases. Repeated margin involvement typically indicates more diffuse disease, making mastectomy a recommended option for optimal oncologic control.

3.6.6 Post-Neoadjuvant Therapy

Management after neoadjuvant therapy (NAT) can be uniquely challenging. While NAT may shrink tumours sufficiently for BCS, residual microscopic disease can remain [38]. Identifying the precise tumour bed can be difficult if the tumour regresses. Hence, before NAT, clip placement is essential if BCS is planned.

A response to NAT may result in tumour bed fibrosis, complicating margin assessment. Positive margins following NAT raise questions about disease biology—particularly in more aggressive phenotypes like triple-negative or HER2-positive tumours—and the completeness of the response.

3.7 Controversies and Future Directions

The ongoing debate surrounding optimal margin width in breast cancer surgery continues to evolve, particularly regarding the universal applicability of the 'no ink on tumor' standard. A recent meta-analysis suggested a 1 mm margin, followed by the update from the NICE guideline [18].

Technological innovations in margin assessment may have an impact on surgical decision-making. New imaging modalities and digital pathology are emerging as transformative forces in margin assessment.

Looking ahead, the field is moving towards increasingly personalized approaches when there is a positive margin. Ongoing research focuses on further specification between various degrees of involvement/close proximity, integration of molecular signatures, patient-specific risk factors, treatment response patterns, and long-term oncological outcomes into decision-making algorithms. The development of frontier in margin assessment technology may also provide a better intraoperative assessment tool to allow immediate additional resection, minimizing the need for second procedure.

References

1. Welch HG, Prorok PC, O'Malley AJ, Kramer BS. Breast-cancer tumor size, overdiagnosis, and mammography screening effectiveness. N Engl J Med. 2016;375(15):1438–47. https://doi.org/10.1056/NEJMoa1600249.
2. Nederend J, Duijm LEM, Louwman MWJ, Groenewoud JH, Donkers-van Rossum AB, Voogd AC. Impact of transition from analog screening mammography to digital screening mammography on screening outcome in The Netherlands: a population-based study. Ann Oncol. 2012;23(12):3098–103. https://doi.org/10.1093/annonc/mds146.
3. Cheung BHH, Co M, Lui TTN, Kwong A. Evolution of localization methods for non-palpable breast lesions: a literature review from a translational medicine perspective. Transl Breast Cancer Res. 2024;5:12.
4. Houssami N, Macaskill P, Luke Marinovich M, Morrow M. The association of surgical margins and local recurrence in women with early-stage invasive breast cancer treated with breast-conserving therapy: a meta-analysis. Ann Surg Oncol. 2014;21:717–30.
5. Baliski C, Bakos B. Patient reported outcomes following breast conserving surgery are improved by minimizing re-excisions and excessive breast tissue removal. Am J Surg. 2022;224(2):716–21. https://doi.org/10.1016/j.amjsurg.2022.03.008.
6. Pleijhuis RG, Kwast AB, Jansen L, et al. A validated web-based nomogram for predicting positive surgical margins following breast-conserving surgery as a preoperative tool for clinical decision-making. Breast. 2013;22(5):773–9.
7. Shirazi S, Hajiesmaeili H, Khosla M, Taj S, Sircar T, Vidya R. Comparison of wire and non-wire localisation techniques in breast cancer surgery: a review of the literature with pooled analysis. Medicina (Kaunas). 2023;59(7):1297. https://doi.org/10.3390/medicina59071297.
8. Bundred JR, Michael S, Stuart B, et al. Margin status and survival outcomes after breast cancer conservation surgery: prospectively registered systematic review and meta-analysis. BMJ. 2022;378:e070346. https://doi.org/10.1136/bmj-2022-070346.
9. Clarke M, Collins R, Darby S, et al. Effects of radiotherapy and of differences in the extent of surgery for early breast cancer on local recurrence and 15-year survival: an overview of the randomised trials. Lancet. 2005;366(9503):2087–106. https://doi.org/10.1016/s0140-6736(05)67887-7.
10. Wazer DE, DiPetrillo T, Schmidt-Ullrich R, et al. Factors influencing cosmetic outcome and complication risk after conservative surgery and radiotherapy for early-stage breast carcinoma. J Clin Oncol. 1992;10(3):356–63. https://doi.org/10.1200/jco.1992.10.3.356.
11. Heil J, Breitkreuz K, Golatta M, et al. Do reexcisions impair aesthetic outcome in breast conservation surgery? Exploratory analysis of a prospective cohort study. Ann Surg Oncol. 2012;19(2):541–7. https://doi.org/10.1245/s10434-011-1947-1.
12. McCahill LE, Single RM, Aiello Bowles EJ, et al. Variability in reexcision following breast conservation surgery. JAMA. 2012;307(5):467–75. https://doi.org/10.1001/jama.2012.43.
13. Oudhoff JP, Timmermans DR, Knol DL, Bijnen AB, van der Wal G. Waiting for elective general surgery: impact on health related quality of life and psychosocial consequences. BMC Public Health. 2007;7:164. https://doi.org/10.1186/1471-2458-7-164.
14. Klassen AF, Dominici L, Fuzesi S, et al. Development and validation of the BREAST-Q breast-conserving therapy module. Ann Surg Oncol. 2020;27(7):2238–47. https://doi.org/10.1245/s10434-019-08195-w.

15. Matar-Ujvary R, Haglich K, Flanagan MR, et al. The impact of breast-conserving surgery re-excision on patient-reported outcomes using the BREAST-Q. Ann Surg Oncol. 2023;30(9):5341–9. https://doi.org/10.1245/s10434-023-13592-3.
16. Moran MS, Schnitt SJ, Giuliano AE, et al. Society of Surgical Oncology-American Society for Radiation Oncology consensus guideline on margins for breast-conserving surgery with whole-breast irradiation in stages I and II invasive breast cancer. Ann Surg Oncol. 2014;21(3):704–16. https://doi.org/10.1245/s10434-014-3481-4.
17. Gradishar WJ, Moran MS, Abraham J, et al. Breast cancer, version 3.2024, NCCN clinical practice guidelines in oncology. J Natl Compr Cancer Netw. 2024;22(5):331–57.
18. National Institute for Health and Care Excellence. Early and locally advanced breast cancer: diagnosis and management (NG101). 2024. https://www.nice.org.uk/guidance/ng101/chapter/Recommendations#surgery-to-the-breast.
19. Dunne C, Burke JP, Morrow M, Kell MR. Effect of margin status on local recurrence after breast conservation and radiation therapy for ductal carcinoma in situ. J Clin Oncol. 2009;27(10):1615–20. https://doi.org/10.1200/jco.2008.17.5182.
20. Morrow M, Van Zee KJ, Solin LJ, et al. Society of Surgical Oncology–American Society for Radiation Oncology–American Society of Clinical Oncology consensus guideline on margins for breast-conserving surgery with whole-breast irradiation in ductal carcinoma in situ. J Clin Oncol. 2016;34(33):4040–6. https://doi.org/10.1200/jco.2016.68.3573.
21. Ezzat A, Shanthakumar D, Laskar N, et al. Impact of resection margin width on local recurrence following breast-conserving surgery and whole breast radiotherapy for pure ductal carcinoma in situ: a systematic review and meta-analysis. BMJ Oncol. 2025;4(1):e000633. https://doi.org/10.1136/bmjonc-2024-000633.
22. Biglia N, Maggiorotto F, Liberale V, et al. Clinical-pathologic features, long term-outcome and surgical treatment in a large series of patients with invasive lobular carcinoma (ILC) and invasive ductal carcinoma (IDC). Eur J Surg Oncol. 2013;39(5):455–60. https://doi.org/10.1016/j.ejso.2013.02.007.
23. Galimberti V, Maisonneuve P, Rotmensz N, et al. Influence of margin status on outcomes in lobular carcinoma: experience of the European Institute of Oncology. Ann Surg. 2011;253(3):580–4. https://doi.org/10.1097/SLA.0b013e31820d9a81.
24. Beck AC, Bayard S, Plitas G, et al. Does non-classic lobular carcinoma in situ at the lumpectomy margin increase local recurrence? Ann Surg Oncol. 2023;30(10):6061–9. https://doi.org/10.1245/s10434-023-13899-1.
25. Langhans L, Jensen MB, Talman MM, Vejborg I, Kroman N, Tvedskov TF. Reoperation rates in ductal carcinoma in situ vs invasive breast cancer after wire-guided breast-conserving surgery. JAMA Surg. 2017;152(4):378–84. https://doi.org/10.1001/jamasurg.2016.4751.
26. Chauhan H, Jiwa N, Nagarajan VR, et al. Clinicopathological predictors of positive resection margins in breast-conserving surgery. Ann Surg Oncol. 2024;31(6):3939–47. https://doi.org/10.1245/s10434-024-15153-8.
27. Christgen M, Steinemann D, Kühnle E, et al. Lobular breast cancer: clinical, molecular and morphological characteristics. Pathol Res Pract. 2016;212(7):583–97. https://doi.org/10.1016/j.prp.2016.05.002.
28. Clough KB, Gouveia PF, Benyahi D, et al. Positive margins after oncoplastic surgery for breast cancer. Ann Surg Oncol. 2015;22(13):4247–53. https://doi.org/10.1245/s10434-015-4514-3.
29. Wanis ML, Wong JA, Rodriguez S, et al. Rate of re-excision after breast-conserving surgery for invasive lobular carcinoma. Am Surg. 2013;79(10):1119–22.
30. Pereslucha AM, Wenger DM, Morris MF, Aydi ZB. Invasive lobular carcinoma: a review of imaging modalities with special focus on pathology concordance. Healthcare. 2023;11(5):746.
31. Chen Y-Y, Hwang E-SS, Roy R, et al. Genetic and phenotypic characteristics of pleomorphic lobular carcinoma in situ of the breast. Am J Surg Pathol. 2009;33(11):1683–94.
32. Lowery AJ, Kell MR, Glynn RW, Kerin MJ, Sweeney KJ. Locoregional recurrence after breast cancer surgery: a systematic review by receptor phenotype. Breast Cancer Res Treat. 2012;133:831–41.

33. Smitt MC, Nowels K, Carlson RW, Jeffrey SS. Predictors of reexcision findings and recurrence after breast conservation. Int J Radiat Oncol Biol Phys. 2003;57(4):979–85. https://doi.org/10.1016/s0360-3016(03)00740-5.
34. Holland R, Connolly JL, Gelman R, et al. The presence of an extensive intraductal component following a limited excision correlates with prominent residual disease in the remainder of the breast. J Clin Oncol. 1990;8(1):113–8. https://doi.org/10.1200/jco.1990.8.1.113.
35. Martins Maia C, Siderides C, Jaffer S, et al. Mastectomy or margin re-excision? A nomogram for close/positive margins after lumpectomy for DCIS. Ann Surg Oncol. 2022;29(6):3740–8. https://doi.org/10.1245/s10434-021-11293-3.
36. Fauveau LR, Dao TN, Wallace LB, et al. Positive surgical margins after breast-conserving surgery for ductal carcinoma in-situ: does histologic grade or estrogen receptor status matter? Breast Cancer Res Treat. 2023;199(2):215–20. https://doi.org/10.1007/s10549-023-06905-3.
37. Patterson R, Guest M, Shenouda M, et al. Predictors of residual disease after breast conservation surgery for ductal carcinoma in situ: a retrospective study. J Cancer Res Ther. 2024;20(3):844–9. https://doi.org/10.4103/jcrt.jcrt_2657_22.
38. Cen C, Chun J, Kaplowitz E, et al. Margin assessment and re-excision rates for patients who have neoadjuvant chemotherapy and breast-conserving surgery. Ann Surg Oncol. 2021;28(9):5142–8. https://doi.org/10.1245/s10434-020-09524-0.
39. Kaplan J, Giron G, Tartter PI, Bleiweiss IJ, Estabrook A, Smith SR. Breast conservation in patients with multiple ipsilateral synchronous cancers. J Am Coll Surg. 2003;197(5):726–9. https://doi.org/10.1016/j.jamcollsurg.2003.06.003.
40. Bauman L, Barth RJ, Rosenkranz KM. Breast conservation in women with multifocal-multicentric breast cancer: is it feasible? Ann Surg Oncol. 2010;17(Suppl 3):325–9. https://doi.org/10.1245/s10434-010-1247-1.
41. Georgescu R, Tutuianu F, Bauer O, et al. Risk factors for positive resection margins in breast-conserving surgery for breast cancer-retrospective analysis. Cancers (Basel). 2024;16(17):2930. https://doi.org/10.3390/cancers16172930.
42. Cantini L, Trapani D, Guidi L, et al. Neoadjuvant therapy in hormone receptor-positive/HER2-negative breast cancer. Cancer Treat Rev. 2024;123:102669. https://doi.org/10.1016/j.ctrv.2023.102669.
43. Walsh SM, Brennan SB, Zabor EC, et al. Does breast density increase the risk of re-excision for women with breast cancer having breast-conservation therapy? Ann Surg Oncol. 2019;26(13):4246–53. https://doi.org/10.1245/s10434-019-07647-7.
44. Jung W, Kang E, Kim SM, et al. Factors associated with re-excision after breast-conserving surgery for early-stage breast cancer. J Breast Cancer. 2012;15(4):412–9. https://doi.org/10.4048/jbc.2012.15.4.412.
45. Burkbauer L, Goldbach M, Hoffman DI, et al. Preoperative MRI and its impact on surgical outcomes in patients with triple negative breast cancer treated with primary surgery: did new margin guidelines or cavity shave margins practice diminish the role of preoperative MRI? Ann Surg Oncol. 2022;29:4079–88. https://doi.org/10.1245/s10434-022-11545-w.
46. Patel BK, Shah NA, Galgano SJ, et al. Does preoperative MRI workup affect mastectomy rates and/or re-excision rates in patients with newly diagnosed breast carcinoma? A retrospective review. Breast J. 2015;21(6):604–9. https://doi.org/10.1111/tbj.12490.
47. McEvoy MP, Landercasper J, Naik HR, Feldman S. Update of the American Society of Breast Surgeons Toolbox to address the lumpectomy reoperation epidemic. Gland Surg. 2018;7(6):536–53. https://doi.org/10.21037/gs.2018.11.03.
48. Chauhan A, Sharma MM. Evaluation of surgical outcomes following oncoplastic breast surgery in early breast cancer and comparison with conventional breast conservation surgery. Med J Armed Forces India. 2016;72(1):12–8. https://doi.org/10.1016/j.mjafi.2015.11.001.
49. Heeg E, Jensen MB, Hölmich LR, et al. Rates of re-excision and conversion to mastectomy after breast-conserving surgery with or without oncoplastic surgery: a nationwide population-based study. Br J Surg. 2020;107(13):1762–72. https://doi.org/10.1002/bjs.11838.

50. Chagpar AB, Killelea BK, Tsangaris TN, et al. A randomized, controlled trial of cavity shave margins in breast cancer. N Engl J Med. 2015;373(6):503–10. https://doi.org/10.1056/NEJMoa1504473.
51. Wang K, Ren Y, He J. Cavity shaving plus lumpectomy versus lumpectomy alone for patients with breast cancer undergoing breast-conserving surgery: a systematic review and meta-analysis. PLoS One. 2017;12(1):e0168705. https://doi.org/10.1371/journal.pone.0168705.
52. Esbona K, Li Z, Wilke LG. Intraoperative imprint cytology and frozen section pathology for margin assessment in breast conservation surgery: a systematic review. Ann Surg Oncol. 2012;19(10):3236–45. https://doi.org/10.1245/s10434-012-2492-2.
53. Garcia MT, Mota BS, Cardoso N, et al. Accuracy of frozen section in intraoperative margin assessment for breast-conserving surgery: a systematic review and meta-analysis. PLoS One. 2021;16(3):e0248768. https://doi.org/10.1371/journal.pone.0248768.
54. Pradipta AR, Tanei T, Morimoto K, Shimazu K, Noguchi S, Tanaka K. Emerging technologies for real-time intraoperative margin assessment in future breast-conserving surgery. Adv Sci (Weinh). 2020;7(9):1901519. https://doi.org/10.1002/advs.201901519.
55. Jorns JM, Visscher D, Sabel M, et al. Intraoperative frozen section analysis of margins in breast conserving surgery significantly decreases reoperative rates: one-year experience at an ambulatory surgical center. Am J Clin Pathol. 2012;138(5):657–69.
56. Jaafar H. Intra-operative frozen section consultation: concepts, applications and limitations. Malays J Med Sci. 2006;13(1):4.
57. Kopicky L, Fan B, Valente SA. Intraoperative evaluation of surgical margins in breast cancer. Semin Diagn Pathol. 2024;41(6):293–300. https://doi.org/10.1053/j.semdp.2024.06.005.
58. Kim JY, Jung YS, Han SH, Sung JH, Hur MH. Indications and methods of intraoperative specimen radiography in breast-conserving surgery. Transl Cancer Res. 2020;9(11):6625–8. https://doi.org/10.21037/tcr-20-2859.
59. Lin C, Wang KY, Chen HL, Xu YH, Pan T, Chen YD. Specimen mammography for intraoperative margin assessment in breast conserving surgery: a meta-analysis. Sci Rep. 2022;12(1):18440. https://doi.org/10.1038/s41598-022-23234-5.
60. Chen KA, Kirchoff KE, Butler LR, et al. Analysis of specimen mammography with artificial intelligence to predict margin status. Ann Surg Oncol. 2023;30(12):7107–15. https://doi.org/10.1245/s10434-023-14083-1.
61. Ivanov V, Dimov R, Marinov B, Ivanov V, Tashkova D. Intraoperative ultrasound for nonpalpable breast lesions – experience and operative time. Folia Med (Plovdiv). 2023;65(1):16–9. https://doi.org/10.3897/folmed.65.e76193.
62. Banys-Paluchowski M, Rubio IT, Karadeniz Cakmak G, et al. Intraoperative ultrasound-guided excision of non-palpable and palpable breast cancer: systematic review and meta-analysis. Ultraschall Med. 2022;43(4):367–79. Intraoperative Sonographie zur Entfernung von nicht-palpablen und palpablen Mammakarzinomen: systematisches review und meta-analyse. https://doi.org/10.1055/a-1821-8559.
63. Hatzipanagiotou ME, Huber D, Thede E, et al. Automated breast ultrasound (ABUS) for intraoperative margin control on surgical specimens in breast conserving surgery. Arch Gynecol Obstet. 2023;307(6):1949–55. https://doi.org/10.1007/s00404-022-06837-1.
64. McClatchy DM, Zuurbier RA, Wells WA, Paulsen KD, Pogue BW. Micro-computed tomography enables rapid surgical margin assessment during breast conserving surgery (BCS): correlation of whole BCS micro-CT readings to final histopathology. Breast Cancer Res Treat. 2018;172:587–95.
65. Kulkarni SA, Kulkarni K, Schacht D, et al. High-resolution full-3D specimen imaging for lumpectomy margin assessment in breast cancer. Ann Surg Oncol. 2021;28(10):5513–24. https://doi.org/10.1245/s10434-021-10499-9.
66. Abel TN, Bourke AG. Can micro-computed tomography imaging improve interpretation of macroscopic margin assessment of specimen radiography in excised breast specimens? J Cancer Res Ther. 2020;16(6):1366–70. https://doi.org/10.4103/jcrt.JCRT_949_19.

67. Streeter SS, Zuurbier RA, diFlorio-Alexander RM, et al. Breast-conserving surgery margin guidance using micro-computed tomography: challenges when imaging radiodense resection specimens. Ann Surg Oncol. 2023;30(7):4097–108. https://doi.org/10.1245/s10434-023-13364-z.
68. Dowling GP, Hehir CM, Daly GR, et al. Diagnostic accuracy of intraoperative methods for margin assessment in breast cancer surgery: a systematic review & meta-analysis. Breast. 2024;76:103749. https://doi.org/10.1016/j.breast.2024.103749.
69. Hanna K, Krzoska E, Shaaban AM, Muirhead D, Abu-Eid R, Speirs V. Raman spectroscopy: current applications in breast cancer diagnosis, challenges and future prospects. Br J Cancer. 2022;126(8):1125–39. https://doi.org/10.1038/s41416-021-01659-5.
70. Rossou C, Alampritis G, Patel B. Reducing re-excision rates in breast conserving surgery with Margin Probe: systematic review. Br J Surg. 2024;111(1):znad335. https://doi.org/10.1093/bjs/znad335.
71. Dixon JM, Renshaw L, Young O, et al. Intra-operative assessment of excised breast tumour margins using ClearEdge imaging device. Eur J Surg Oncol. 2016;42(12):1834–40. https://doi.org/10.1016/j.ejso.2016.07.141.
72. Duan Y, Guo D, Zhang X, et al. Diagnostic accuracy of optical coherence tomography for margin assessment in breast-conserving surgery: a systematic review and meta-analysis. Photodiagn Photodyn Ther. 2023;43:103718. https://doi.org/10.1016/j.pdpdt.2023.103718.
73. Inc. DT. MarginProbe®. Dilon Technologies Inc. https://dilon.com/marginprobe/. Accessed 13 Jan 2024.
74. Inc. LB. Solution – ClearEdge. LS BioPath Inc. https://lsbiopath.com/solution/. Accessed 13 Jan 2024.
75. Smith BL, Lanahan CR, Specht MC, et al. Feasibility study of a novel protease-activated fluorescent imaging system for real-time, intraoperative detection of residual breast cancer in breast conserving surgery. Ann Surg Oncol. 2020;27(6):1854–61. https://doi.org/10.1245/s10434-019-08158-1.
76. Saini KS, Taylor C, Ramirez AJ, et al. Role of the multidisciplinary team in breast cancer management: results from a large international survey involving 39 countries. Ann Oncol. 2012;23(4):853–9. https://doi.org/10.1093/annonc/mdr352.
77. Angarita FA, Acuna SA, McCready DR, Escallon J. Management of positive margins after initial lumpectomy in elderly women with breast cancer. Eur J Surg Oncol. 2018;44(7):1048–53. https://doi.org/10.1016/j.ejso.2018.02.011.
78. O'Connell L, Walsh S, Evoy D, et al. The approach to an isolated close anterior margin in breast conserving surgery. Ann R Coll Surg Engl. 2019;101(4):268–72. https://doi.org/10.1308/rcsann.2019.0017.
79. Ang SC, Tapia G, Davidson EJ, et al. Positive anterior margins in breast conserving surgery: does it matter? A systematic review of the literature. Breast. 2016;27:105–8. https://doi.org/10.1016/j.breast.2015.12.013.
80. Piper ML, Wong J, Fahrner-Scott K, et al. Success rates of re-excision after positive margins for invasive lobular carcinoma of the breast. NPJ Breast Cancer. 2019;5(1):29. https://doi.org/10.1038/s41523-019-0125-7.
81. O'Sullivan MJ, Li T, Freedman G, Morrow M. The effect of multiple reexcisions on the risk of local recurrence after breast conserving surgery. Ann Surg Oncol. 2007;14(11):3133–40. https://doi.org/10.1245/s10434-007-9523-4.
82. Coopey S, Smith BL, Hanson S, et al. The safety of multiple re-excisions after lumpectomy for breast cancer. Ann Surg Oncol. 2011;18(13):3797–801. https://doi.org/10.1245/s10434-011-1802-4.
83. Martin TA, Choudhry S, Holton LH, et al. Outcomes of margin reexcision after oncoplastic breast reduction. Plast Reconstr Surg Glob Open. 2022;10(9):e4509. https://doi.org/10.1097/gox.0000000000004509.

84. Quinn EM, Burrah R, O'Ceallaigh S, Highton L, Murphy J. Six-year experience of oncoplastic volume replacement using local perforator flaps. J Plast Reconstr Aesthet Surg. 2021;74(9):2184–93. https://doi.org/10.1016/j.bjps.2020.12.083.
85. Jorns JM, Daignault S, Sabel MS, Wu AJ. Is intraoperative frozen section analysis of reexcision specimens of value in preventing reoperation in breast-conserving therapy? Am J Clin Pathol. 2014;142(5):601–8. https://doi.org/10.1309/ajcprsoa2g8rlexy.
86. Shen JG, Wang LB, Jiang ZN, Yuan XM, Zhao WH, Shen J. Value of intraoperative frozen section analysis in re-excision margin evaluation in breast-conserving surgery for cancer: a single institution experience. Indian J Surg. 2022;84(3):733–8. https://doi.org/10.1007/s12262-021-02952-6.
87. O'Donnell ME, Salem A, Badger SA, Sharif MA, Lioe T, Spence RA. Completion mastectomy after breast conserving surgery. Breast. 2008;17(2):199–204. https://doi.org/10.1016/j.breast.2007.10.001.
88. Rochlin DH, Sheckter CC, Momeni A. Failed breast conservation therapy predicts higher frequency of revision surgery following mastectomy with reconstruction. Plast Reconstr Surg. 2022;149(4):811–8. https://doi.org/10.1097/prs.0000000000008896.
89. Pahmeyer C, Schablack A, Ratiu D, et al. Occurrence of residual cancer within re-excisions after subcutaneous mastectomy of invasive breast cancer and ductal carcinoma in situ – a retrospective analysis. In Vivo. 2020;34(4):2015–9. https://doi.org/10.21873/invivo.12000.
90. Bartelink H, Maingon P, Poortmans P, et al. Whole-breast irradiation with or without a boost for patients treated with breast-conserving surgery for early breast cancer: 20-year follow-up of a randomised phase 3 trial. Lancet Oncol. 2015;16(1):47–56. https://doi.org/10.1016/s1470-2045(14)71156-8.
91. Monteau A, Sigal-Zafrani B, Kirova YM, et al. Ductal carcinoma in situ of the breast with close or focally involved margins following breast-conserving surgery: treatment with reexcision or radiotherapy with increased dosage. Int J Radiat Oncol Biol Phys. 2009;75(4):1021–8. https://doi.org/10.1016/j.ijrobp.2008.12.014.
92. Kim H, Kim TG, Park B, et al. Tailored radiation dose according to margin width for patients with ductal carcinoma in situ after breast-conserving surgery. Sci Rep. 2024;14(1):300. https://doi.org/10.1038/s41598-023-50840-8.
93. Kim H, Kim TG, Park B, et al. Effect of high-dose radiation therapy on positive margins after breast-conserving surgery for invasive breast cancer. Breast. 2023;71:106–12. https://doi.org/10.1016/j.breast.2023.08.003.
94. Jones HA, Antonini N, Hart AA, et al. Impact of pathological characteristics on local relapse after breast-conserving therapy: a subgroup analysis of the EORTC boost versus no boost trial. J Clin Oncol. 2009;27(30):4939–47. https://doi.org/10.1200/jco.2008.21.5764.
95. Gentilini O, Botteri E, Rotmensz N, et al. Conservative surgery in patients with multifocal/multicentric breast cancer. Breast Cancer Res Treat. 2009;113(3):577–83. https://doi.org/10.1007/s10549-008-9959-7.
96. Mactier M, Mansell J, Arthur L, Doughty J, Romics L. Survival after standard or oncoplastic breast-conserving surgery versus mastectomy for breast cancer. BJS Open. 2025;9(2):zraf002. https://doi.org/10.1093/bjsopen/zraf002.
97. Tokui R, Ishitobi M, Kurita T, et al. A comparison of the oncological outcomes after breast-conserving surgery with or without latissimus dorsi myocutaneous flap reconstruction for breast cancer. Clin Breast Cancer. 2022;22(2):e184–90. https://doi.org/10.1016/j.clbc.2021.06.005.

Chapter 4
Current Trends in Axillary Management

Christopher D. Vetter and Judy C. Boughey

Contents

C. D. Vetter · J. C. Boughey (✉)
Division of Breast and Melanoma Surgical Oncology, Mayo Clinic, Rochester, MN, USA
e-mail: Boughey.Judy@mayo.edu

R. Vidya, N. Sharma (eds.), *Breast and Axilla Localisation Techniques*,
https://doi.org/10.1007/978-3-032-17995-1_4

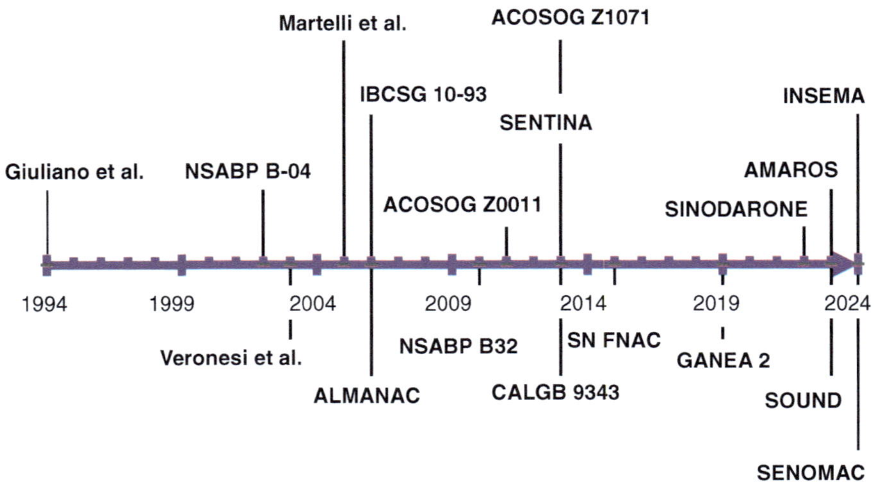

Fig. 4.1 Timeline of landmark clinical trials in axillary management

4.1 Introduction

Axillary surgery for breast cancer has seen a significant shift over the last 30 years, from axillary lymph node dissection (ALND) to sentinel lymph node (SLN) surgery for axillary staging for clinically node-negative breast cancer, followed by progressive de-escalation of axillary surgery with increasing indication for SLN surgery even in node-positive disease. Recently some studies have led to complete omission of axillary surgery in select patients. Figure 4.1 illustrates the timeline of important clinical trials that will be referenced throughout the ensuing section.

4.2 The Role of Axillary Surgery in Breast Cancer Treatment

When considering the role of axillary surgery, this must be done within the context of the goals of axillary surgery and the impact on the overall breast cancer treatment. In the era of the Halsted radical mastectomy, the primary goal of axillary surgery was locoregional disease control. However, the findings of the National Surgical Adjuvant Breast and Bowel Project (NSABP) B-04 demonstrated that axillary lymph node dissection (ALND) does not improve survival as there was no difference in overall survival (OS), disease-free survival (DFS), relapse free survival (RFS), or distant disease-free survival (DDFS) between women who underwent mastectomy and no axillary surgery versus modified radical mastectomy

(mastectomy and ALND) [25]. Thus, the primary role of axillary surgery is to provide critical staging information. Pathologic axillary staging information has been a cornerstone of adjuvant therapy decision-making, guiding recommendations for adjuvant chemotherapy and adjuvant radiation for decades. However, this is becoming less important for select patients, such as early-stage ER-positive, HER2-negative disease where the decision for chemotherapy is increasingly based on genomic information [84]. Consequently, the role of axillary surgery continues to evolve.

4.3 The Development of SLN Surgery

As improvements in screening resulted in diagnosis at earlier stage, the rate of node-positive disease at presentation decreased. To decrease the morbidity from axillary surgery in patients without axillary nodal disease, a variety of strategies were explored to identify the status of the axillary nodes without requiring ALND for all patients. Ultimately SLN surgery emerged as the standard of care for nodal staging.

SLN surgery for breast cancer was first described in the early 1990s by Armando Giuliano and David Krag [31, 49]. Initial studies used either technetium sulphur colloid or isosulphan blue (lymphazurin). Veronesi et al. reported on a randomized trial of SLN surgery and ALND versus SLN surgery and only proceeding with ALND if any of the SLNs were positive [96]. This trial demonstrated a false negative rate (FNR) of SLN surgery of 8.8%. Concerns regarding oncologic safety remained and the NSABP B-32 trial was conducted, which found no difference in OS, DFS, or regional control with omission of ALND in patients with negative SLNs [50, 51]. Another important finding was that 4% of SLNs were identified by palpation and 23% of these contained metastatic disease, resulting in subsequent guidelines recommending that palpably abnormal nodes as well as blue or radioactive nodes be removed at the time of SLN surgery.

Further studies contributed to refinement of the technique. Utilization of preoperative lymphoscintigraphy was reduced when no difference in SLN detection or FNR was found [66]. Intradermal injection was found to have more success with SLN identification than peritumoural administration [57] and decreased time to SLN identification [74]. Dual tracer, with both a vital blue dye and a radioactive tracer, was shown to increase the rate of SLN detection in NSABP B-32 and the subsequent Axillary Lymphatic Mapping Against Nodal Axillary Clearance (ALMANAC) and After Mapping of the Axilla Radiation or Surgery (AMAROS) trials [61, 23, 87].

SLNs can be mapped using a radiotracer, a visual dye, both a visual dye and a radiotracer, or a single tracer that combines properties of both a visual tracer and a radiotracer. Technetium-99 bound to a colloid molecule is the most common radiotracer [2].

Multiple blue dyes have been investigated, including isosulphan blue, methylene blue, and patent blue V with no demonstrable difference in SLN identification rates between them [65]. Alternative visual dyes are currently being investigated. Carbon nanoparticle suspensions are currently in use in China [42] and indocyanine green has also demonstrated promise for SLN mapping [1].

Superparamagnetic iron oxide (SPIO) is another tracer that functions as both a visual and radio-guided dye as it causes a dark staining of lymph nodes and can be detected by a probe. SPIO also remains in the nodes for up to 30 days after injection, so it can also be used for delayed SLN surgery if there is not an indication for SLN surgery at the time of mastectomy, such as in patients with DCIS or undergoing prophylactic mastectomy [47].

While SLN surgery has a very high node identification rate, it is not infallible and in a small percentage of cases there is failure of lymphatic mapping and a SLN cannot be identified. A single centre experience of failure of SLN identification in which subsequent ALND was performed demonstrated axillary nodal metastasis in 48.5% of these patients compared to 23.6% of patients in whom a SLN was identified [71]. Patients without an identifiable SLN were also found to have higher rates of extracapsular extension (68.4% vs. 41.7%). In addition, 22.1% were pN2 and 33.7% were pN3. This would suggest that ALND should be considered when a SLN cannot be identified; however, alternatives include axillary sampling or omission of axillary surgery. Evaluation of the axilla with intraoperative palpation for palpably abnormal nodes is important as one of the reasons for failure of lymphatic mapping is tumour replacement of the lymph node and prevention of uptake of tracer or tumour obstruction of lymphatic pathways. A Dutch nationwide survey of surgical oncologists found that, when unable to identify a SLN, most would not routinely proceed on to ALND but would make a judgement based on individual patient and tumour characteristics [95].

With refinement of the technique of SLN surgery, establishment of the quality-of-life benefits of SLN surgery over ALND, and validation of the oncologic safety, SLN surgery developed sufficient evidentiary support to be considered the standard of care for cN0 disease in the upfront surgery setting both in patients undergoing Breast-Conserving Surgery (BCS) and mastectomy. As evidence mounted, this resulted in a gradual increase in SLN surgery over ALND from 2003 to 2010 in both Europe and the United States. In a review of population-based and institution-specific databases across Europe, SLN surgery utilization ranged from 26% to 81% for T1 tumours in 2003 and increased to 79%–96% in 2010 [34]. There was a corresponding decrease in ALND for pT1 tumours from 27%–75% in 2003 to 12%–47% in 2010. In the United States, review of the National Cancer Database (NCDB) for patients with T1–2N0 breast cancer showed an increase in SLN surgery utilization from 26.8% in 1998 to 65.5% in 2005 [16]. Today, SLN surgery, rather than ALND, is standard of care for most patients presenting with clinically node-negative breast cancer, apart from those in whom surgical axillary staging is being omitted.

4.4 De-escalation of ALND in the Setting of Upfront Surgery

While SLN surgery was initially used to identify patients who had no axillary disease (i.e. were pathologic node-negative) and could therefore be spared ALND, the significant morbidity of ALND prompted development of the ACOSOG Z0011 trial to assess whether ALND was needed in patients with low volume SLN disease [32, 33]. This was designed to determine whether patients with cT1–2 tumours who were clinically node-negative by physical examination, undergoing BCS, and found to have low volume axillary disease (1 or 2 positive SLNs) could safely be treated with lumpectomy, whole breast radiation, and adjuvant systemic therapy, if indicated, without completion ALND. At 10 years, there was no difference in OS, DFS, and locoregional recurrence (LRR) between patients treated with SLN surgery and ALND and those who underwent SLN surgery alone and omitted ALND. These findings were echoed by the International Breast Cancer Study Group (IBCSG) 23-01 trial which included patients with cT1–2 tumours with no palpable adenopathy, one or more SLNs with micrometastasis (<2 mm), and no extracapsular extension [27]. In contrast to Z0011, patients undergoing mastectomy were included but only accounted for 9% of the study population. At 5 years, there was no difference in OS or DFS with the addition of ALND to SLN surgery. The Omitting Axillary Dissection in Breast Cancer with SEntinel-NOde MACrometastases trial (SENOMAC) expanded the population of Z0011 and IBCSG 23-01 to include T3 tumours and 1–2 lymph nodes with macrometastasis [21]. Similarly, it reported no difference in RFS or OS.

These trials were designed for patients undergoing BCS with planned subsequent whole breast radiation. While the Z0011 protocol recommended against definitive axillary radiation (AxRT), the radiation fields were not reviewed on all patients. In a separate study, details of the radiation therapy records that were able to be obtained from the Z0011 trial patients (228/589 patients) were reviewed [40]. High tangents were used in 50% of patients assigned to ALND and 52.6% of patients assigned to SLN surgery. Similarly, there were 16.9% of SLN surgery patients who received directed regional nodal RT compared to 21.2% of ALND patients, indicating that there was no escalation of RT in the SLN surgery group to compensate for the omission of ALND. Following publication of Z0011, omission of ALND in patients with axillary LN metastases meeting Z0011 criteria reached 89.2% by 2015 [75].

In addition, two trials have compared ALND to AxRT in patients with clinically node-negative, but low volume histologically node-positive disease, both finding that AxRT provides similar oncologic outcomes with less morbidity. The AMAROS trial randomized 1425 patients with cT1–2, cN0 breast cancer with one or more positive SLNs to ALND versus AxRT [5]. The AMAROS trial was underpowered and did not meet its primary endpoint of non-inferiority due to a very low event rate. At 10 years, axillary recurrence was 0.93% after ALND and 1.82% after AxRT, which was not statistically significant. OS and DFS were also similar between groups, but ALND was associated with significantly higher lymphoedema at all time points (5-years: 24.5% vs. 11.9%, $p < 0.001$), showing that AxRT is an acceptable treatment with less morbidity for women with a low nodal burden. Importantly, 70% of patients had only one to two positive SLNs and only 9.7% had four or more positive LNs, which limits the application of this result to patients with higher nodal burden. The Optimal Treatment of the Axilla-Surgery or Radiation (OTOASOR) trial reported on patients with tumours less than 3 cm in size and clinically node-negative who underwent BCS or mastectomy and had at least one positive SLN (60% >2 mm, 34% <2 mm, 6% ITCs) who were then randomized to regional nodal irradiation (RNI) or ALND (23.3% underwent both ALND and RNI in the ALND group) [80]. At 8 years, there was no difference in DFS, OS, or axillary recurrence, again confirming the safety of ALND omission in place of AxRT in early breast cancer with low nodal burden.

For many years this led to the situation where patients with cT1 or cT2 disease with one or two positive SLNs were able to be spared ALND if treated with BCS, but generally underwent ALND if they chose mastectomy. Over time the practice of axillary conservation in patients treated with mastectomy has expanded, albeit without a large prospective randomized trial demonstrating the oncologic safety, and many of these patients were treated with adjuvant radiation [98]. There was a growing body of retrospective data showing no difference in LRR or DFS with omission of ALND in patients treated with mastectomy who would otherwise meet Z0011 criteria and who were subsequently treated with post-mastectomy radiation therapy (PMRT) and AxRT [46]. A systematic review and meta-analysis of ten retrospective studies of patients with ≤3 SLN with metastases undergoing mastectomy did not find a benefit from ALND regarding OS, DFS, LRFS, or DRFS ($p > 0.05$) despite more advanced disease including larger tumours, a higher percentage of LVI, higher grade, extranodal extension (ENE), and more positive surgical margins in patients treated with ALND [17]. However, no randomized trials had addressed this question until recently.

The SINODAR-ONE trial was a multicentre randomized controlled non-inferiority trial comparing completion ALND to no further axillary surgery in women 40–75 years old with T1–2, cN0 breast cancer who were found to have one to two SLNs with macrometastases at the time of SLN surgery [92]. Both patients undergoing Breast-Conserving Therapy (BCT) and mastectomy were enrolled. A subset analysis in the 218 patients treated with mastectomy found no difference in

OS or RFS at 5 years, with 5.6% recurrence in the ALND group and 6.1% in the SLN surgery-only group [93]. In the mastectomy group, 17.4% underwent adjuvant radiotherapy. A re-analysis of the radiotherapy treatment data in SINODAR-ONE found 17 cases of locoregional radiotherapy among the 355 patients for whom the radiotherapy data were available and no difference in locoregional radiotherapy use between the two arms [85]. Table 4.1 summarizes the key characteristics of these trials.

There are two ongoing trials comparing ALND to omission of ALND with one to two positive nodes and include patients treated with mastectomy. The POsitive Sentinel NOde: Adjuvant Therapy Alone Versus Adjuvant Therapy Plus Clearance or Axillary Radiotherapy (POSNOC) trial (NCT02401685) has a planned completion in 2026 and is comparing adjuvant systemic therapy alone to adjuvant systemic therapy in conjunction with axillary treatment (axillary node clearance and/or AxRT). The SERC trial (NCT01717131) is a multicentre randomized controlled trial comparing ALND to no ALND in cN0 patients with T1–2 breast cancer who are found to have positive SLNs with a planned completion in 2031. Both BCT and mastectomy are included with mastectomy currently accounting for 19.9% of patients [36]. Radiotherapy is left to the discretion of the treating team and has been utilized in >90% of patients thus far.

Overall, there has remained significant heterogeneity in the speed of trial data implementation into practice across the United States and Europe, with many surgeons slowly changing practice in response to trial results and a small subset extrapolating trial results to additional populations. Omission of ALND in the setting of one to two positive SLNs after mastectomy lagged behind BCT with 45.7% of patients with one to two positive SLNs after mastectomy undergoing completion ALND compared to 12.4% after BCT in the NCDB in 2018 [86]. A review of the NCDB from 2010 to 2017 found that among 20,001 patients with cT1–2cN0 breast cancer treated with mastectomy, 42.1% had SLN surgery alone and 57.9% had completion ALND after SLN surgery and that as time went on, patients were less likely to undergo ALND [81]. A survey of breast surgeons and radiation oncologists in the United States in 2020 found that 52% of surgeons routinely sent SLNs for frozen section during mastectomy and 78% of them would then proceed to ALND if positive, indicating some extrapolation of the Z0011 findings to this population prior to publication of SINODAR-ONE [20].

Table 4.1 Characteristics of clinical trials related to axillary management in the setting of upfront surgery

Trial	Year	Design	Inclusion criteria	Arms	Outcomes	Significance
ACOSOG Z0011	2011	Multicentre RCT	891 Women with cT1–2 N0 BC and 1–2 SLN with metastases	SLN surgery alone vs. ALND	No difference in OS, DFS, or LRR	In women >50 year with T1–2 HR+ BC, no palpable nodes, and 1–2 positive SLNs, treated with BCS, no benefit to ALND
SINODAR-ONE	2022	Multicentre RCT	889 Women with T1–2 BC and 1–2 macrometastatic SLN treated with BCS or mastectomy	ALND vs. no further axillary surgery	No difference in OS, RFS, ARR, DDFS. Subset analysis in the mastectomy group found the same	Confirms Z0011 findings, supports ALND omission patients 1–2 macromets treated with BCS or mastectomy
AMAROS	2023	Multicentre RCT	1425 Women with cT1–2cN0 BC with 1+ SLN metastases	ALND (RT allowed if ≥4 positive LNs) vs. axillary RT	No difference in OS. Axillary recurrence 0.93% (95% CI, 0.18–1.68) after ALND and 1.82% (95% CI, 0.74–2.94) after ART. Higher lymphoedema rate in ALND (24.5% v. 11.9%, $p < 0.001$)	Axillary RT associated with good disease control and less lymphoedema than ALND in cT1–2 patients with cN0 disease at diagnosis and 1–2 positive LNs

SOUND	2023	Multicentre RCT	1405 Women with T1 BC and (−) AxUS or (−) FNA	SLN surgery vs. no axillary surgery	Omission of axillary surgery was non-inferior to SLN surgery (hazard ratio, 0.84; 90% CI, 0.45–1.54; noninferiority $p = 0.02$)	Postmenopausal women with G1–2 HR+ T1 BC and a negative axillary US may safely omit SLN surgery
INSEMA	2024	Multicentre RCT	4858 Women with cT1–2 N0 BC with planned BCS	4:1 SLN vs. no axillary surgery, SLN group randomized to SLN alone or ALND if macrometastasis	No difference in 5-year IDFS with SLN omission. HER2+ (3.6%), TNBC (1.2%), G3 (3.6%), Ki-67 ≥ 20% (12.9%), and ILC/MIDLC (12.7%) not well represented. Lower complication rate and arm/shoulder restriction in SLN omission group	Omission of SLN surgery in pts. >50 with cT1N0 G1–2 ER+ HER2− BC with Ki-67 ≤ 20% treated with BCS and RT is non-inferior to SLN surgery with less complications/morbidity
SENOMAC	2024	Multicentre RCT	2540 Men and women with cT1–3 N0 undergoing mastectomy or BCS	SLN surgery alone vs. completion ALND	No difference in 5-year OS, BCSS, RFS in patients with 1–2 SLN macromets. >1/3 of patients in both groups treated with mastectomy and 1/3 had ENE	Confirms safety of ALND omission in patients with cT1–2 N0 BC with 1–2 SLN macromets treated with mastectomy and those with ENE

4.5 Axillary Management After NAC

4.5.1 SLN Surgery in Patients with Clinically Node-Negative (cN0) Disease Treated with NAC

While SLN surgery was adopted in patients undergoing surgical resection first, the adoption of SLN surgery in patients treated with NAC was significantly later, due to concern that the fibrotic reaction might alter the lymphatic mapping in this setting, resulting in a higher FNR. Furthermore, adjuvant radiation therapy recommendations were historically based on pathologic nodal staging information from surgery prior to neoadjuvant systemic therapy and thus SLN surgery after NAC was not supported by many multidisciplinary teams.

Data regarding the feasibility and accuracy of SLN surgery after NAC slowly emerged. The National Surgical Adjuvant Breast and Bowel Project (NSABP) B-27 trial, which was designed to evaluate the impact of the addition of taxotere to adriamycin and cyclophosphamide, had a subgroup of patients in whom SLN surgery was performed prior to ALND after NAC [59]. This demonstrated a FNR of 10.7% for SLN surgery after NAC in cN0 patients. A large retrospective review from MD Anderson found successful identification of SLN in 97.4% of 575 patients after NAC with a similar FNR to upfront SLN surgery (5/84, 5.8% vs. 22/542, 4.1%, $p = 0.39$) and fewer patients with positive SLNs in the NAC group [38]. After adjusting for clinical stage, there was no difference in LRR, DFS, or OS between upfront SLN surgery or NAC followed by SLN surgery. Thus, it was concluded that SLN after NAC could provide similar staging information and reduce the number of patients requiring ALND. Several meta-analyses have demonstrated the oncologic safety of SLN surgery in this setting [90, 100, 101].

The Ganglion sentinel apres chimiotherapie NEoAdjuvante (GANEA) 2 trial evaluated the accuracy and safety of SLN after NAC in clinically node-negative patients [18]. At least one SLN was identified in 97.6% of patients (575/589). In the subgroup of 419 patients treated with only SLN surgery (i.e. pN0 and no ALND), at a median 36 months of follow-up, there was a 97.2% 3-year OS and 97.8% EFS with only one patient with axillary recurrence.

Collectively, these studies established the oncologic safety of SLN surgery after NAC with the associated benefit of reduced need for ALND. In addition, SLN surgery after NAC allows for response assessment, which is now critically important to guide adjuvant therapy decisions.

A review of the I-SPY2 data of patients treated with NAC demonstrated a decrease in ALND only from 20% in 2011 to 6.25% in 2021 and an increase in SLN-only from 70.0% to 87.5% in cN0 patients treated with NAC, indicating both implementation of SLN surgery after NAC and subsequent omission of ALND in the absence of nodal disease has wide acceptance [11].

4.5.2 SLN Surgery in Patients with Clinically Node-Positive (cN+) Disease Treated with NAC

While SLN surgery was getting adopted for patients presenting with cN0 disease who were treated with NAC, ALND remained the standard of care for those patients with cN+ disease at diagnosis. As advancements in systemic therapy evolved, including the introduction of HER2 directed therapy for HER2+ breast cancer, the nodal pathologic complete response rates increased, resulting in final pathology increasingly reflecting all resected nodes from ALND were negative. This led to evaluation of SLN surgery after NAC in the setting of clinically node-positive disease prior to chemotherapy. The ACOSOG Z1071 trial was a prospective multicentre trial designed to determine the FNR of SLN surgery in breast cancer patients with biopsy-proven nodal metastasis and no prior axillary surgery treated with NAC. SLN identification rate was 92.9% in patients with cN1 disease. The FNR was found to be 12.6% in women with two or more SLNs removed, and 9.1% with three or more SLNs removed. When dual tracers were used, the FNR was 10.8% [9].

The SENTINA trial was a four-arm multicentre cohort trial that evaluated SLN surgery before and after NAC; it found that in patients who converted from cN+ to cN0, the SLN identification rate after NAC was 80% and the FNR was 14.2%, which improved to 12% with dual tracer and 9.6% if two or more nodes were removed [53]. The Sentinel Node Following NeoAdjuvant Chemotherapy (SN FNAC) study, which was similarly designed, but included immunohistochemistry on the SLN and included isolated tumour cells (ITCs) (i.e. ypN0(i+) as node-positive) reported similar outcomes with a FNR of 8.4% [7]. Across all three trials, retrieval of one SLN was associated with a higher FNR, ACOSOG Z1071 (31.5%), SENTINA (24.3%), and SN FNAC (18.2%). Additionally, the trials reported a two- to threefold decrease in FNR when two tracers were used.

In GANEA2, a FNR of 11.9% was found in the patients with biopsy-proven disease prior to NAC. Residual breast tumour size ≥5 mm and lymphovascular invasion predicted additional node involvement at the time of ALND. In patients that did not have these factors and had a negative SLN, the FNR was 3.7% regardless of the number of SLN removed.

An unplanned subset analysis of ACOSOG Z1071 was performed on the patients where a clip was placed in the positive node at the time of percutaneous biopsy. When the clipped node was retrieved at the time of SLN surgery, the FNR was 7.4% [10]. The clipped node was one of the SLNs in approximately 75% of cases. In order to increase the likelihood of resection of the clipped node, the clipped node can be localized preoperatively. Combination of SLN surgery along with localization of the clipped node is often called 'targeted axillary dissection' and has been shown to significantly increase clipped node retrieval [22] and decrease the false negative rate to as low as 2.4% [14] (Table 4.2).

Other approaches to axillary staging in this setting have been explored. Marking the axilla with radioactive iodine seed (MARI) was first described by Vrancken Peeters et al. [97]. This procedure involves placement of an I-125 seed prior to NAC

Table 4.2 Comparison of trials examining sentinel lymph node surgery after NAC

Trial	ACOSOG Z1071	SENTINA	SN FNAC	GANEA 2
Year	2013	2013	2015	2019
Design	Multicentre prospective phase II	Multicentre prospective cohort	Multicentre prospective phase II	Multicentre prospective cohort
Inclusion	756 Women with cT0–4 N1–2 BC treated with NAC	1737 Women with cN0 BC and planned NAC	153 Patients with cT0–3 N1–2 biopsy-proven node-positive BC receiving NAC	957 Women with cT1–3 N0–2 BC treated with NAC with planned mastectomy or BCS
Arms	SLN surgery followed by ALND	Arm A: cN0 pts. SLN before NAC arm B: pN1 pts. before NAC underwent second SLN after NAC arm C: pN1 patients who became ycN0 treated with SLN surgery and ALND arm D: pN1 pts. who were ycN+ after NAC treated with ALND alone	Axillary US prior and after NAC followed by SLN surgery and completion ALND	Pts cN0 prior to NAC treated with SLN surgery, ALND only if micro- or macro-metastasis or SLN mapping failure. cN1 pts. prior to NAC treated with SLN surgery and completion of ALND
SLN identification (%)	92.9	80	87.6	97.6
FNR (%)	12.6	14.2	13.3	11.9
Results	SLN identification rate 92.9% in cN1 pts. FNR 12.6% with ≥2 SLNs removed, and 9.1% when ≥3 SLNs removed. With dual tracer, FNR was 10.8%	In pts. who converted from cN+ to cN0 (arm C), SLN identification rate was 80% and FNR was 14.2% which improved to 12% with dual tracer and 9.6% if ≥2 nodes were removed	SLN identification rate 87.6%, FNR 8.4% (with ypN0(i-). If ypN0(i+) considered negative, FNR 13.3%	SLN identification rate after NAC 97.6%. FNR in cN1 pts. 11.9%. FNR 3.7% when residual breast tumour ≤5 mm and no LVI. In cN0 pts., only 1/419 axillary recurrence
Significance	Established FNR of SLN surgery after NAC. SLN FNR can be acceptably low if ≥2 nodes removed after NAC	SLN FNR can be acceptably low if ≥2 nodes are removed after NAC	SLN with IHC after NAC has acceptable FNR	SLN surgery after NAC in women with cN0 disease at diagnosis treated with NAC has low LRR risk

and resection of the node with the seed without SLN surgery. It was shown to have a 97% node identification rate and 7% FNR when just the node containing the seed was removed [24]. Radioactive Iodine Seed Localization in Axilla with Sentinel Node Biopsy (RISAS) was investigated as a modification of the MARI procedure and found a FNR of 3.5% compared to FNR of 17.9% for SLN surgery alone and a FNR of 7.0% for MARI [82]. The Ideal Marker for Targeted Axillary Dissection (IMTAD) study evaluated three different localization markers (clip + radioactive seed, magnetic seed, and carbon suspension) for localization of the biopsied node after NAC and found no statistically significant difference with regard to complications, node detection, and marker dislodgement between the three markers [102].

Overall multiple techniques to decrease the FNR of SLN surgery after NAC have been identified and surgeons and institutions can use a variety of these in their practice. These include use of dual tracer for lymphatic mapping, retrieval of at least two and, when possible, three or more nodes, retrieval of the index biopsy-proven positive node, and the use of IHC on SLNs [26]. While the use of IHC may decrease the technical FNR, the clinical significance of identification of ITCs is limited, with most experts at the St. Gallen International Consensus Conference recommending no ALND for ITCs alone [13].

Institutional data from the Mayo Clinic demonstrated uptake of SLN surgery in the setting of node-positive disease treated with NAC and reduction in ALND in those with negative SLNs [70, 73]. A review of the I-SPY2 data on patients treated with NAC demonstrated an increase in ALND omission in patients with cN+ disease at presentation from 14.6% in 2011 to 56.5% in 2021 [11]. A survey of the American Society of Breast Surgeons members in 2017 found that 45% of surgeons offered SLN surgery prior to publication of the Z1071, SENTINA, and SN-FNAC trials and that increased to 85% following publication [15].

While no prospective trials have compared outcomes between ALND and SLN surgery without ALND in patients with node-positive disease treated with NAC who convert to pathologic node-negative disease, both retrospective series and prospective cohort studies have shown good long-term outcomes with omission of ALND in this population. Multiple retrospective single-institution series have shown equivalent freedom from local recurrence with short-term follow-up in patients who convert from cN1–2 to ypN0 after NAC and did not have ALND [28, 43, 73]. In a multicentre retrospective cohort study of 1144 patients with stage II-III breast cancer who achieved nodal pCR after NAC and then did not undergo ALND, the axillary recurrence rate was 0.65% at 3 years and 1% at 5 years [67, 68]. A prospective cohort study was designed for patients with cN1 breast cancer who have three or more pathologically negative SLNs after NAC who would then be spared ALND [3]. At 40 months median follow-up, only one axillary recurrence was identified in a patient who refused RT among the 234 participants. Martelli et al. undertook a prospective cohort study of cT2 cN0/1 patients treated with NAC and found equivalent 10-year OS and DFS between propensity score matched ypN0 patients who underwent SLN surgery alone and ypN1 patients who were treated with ALND [64].

There is limited guidance when a SLN cannot be identified after NAC. In the SN FNAC trial, when no SLN was identified, 12 of 18 patients (66.7%) had nodal disease, indicating that ALND should be considered when a SLN is not able to be identified after NAC [7].

There is limited data on SLN surgery after neoadjuvant endocrine therapy (NET). A retrospective review of the NCDB found that nodal pCR was uncommon (10%) among cN1 patients and that outcomes based on node status after NET are similar to patients treated with upfront surgery [44]. Another retrospective review of patients with cT1-4 N0–1M0 HR+/HER2− breast cancer who were treated with NET found that in patients with cN0 disease, >90% had fewer than three positive nodes at surgery and that 5-year OS did not differ between SLN surgery and ALND regardless of number of positive SLNs ($p > 0.10$) [45]. In a review of 186 patients with both cN0 and cN+ disease treated with NET, 21.3% (23/108) of patients with ypN+ disease had SLN surgery alone [69]. After a median follow-up of 35 months, there were no regional recurrences. Collectively, these studies suggest that patients treated with NET may be treated similarly to the upfront surgery setting.

In addition to de-escalation of axillary surgery, the question of de-escalation of AxRT in patients with eradication of disease in the axillary nodes is important. The NRG Oncology NSABP B-51 RTOG 1304 clinical trial investigated whether radiation can be de-escalated in patients who are clinically node-positive at presentation but convert to ypN0 after NAC by SLN surgery or ALND. Patients undergoing mastectomy were randomly assigned to no radiation or chest wall radiation with regional nodal irradiation and patients undergoing BCS were randomized to whole breast RT versus WBRT + RNI. Analysis demonstrated no difference in distant recurrence, DFS, LRR, or OS [60]. The results of this trial are slow to be implemented into practice. The ATNEC trial is investigating whether omission of axillary treatment in cT1–3 patients with biopsy-confirmed nodal disease who convert to ypN0 is non-inferior to the control arm receiving either ALND or RNI [35]. This trial is currently recruiting with a planned completion in 2030.

4.5.3 Management of SLN-Positive Disease After NAC

Use of SLN surgery after NAC was initially undertaken to identify patients who convert to pN0 to allow omission of ALND, while ALND was recommended for patients with pN+ disease. However, axillary management has continued to evolve and, given that patients with pN+ disease after NAC are recommended AxRT, the question arises whether definitive management of the axilla could be with AxRT without ALND.

The Alliance A011202 is investigating whether axillary nodal irradiation alone is not inferior to ALND and nodal irradiation in patients with cN1 non-inflammatory breast cancer (NCT01901094). Women with cT1–3 N1 M0 breast cancer treated with NAC and one or more positive lymph nodes at SLN surgery were randomized to ALND + Nodal XRT versus axillary and nodal XRT with no ALND. It has completed accrual and results are awaited. The TAXIS trial is investigating whether 'tailored axillary surgery' (TAS) can decrease the axillary tumour burden to the point where AxRT can control it by randomizing patients with STAGE II-III breast cancer and histologically confirmed nodal disease undergoing both upfront surgery and NAC to TAS + RNI or completion ALND and RNI and has a projected completion in 2029 (NCT03513614). The MINIMAX study is a prospective registry for female patients with pathologically proven axillary lymph node disease planned to undergo NAC followed by axillary staging and will evaluate DFS, BCSS, OS, ARR, and QoL with a planned completion in 2027 (NCT04486495).

Isolated Tumour Cells: ypN(0i+)

ITCs in the SLN were associated with additional positive nodes at the time of ALND in 57% (4/7 patients) after NAC in the SN FNAC trial and 36.4% (4/11 patients) in Z1071; however these were small patient cohorts. In a large international retrospective study of patients with cN0–3 disease at diagnosis treated with NAC and found to have ITCs in the SLN(s), the rate of additional positive nodes was 30% in the 182 patients treated with ALND, but only 5% were found to have macrometastases [68]. This study showed there was no difference in 3-year IDFS and LRR between those patients with ITCs in the SLN treated with ALND and those without further axillary surgery, indicating that it may be reasonable to omit ALND in patients with ypN0(i+) disease.

Micrometastases: ypN1mi

A review of the NCDB identified patients between 2004 and 2016 with cT1–3 who had ypN0i + and ypN1mi disease after NAC and mastectomy found that PMRT was utilized in 51.8% of patients with ypN0i+ and 61.9% with ypN1mi disease with increasing frequency in the latter half of the review period [48]. Five-year OS was 84.3% in ypN0i+ patients compared to 79.9% in ypN1mi patients (HR 1.23 [0.97–1.55], $p = 0.092$). There was no association between PMRT use and OS.

In a single institution retrospective study, 14 (30%) of the 47 patients with ypN1mi on SLN surgery were found to have additional macrometastases with ALND and 10 (21%) were found to have additional micrometastases [54]. Final pathology of ypN1mi, as determined by ALND was not associated with a difference in RFS or OS compared to ypN0 (HR 1.02, 95% CI 0.42–2.49, $p = 0.958$). However, SLNs with micrometastasis was associated with significantly worse 5-year RFS than SLN-negative disease (76.6% vs. 89.5%, $p = 0.023$). Interestingly, upstaging to ypN+ was not a significant contributor to the difference on multivariate analysis. Risk factors for additional metastases in patients with micrometastases in their SLNs included T2+, ER+/HER2−, and low Ki-67 (<14%). Only 13% of patients with TNBC and SLN micrometastases had additional positive nodes and 30% of patients with HER2-enriched cancer had additional positive nodes compared to 73.1% of patients with HR+/HER2− cancer.

The AXSANA study (EUBREAST 03) is a prospective cohort study to evaluate the IDFS, Axillary Recurrence Rate (ARR), health-related quality of life (QoL), and arm morbidity in patients who convert from cN+ to ycN0 who undergo any form of axillary staging after NAC and has an anticipated completion in 2030 (NCT04373655). Upgrade rates at the time of ALND for ITC and micrometastases within the study were reported at SABCS 2024, with 1/16 patients with ypN0(i+) having macrometastasis identified on completion ALND and no patient that had a breast pCR and ypN0(i+) was found to upgrade on completion ALND [52]. Among patients with ypN1(mi), only 1/18 (6%) with breast pCR had macrometastases identified on completion ALND. Conversely, 17% of patients without breast pCR were ultimately found to have ypN2–3 disease.

Macrometastases: ypN+ Disease

While data from prospective trials is awaited, omission of ALND in patients with low-volume residual axillary disease after NAC is increasing within the United States, despite the lack of trial data to support this practice. A survey of the members of the American Society of Breast Surgeons demonstrated that 60.7% of surgeons always offer SLN surgery to cN1 patients who respond to NAC and 43.9% sometimes omit ALND in the setting of residual nodal disease [99]. Review of data from patients treated in the I-SPY2 clinical trial also indicated a decrease in ALND for patients with ypN+ disease with 69% undergoing ALND in 2011 compared to 39% in 2021 [11]. This is predominantly based on the belief (in the absence of trial data) that ALND would not improve locoregional control, distant recurrence, or survival outcomes when AxRT is administered. A multicentre retrospective study from Korea (KROG 21-06) found no difference in 5-year DFS or OS between the 258 women with ypN+ disease after NAC who were treated with ALND and the 136 who underwent SLN surgery alone [72]. A review of the NCDB found that the rate of ALND omission in patients found to have ypN+ disease after NAC has increased from 28% in 2012 to 40% by the end of 2021 [56], indicating increasing use of SLN after NAC and omission of ALND in some cases of ypN+ disease ahead of results from randomized controlled trials.

Factors associated with additional nodal disease and pathologic nodal upstaging in patients with residual nodal disease after NAC on the Alliance A011202 trial were presented at the San Antonio Breast Cancer Symposium in 2024 [8]. Among the 841 patients randomized to ALND, 53.6% had no additional disease on ALND and 16.8% had one additional positive node; however, 15.1% had 4+ additional positive nodes. SLN macrometastases had additional positive LNs in 47.8% compared to micrometastases at 38.4% ($p = 0.064$). Patients with TNBC and HER2+ tumours had additional positive LNs 39.8% and 40.3%, respectively, compared to

49.1% for HR+/HER2− ($p = 0.053$). The rate of additional positive LNs on ALND also increased with the number of positive SLNs, from 33.2% for one positive SLN to 83.9% for four or more positive SLNs. In addition, patients with ypT3 tumours were more likely to have additional positive LNs and this persisted on MVA. ALND resulted in pathologic nodal upstaging in 25.4% of patients with the majority increasing from ypN1 to ypN2. However, 3.8% of patients increased from ypN1 to ypN3 and 2.4% from ypN2 to ypN3. Given the high rate of upstaging and the significant proportion of patients with four or more additional positive nodes at the time of ALND, ALND is indicated in the setting of residual axillary disease after NAC until oncologic outcomes have been verified with prospective clinical trial results.

4.5.4 Other Patient Populations Treated with NAC

Research on post-NAC SLN has been predominantly focused on cN1 disease and therefore there is limited data to support the use of SLN surgery in the setting of cN2/3 disease. However, nodal pathologic complete response (pCR) rates are high among some tumour subtypes (around 60% for HER2-positive breast cancer and 48% for TNBC), suggesting that SLN surgery may be worth pursuing in this population [79]. In addition, patients with cN2–3 disease secondary to internal mammary node involvement with minimal axillary node involvement would not be expected to benefit from ALND in the same way that a patient with extensive axillary disease burden would. Thus, they may potentially be treated similar to cN1 disease, although data regarding outcomes in this setting are lacking.

Likewise, patients with inflammatory breast cancer have been excluded from most studies, but a single institution retrospective study found a FNR for the clipped node of 4% (1/28), suggesting further investigation of SLN surgery in this population is warranted [58].

4.6 Omission of SLN Surgery

4.6.1 In the Upfront Surgery Setting

The Choosing Wisely statement by the Society of Surgical Oncology in 2016 recommended avoiding routine SLN surgery in patients ≥70 years old with early-stage hormone receptor-positive HER2-negative breast cancer [83]. This is based on the results of several trials, including the Cancer and Leukaemia Group B (CALGB) 9343 [37], the International Breast Cancer Study Group (IBCSG) 10-93 [39], and a 2005 study by Martelli et al. [64].

Martelli et al. found that there was no difference in OS or breast cancer-specific survival (BCSS) at 5 years in women >65 years with cT1N0 breast cancer who were randomized to ALND versus no axillary surgery and subsequently received adjuvant endocrine therapy [62]. At 15 years of follow-up of a larger non-randomized cohort, there was no difference in BCSS with the use of ALND [63]. Interestingly, in the women with T1 disease who underwent ALND, 29% were found to have nodal metastasis. Despite this, only 3.7% of women who did not have axillary surgery developed overt axillary disease at 15 years.

IBCSG 10-93 randomized women ≥60 years with cT1–3 N0 operable breast cancer to either primary surgery alone or primary surgery with ALND [27]. Adjuvant tamoxifen was given in both groups and 45% of patients were treated with mastectomy, 33% BCS with RT, and 23% had BCS without RT. 28% of patients who had axillary surgery were found to have node-positive disease. At a median follow-up of 6.6 years, there was no difference in DFS or OS, but there were better QoL scores among patients in the no axillary surgery group, although the difference disappeared by 6–12 months.

Finally, CALGB 9343 evaluated omission of adjuvant RT in cT1N0 ER-positive breast cancer; however, 62% ($n = 395$) of patients had no axillary surgery performed [37]. In the 195 women without axillary surgery who were treated with tamoxifen and WBRT including tangents covering levels I and II, there were no axillary recurrences at 10 years and only 3% (6/200) of women treated with tamoxifen alone experienced an axillary recurrence. Overall the 2016 Choosing Wisely statement led to a decrease in the use of SLN surgery for women aged 70 and older with ER+ HER2- disease.

The potential for omission of SLN surgery has been further expanded to younger patients with the results of the Sentinel Node vs. Observation After Axillary Ultra-Sound (SOUND) trial, which was a prospective randomized multicentre trial comparing SLN surgery with subsequent ALND in cases of macrometastasis to complete omission of axillary surgery in patients with cT1N0 breast cancer with either a negative axillary US or a negative FNA if concerning lymph nodes were identified on US [29]. While the SOUND trial had broad inclusion criteria, there was clearly selection in which patients were enrolled in the trial, with only 12% of participants having triple-negative or HER2-positive disease, only 4.4% with T2 tumours, and 20.6% premenopausal in the SLN surgery-only group. Thus, there has been variance in how the trial is applied in clinical practice. A retrospective review of factors associated with nodal positivity in an institutional database found that axillary tail and centrally located tumours, younger age, black race, increasing tumour size, high grade, higher ER/PR expression, lobular histology, and increasing Ki-67 were associated with higher risk of nodal metastasis [6]. Overall there has been selective implementation of SOUND trial within a subset of patients who are at lower risk. There is also concern regarding the loss of definitive nodal staging information to inform adjuvant radiation and medical oncology plans. Another retrospective review of an institutional database for hormone receptor positive, HER2-negative, 'SOUND eligible' patients found that the population had a similar distribution of patient and disease characteristics to the SOUND trial population and that the SLN was positive in 12.2% (38/318) of patients who had a negative axillary ultrasound [30]. Only 3 of the 318 patients had 4 or more positive nodes. At a median follow-up of 26.2 months, there were no axillary recurrences and one distant recurrence. Among postmenopausal women with low recurrence scores, chemotherapy recommendations would not have been changed by the finding of positive nodes within the study population, suggesting that there is a subset of the SOUND trial population in whom omission of SLN surgery will not negatively impact adjuvant therapy decisions.

The INtergroup-SEntinel-MAmma (INSEMA) trial randomized patients with cT1–2 breast cancer, which were node-negative by physical exam and imaging with planned BCS to SLN surgery or no axillary surgery in a 4:1 ratio [76]. Patients undergoing SLN surgery were subsequently randomized to SLN alone or completion ALND if they had macrometastasis in a SLN, otherwise they were treated with SLN alone. After a median follow-up of 73.6 months, 5-year IDFS was 91.9% in the SLN omission group versus 91.7% in the SLN surgery group with a slightly higher rate of axillary recurrence in the SLN omission group (1.0% vs. 0.3%). The INSEMA patient characteristics were notable for low percentages of HER2+ (3.6%), TNBC (1.2%), grade 3 (3.6%), Ki-67 ≥ 20% (12.9%), and ILC/MIDLC histology (12.7%), leading to the recommendation from the authors that omission of SLN surgery may be appropriate in women ≥50 years old with T1, grade 1–2, HR-positive, HER2-negative breast cancer.

There are multiple ongoing clinical trials exploring omission of cSLN surgery in patients undergoing BCS in both the upfront surgery setting and after NAC. Results from BOOG 13–38 (NCT02271828), NAUTILUS (NCT04303715), and SOAPET (NCT04072653) are expected in the next couple of years.

BOOG 2013-08 (Netherlands) is a non-inferiority randomized controlled multicentre trial in which cT1–2 N0 patients with planned BCS are randomized to SLN surgery versus no SLN surgery. This trial notably is including patients undergoing NAC. It is currently enrolling and has a planned completion in 2027. There are also two ongoing Asian trials SOAPET (China) and NAUTILUS (Korea). SOAPET is a two-stage trial with the first stage evaluating the NPV of preoperative axillary assessment (PET, MRI, US, and physical exam) and the second stage in which SLN will be omitted in patients with negative imaging. SOAPET has reported the outcomes of the first stage, with a NPV of 86.3% for US alone, 87.8% for LymphPET, and 91% for the combination of US and LymphPET for macrometastatic disease [55]. SOAPET has a planned completion in 2027. NAUTILUS has a similar design to INSEMA, however, will have a 1:1 randomization between groups and has a planned completion in 2027.

4.6.2 Omission of SLN Surgery After NAC

While no study has evaluated omission of SLN surgery after NAC, there are some populations in whom omission may be safe. In a retrospective study of 116 patients with T1–2 cN0 triple-negative or HER2-positive breast cancer with a breast pCR after NAC, who subsequently underwent SLN surgery, none had evidence of axillary metastasis [88]. In a review of the NCDB, patients with cN0 HER2-positive and triple-negative breast cancer (TNBC) who achieved a breast pCR had positive nodes in only 1.6% of cases [4]. However, nodal positivity was considerably higher in patients with HR-positive disease, cN1 at diagnosis, and those with cN1 disease without breast pCR indicating that SLN omission may not be appropriate in this setting [4]. Another retrospective study from the Netherlands showed that nodal positivity was 3% in patients with cT1–3 N0 triple-negative or HER2-positive breast cancer after NAC and 0% in patients with breast pCR with any histology [94]. However, the identification of breast pCR preoperatively is not reliable and intraoperative frozen section of the breast specimen is not widely available. Preoperative determination of breast pCR using vacuum-assisted biopsy has been shown to have an acceptable FNR within patients with a tumour bed ≤2 cm with six or more representative samples [89].

There are three prospective single-arm trials, EUBREAST-01 (NCT04101851), ASICS (NCT04225858), and ASLAN (NCT04101851), evaluating the possibility of SLN surgery omission in triple-negative and HER2-positive breast cancer. EUBREAST-01 is a prospective single-arm trial evaluating axillary recurrence-free survival in patients with cN0 HER2-positive or TNBC with breast pCR (ypT0 or ypTis) who undergo lumpectomy alone with postoperative WBRT. It is currently recruiting and has a planned completion in 2028. ASICS is another prospective single-arm study evaluating 5-year axillary recurrence in patients with HER2-positive or TNBC, are cN0 by physical exam, axillary US, and PET scan, and who achieve radiographic complete response who are subsequently treated with either BCT or mastectomy without axillary surgery. ASLAN is a prospective multicentre single-arm trial in Korea evaluating recurrence-free survival in cT1–3 N0–1 patients with HER2-positive or TNBC who achieve pCR on BCT specimen and then omit axillary surgery [77]. The clinicopathologic characteristics from the ASLAN trial were reported at the San Antonio Breast Cancer Symposium (SABCS) in 2024, with a breast pCR rate of 75.1% for cT1–2 cN0–1 patients with HER2+ or TNBC. In patients with cN0 at diagnosis and non-pCR in the breast, only one patient (2.1%) had SLN-positive disease and was ypN1mic. In patients with cN1 at diagnosis and non-pCR in the breast, 14 (87.5%) were ypN0, one (6.3%) was ypN1mic, and one (6.3%) was ypN2. ASLAN has a planned completion in 2028. These are summarized alongside the other ongoing clinical trials of axillary management in Table 4.3.

Table 4.3 Ongoing clinical trials pertinent to axillary management

Trial	Planned completion	Aim	Inclusion	Arms	Outcome measures
Alliance A011202 (NCT01901094)	2025	Assess whether radiation to the undissected axilla and regional LNs is non-inferior to ALND + RNI	cT1–3N1M0 BC treated with NAC who are clinically node-negative by physical exam (PE) after NAC	1. ALND + RNI 2. Axillary and nodal RT without ALND	Primary: IBC-RFI Secondary, OS, LRR, lymphoedema
POSNOC (NCT02401685)	2026	Assess whether adjuvant therapy alone is non-inferior to adjuvant therapy plus axillary treatment for women with early-stage breast cancer and 1–2 sentinel lymph node (SLN) macrometastases	cT1–2 BC with 1–2 macrometastases on SLN	1. Adjuvant systemic therapy alone 2. Adjuvant systemic therapy + axillary treatment (axillary node clearance and/or AxRT)	Primary: 5-year ARR Secondary: Arm morbidity, QoL, LRR, DFS, OS
MINIMAX (NCT04486495)	2027	Assess oncologic safety and impact on QoL of the current axillary staging and treatment strategies in women with node-positive disease treated with neoadjuvant chemotherapy (NAC)	Women with unilateral invasive BC and cN1–3, pathologically proven LNs, and planned NAC	Single cohort	Primary: 5-year DFS, BCSS, OS, ARR, QoL

(continued)

Table 4.3 (continued)

Trial	Planned completion	Aim	Inclusion	Arms	Outcome measures
BOOG 2013-08 (NCT02271828)	2027	Determine whether SLN omission is non-inferior to SLN surgery with regard to regional recurrence	Women with cT1–2 N0 (by US and PE) BC patients with planned BCS	1. SLN surgery 2. No SLN surgery	Regional recurrence rate
SOAPET (NCT04072653)	2027	Two-stage trial with the first stage evaluating the NPV of preoperative axillary assessment (PET, MRI, US, and physical exam) and the second stage in which SLN will be omitted in patients with negative imaging	Stage 1: Women with T1–2 IDC or DCS and negative LNs by PE, US, and MRI Stage 2: Invasive breast cancer, planned BCS and RT, negative LNs by PE, US, axillary PET	Single cohort SLN surgery omission	Primary: 5-year D-DFS, LRFS Secondary: 5-year DFS, OS, adverse events, BREAST-Q
NAUTILUS (NCT04303715)	2027	Assess safety of omission of SLN surgery in cT1–2 N0 BC	cT1–2 breast cancer which was node-negative by physical exam and imaging with planned BCS	1. SLN surgery 2. No axillary surgery	Primary: 5-year IDFS Secondary: 5-year OS, DDFS, ARR, AE, QoL
ASICS (NCT04225858)	2027	Assess whether SLN surgery can be safely omitted in HER2+ and TNBC with radiographic complete response (rCR)	-cT1–3 N0 HER2+ or TNBC treated with NAC Tumour stage assessed with breast MRI before start NAC MRI after or during NAC shows rCR	Single cohort SLN surgery omission	Primary: 5-year axillary recurrence Secondary: RFS, OS, DSS, BCSQoL

NSABP B-51 (NCT01872975)	2028	Determine if radiation improves IBC-RFI in cN+ patients who convert to ypN0 after NAC	cT1–3 N1 confirmed by biopsy, treated with NAC, and converted to ypN0 (i + and Mol + are eligible)	Mastectomy: 1. No radiation vs. 2. Chest wall radiation with RNI BCS: 1. WBRT vs. 2. WBRT + RNI	Primary: IBC-RFI Secondary, OS, LRRFI, DRFI, DFS-DCIS, QoL, AE
EUBREAST-01 (NCT04101851)	2028	Assess axillary RFS in patients with cN0 HER2-positive or TNBC with breast pCR (ypT0 or ypTis) who undergo BCS alone with postoperative WBRT	cT1–3 N0 (by PE and imaging) HER2+ or TNBC treated with NAC and rCR, planned BCS and WBRT	Single cohort SLN surgery omission	Primary: 3-year axillary RFS Secondary: 5-year INV-DFS, OS, LR-DFS, DDFS, diagnostic accuracy of rCR for pCR
ASLAN (NCT04101851)	2028	Evaluate RFS in cT1–3 N0–1 patients with HER2+ or TNBC who achieve pCR on BCT specimen and then omit axillary surgery	cT1–3 N0–1 patients with HER2+ or TNBC who achieve pCR on BCT specimen after NAC	Single cohort SLN surgery omission	Primary: 3-year axillary RFS Secondary: 5-year INV-DFS, OS, LR-DFS, DDFS, diagnostic accuracy of rCR for pCR
TAXIS (NCT03513614)	2029	Assess whether 'tailored axillary surgery' (TAS) can decrease the axillary tumour burden to the point where AxRT can control it	Stage II–III breast cancer and histologically confirmed nodal disease undergoing both upfront surgery and NAC	1. TAS + RNI 2. Completion ALND and RNI	Primary: DFS Secondary: OS, BCSS, TTLR, TTDR, AE

(continued)

Table 4.3 (continued)

ATNEC (NCT04109079)	2030	Determine whether omission of axillary treatment is non-inferior to axillary lymph node dissection (ALND) or regional nodal irradiation (RNI) in women who convert to ypN0	T1–3N1M0 with biopsy-proven nodal metastases, who convert to ypN0 after NAC and have removal of at least 3 SLN	1. Omission of axillary treatment 2. ALND and/or RNI per local guidelines	Primary: 5-year DFS, lymphoedema Secondary: Arm function, HR-QoL, axillary RFI, OS, LRR
AXSANA (EUBREAST 03) (NCT04373655)	2030	Evaluate outcomes in patients who convert from cN+ to ycN0 who undergo any form of axillary staging after NAC	Women with cT1-4cN+ primary invasive BC and planned NAC	Single cohort of patients who convert from cN+ to ycN0 with NAC	Primary: 5-year iDFS, ARR, HR-QoL, arm morbidity
SERC (NCT01717131)	2031	Assess whether omission of ALND is non-inferior to ALND for pathologically positive SLNs in patients who are cN0	Women with cN0 patients with T1–2 breast cancer who are found to have positive SLNs	1. ALND 2. No ALND	Primary: DFS Secondary: ARR, OS

4.7 Axillary Reverse Mapping

Axillary reverse mapping was introduced as a method of identifying, in order to subsequently spare, the lymphatics that drain the arm [91]. In the initial paper, Klimberg and colleagues used lymphazurin injected into the upper arm and identified blue lymphatics draining from the arm within the axillary contents in 61% of patients. This has subsequently been described using alternative radiotracers [12] and ICG [78] so that arm nodes can be differentiated from SLNs.

In addition, axillary reverse mapping allows identification of lymphatics, that, when divided, can be used for prophylactic lymphovenous (LV) bypass. There have been mixed results on LV bypass, with some studies showing it is not associated with a decrease in lymphoedema [41], and some showing that prophylactic LV bypass significantly decreases the rate of lymphoedema [19].

4.8 Conclusion

Axillary surgery has undergone major changes over the last 20+ years, from routine ALND to use of SLN surgery in clinically node-negative breast cancer, to SLN surgery with omission of ALND in patients with one or two positive SLNs treated with breast conservation or mastectomy. Now, most recently, axillary surgical staging is being increasingly omitted in patients with small favourable breast cancer (cT1 HR+/Her2− disease with negative axillary ultrasound). In the setting of NAC there has also been a major shift away from ALND to SLN surgery both in patients with clinically node-negative disease at presentation, as well as those with clinically node-positive disease at presentation. Data is eagerly awaited regarding oncologic safety of omission of ALND in the setting of ypN+ disease after NAC. Ultimately axillary surgery is adjusting to ensure the appropriate information is obtained to guide adjuvant therapies, while minimizing the number of patients undergoing ALND and being put at risk of the morbidity associated with ALND.

References

1. Akrida I, Michalopoulos NV, Lagadinou M, et al. An updated review on the emerging role of indocyanine green (ICG) as a sentinel lymph node tracer in breast cancer. Cancers (Basel). 2023;15(24):5755. https://doi.org/10.3390/cancers15245755.
2. Alazraki NP, Styblo T, Grant SF, et al. Sentinel node staging of early breast cancer using lymphoscintigraphy and the intraoperative gamma-detecting probe. Semin Nucl Med. 2000;30(1):56–64.
3. Barrio AV, Montagna G, Mamtani A, et al. Nodal recurrence in patients with node-positive breast cancer treated with sentinel node biopsy alone after neoadjuvant chemotherapy—a rare event. JAMA Oncol. 2021;7(12):1851–5. https://doi.org/10.1001/jamaoncol.2021.4394.

4. Barron AU, Hoskin TL, Day CN, et al. Association of low nodal positivity rate among patients with ERBB2-positive or triple-negative breast cancer and breast pathologic complete response to neoadjuvant chemotherapy. JAMA Surg. 2018;153(12):1120–6.
5. Bartels SA, Donker M, Poncet C, et al. Radiotherapy or surgery of the axilla after a positive sentinel node in breast cancer: 10-year results of the randomized controlled EORTC 10981-22023 AMAROS trial. J Clin Oncol. 2023;41(12):2159–65. https://doi.org/10.1200/JCO.22.01565.
6. Black DM, Day CN, Boughey JC. Predicting nodal positivity in women 50-70 years of age with cT1N0 estrogen receptor positive, HER2 negative breast cancer to aid implementation of the SOUND trial into clinical practice. In: 25th Annual meeting of the American Society of Breast Surgeons. 2024 Annual meeting official proceedings—scientific session abstracts, vol. XXV. Orlando; 2024. p. 357–8.
7. Boileau JF, Poirier B, Basik M, et al. Sentinel node biopsy after neoadjuvant chemotherapy in biopsy-proven node-positive breast cancer: the SN FNAC study. J Clin Oncol. 2015;33(3):258–64. https://doi.org/10.1200/JCO.2014.55.7827.
8. Boughey JC. Factors influencing additional nodal disease and pathologic nodal upstaging with axillary dissection in patients with residual node-positive breast cancer after neoadjuvant chemotherapy enrolled on Alliance A011202 clinical trial. Clin Cancer Res. 2025;31(12_Supplement):RF2-01.
9. Boughey JC, Suman VJ, Mittendorf EA, et al. Sentinel lymph node surgery after neoadjuvant chemotherapy in patients with node-positive breast cancer: the ACOSOG Z1071 (Alliance) clinical trial. JAMA. 2013;310(14):1455–61. https://doi.org/10.1001/jama.2013.278932.
10. Boughey JC, Ballman KV, Le-Petross HT, et al. Identification and resection of clipped node decreases the false-negative rate of sentinel lymph node surgery in patients presenting with node-positive breast cancer (T0-T4, N1-N2) who receive neoadjuvant chemotherapy: results from ACOSOG Z1071 (Alliance). Ann Surg. 2016;263(4):802–7. https://doi.org/10.1097/SLA.0000000000001375.
11. Boughey JC, Yu H, Dugan CL, Piltin MA, Postlewait L, Son JD, et al. Changes in surgical management of the axilla over 11 years—report on more than 1500 breast cancer patients treated with neoadjuvant chemotherapy on the prospective I-SPY2 trial. Ann Surg Oncol. 2023;30(11):6401–10.
12. Britton TB, Solanki CK, Pinder SE, et al. Lymphatic drainage pathways of the breast and the upper limb. Nucl Med Commun. 2009;30(6):427–30.
13. Burstein HJ, Curigliano G, Thürlimann B, et al. Customizing local and systemic therapies for women with early breast cancer: the St. Gallen International Consensus Guidelines for treatment of early breast cancer 2021. Ann Oncol. 2021;32(10):1216–35. https://doi.org/10.1016/j.annonc.2021.06.023.
14. Caudle AS, Yang WT, Krishnamurthy S, et al. Improved axillary evaluation following neoadjuvant therapy for patients with node-positive breast cancer using selective evaluation of clipped nodes: implementation of targeted axillary dissection. J Clin Oncol. 2016;34(10):1072–8. https://doi.org/10.1200/JCO.2015.64.0094.
15. Caudle AS, Bedrosian I, Milton DR, et al. Use of sentinel lymph node dissection after neoadjuvant chemotherapy in patients with node-positive breast cancer at diagnosis: practice patterns of American Society of Breast Surgeons Members. Ann Surg Oncol. 2017;24(10):2925–34. https://doi.org/10.1245/s10434-017-5958-4.
16. Chen AY, Halpern MT, Schrag NM, et al. Disparities and trends in sentinel lymph node biopsy among early-stage breast cancer patients (1998–2005). J Natl Cancer Inst. 2008;100(7):462–74. https://doi.org/10.1093/jnci/djn057.
17. Chen F, Li X, Lin X, et al. Can axillary lymph node dissection be omitted in breast cancer patients with metastatic sentinel lymph nodes undergoing mastectomy? A systematic review and meta-analysis of real-world evidence. World J Surg. 2023;47(10):2446–56. https://doi.org/10.1007/s00268-023-07072-8.

18. Classe JM, Loaec C, Gimbergues P, et al. Sentinel lymph node biopsy without axillary lymphadenectomy after neoadjuvant chemotherapy is accurate and safe for selected patients: the GANEA 2 study. Breast Cancer Res Treat. 2019;173(2):343–52. https://doi.org/10.1007/s10549-018-5004-7.
19. Coriddi M, Dayan J, Bloomfield E, et al. Efficacy of immediate lymphatic reconstruction to decrease incidence of breast cancer-related lymphedema: preliminary results of randomized controlled trial. Ann Surg. 2023;278(4):630–7. https://doi.org/10.1097/SLA.0000000000005952.
20. Cortina CS, Bergom C, Craft MA, et al. A national survey of breast surgeons and radiation oncologists on contemporary axillary management in mastectomy patients. Ann Surg Oncol. 2021;28(10):5568–79. https://doi.org/10.1245/s10434-021-10441-z.
21. de Boniface J, Filtenborg Tvedskov T, Rydén L, et al. Omitting axillary dissection in breast cancer with sentinel-node metastases. N Engl J Med. 2024;390(13):1163–75. https://doi.org/10.1056/NEJMoa2313487.
22. Diego EJ, McAuliffe PF, Soran A, et al. Axillary staging after neoadjuvant chemotherapy for breast cancer: a pilot study combining sentinel lymph node biopsy with radioactive seed localization of pre-treatment positive axillary lymph nodes. Ann Surg Oncol. 2016;23(5):1549–53. https://doi.org/10.1245/s10434-015-5052-8.
23. Donker M, van Tienhoven G, Straver ME, et al. Radiotherapy or surgery of the axilla after a positive sentinel node in breast cancer (EORTC 10981-22023 AMAROS): a randomised, multicentre, open-label, phase 3 non-inferiority trial. Lancet Oncol. 2014;15(12):1303–10. https://doi.org/10.1016/S1470-2045(14)70460-7.
24. Donker M, Straver ME, Wesseling J, et al. Marking axillary lymph nodes with radioactive iodine seeds for axillary staging after neoadjuvant systemic treatment in breast cancer patients: the MARI procedure. Ann Surg. 2015;261(2):378–82. https://doi.org/10.1097/SLA.0000000000000558.
25. Fisher B, Jeong JH, Anderson S, et al. Twenty-five-year follow-up of a randomized trial comparing radical mastectomy, total mastectomy, and total mastectomy followed by irradiation. N Engl J Med. 2002;347(8):567–75.
26. Fu JF, Chen HL, Yang J, et al. Feasibility and accuracy of sentinel lymph node biopsy in clinically node-positive breast cancer after neoadjuvant chemotherapy: a meta-analysis. PLoS One. 2014;9(9):e105316. https://doi.org/10.1371/journal.pone.0105316.
27. Galimberti V, Cole BF, Zurrida S, et al. Axillary dissection versus no axillary dissection in patients with sentinel-node micrometastases (IBCSG 23-01): a phase 3 randomised controlled trial. Lancet Oncol. 2013;14(4):297–305. https://doi.org/10.1016/S1470-2045(13)70035-4.
28. Galimberti V, Ribeiro Fontana SK, Maisonneuve P, et al. Sentinel node biopsy after neoadjuvant treatment in breast cancer: five-year follow-up of patients with clinically node-negative or node-positive disease before treatment. Eur J Surg Oncol. 2016;42(3):361–8. https://doi.org/10.1016/j.ejso.2015.11.019.
29. Gentilini OD, Botteri E, Sangalli C, et al. Sentinel lymph node biopsy vs no axillary surgery in patients with small breast cancer and negative results on ultrasonography of axillary lymph nodes: the SOUND randomized clinical trial. JAMA Oncol. 2023;9(11):1557–64. https://doi.org/10.1001/jamaoncol.2023.3759.
30. Giannakou A, Kantor O, Park KU, et al. Real-world implications of the SOUND trial. Ann Surg Oncol. 2024;31(13):8776–85. https://doi.org/10.1245/s10434-024-16354-x.
31. Giuliano AE, Kirgan DM, Guenther JM, Morton DL. Lymphatic mapping and sentinel lymphadenectomy for breast cancer. Ann Surg. 1994;220(3):391–401. https://doi.org/10.1097/00000658-199409000-00015.
32. Giuliano AE, Hunt KK, Ballman KV, et al. Axillary dissection vs no axillary dissection in women with invasive breast cancer and sentinel node metastasis: a randomized clinical trial. JAMA. 2011;305(6):569–75. https://doi.org/10.1001/jama.2011.90.
33. Giuliano AE, Ballman KV, McCall L, et al. Effect of axillary dissection vs no axillary dissection on 10-year overall survival among women with invasive breast cancer

and sentinel node metastasis: the ACOSOG Z0011 (Alliance) randomized clinical trial. JAMA. 2017;318(10):918–26. https://doi.org/10.1001/jama.2017.11470.
34. Gondos A, Jansen L, Heil J, et al. Time trends in axilla management among early breast cancer patients: persisting major variation in clinical practice across European centers. Acta Oncol. 2016;55(6):712–9. https://doi.org/10.3109/0284186X.2015.1136751.
35. Goyal A, Cramp S, Marshall A, et al. Abstract OT1-04-01: ATNEC: a multi-Centre, randomised trial investigating whether axillary treatment can be avoided in T1-3N1M0 breast cancer patients with no residual cancer in the lymph glands after neoadjuvant chemotherapy (clinicaltrials.gov: nct04109079). Cancer Res. 2022;82(4_Supplement):OT1-04-01. https://doi.org/10.1158/1538-7445.SABCS21-OT1-04-01.
36. Houvenaeghel G, Cohen M, Raro P, et al. Sentinel node involvement with or without completion axillary lymph node dissection: treatment and pathologic results of randomized SERC trial. NPJ Breast Cancer. 2021;7(1):133. https://doi.org/10.1038/s41523-021-00336-3.
37. Hughes KS, Schnaper LA, Bellon JR, et al. Lumpectomy plus tamoxifen with or without irradiation in women age 70 years or older with early breast cancer: long-term follow-up of CALGB 9343. J Clin Oncol. 2013;31(19):2382–7. https://doi.org/10.1200/JCO.2012.45.2615.
38. Hunt KK, Yi M, Mittendorf EA, et al. Sentinel lymph node surgery after neoadjuvant chemotherapy is accurate and reduces the need for axillary dissection in breast cancer patients. Ann Surg. 2009;250(4):558–66.
39. International Breast Cancer Study Group, Rudenstam CM, Zahrieh D, et al. Randomized trial comparing axillary clearance versus no axillary clearance in older patients with breast cancer: first results of international breast cancer study group trial 10-93. J Clin Oncol. 2006;24(3):337–44. https://doi.org/10.1200/JCO.2005.01.5784.
40. Jagsi R, Chadha M, Moni J, et al. Radiation field design in the ACOSOG Z0011 (Alliance) trial. J Clin Oncol. 2014;32(32):3600–6. https://doi.org/10.1200/JCO.2014.56.5838.
41. Jakub JW, Boughey JC, Hieken TJ, et al. Lymphedema rates following axillary lymph node dissection with and without immediate lymphatic reconstruction: a prospective trial. Ann Surg Oncol. 2024;31(11):7349–59. https://doi.org/10.1245/s10434-024-15715-w.
42. Jiang Y, Li J, Chen B, et al. Sentinel lymph node biopsy mapped with carbon nanoparticle suspensions in patients with breast cancer: a systematic review and meta-analysis. Front Oncol. 2022;12:818812. https://doi.org/10.3389/fonc.2022.818812.
43. Kahler-Ribeiro-Fontana S, Pagan E, Magnoni F, et al. Long-term standard sentinel node biopsy after neoadjuvant treatment in breast cancer: a single institution ten-year follow-up. Eur J Surg Oncol. 2021;47(4):804–12. https://doi.org/10.1016/j.ejso.2020.10.014.
44. Kantor O, Wong S, Weiss A, et al. Prognostic significance of residual nodal disease after neoadjuvant endocrine therapy for hormone receptor-positive breast cancer. NPJ Breast Cancer. 2020;6:35. https://doi.org/10.1038/s41523-020-00177-6.
45. Kantor O, Wakeman M, Weiss A, et al. Axillary management after neoadjuvant endocrine therapy for hormone receptor-positive breast cancer. Ann Surg Oncol. 2021;28(3):1358–67. https://doi.org/10.1245/s10434-020-09073-6.
46. Kantor O, Means J, Grossmith S, et al. Optimizing axillary management in clinical T1-2N0 mastectomy patients with positive sentinel lymph nodes. Ann Surg Oncol. 2022;29(2):972–80. https://doi.org/10.1245/s10434-021-10726-3.
47. Karakatsanis A, Eriksson S, Pistiolis L, et al. Delayed sentinel lymph node dissection in patients with a preoperative diagnosis of ductal cancer in situ by preoperative injection with superparamagnetic iron oxide (SPIO) nanoparticles: the SentiNot study. Ann Surg Oncol. 2023;30(7):4064–72. https://doi.org/10.1245/s10434-022-13064-0.
48. Kim JK, Karp JM, Gerber NK. Isolated tumor cells and micrometastatic nodal disease in breast cancer patients after neoadjuvant chemotherapy: is post mastectomy radiation therapy indicated? Int J Radiat Oncol Biol Phys. 2021;111(3):e196. https://doi.org/10.1016/j.ijrobp.2021.07.708.

49. Krag DN, Weaver DL, Alex JC, Fairbank JT. Surgical resection and radiolocalization of the sentinel lymph node in breast cancer using a gamma probe. Surg Oncol. 1993;2(6):335–40. https://doi.org/10.1016/0960-7404(93)90064-6.
50. Krag DN, Anderson SJ, Julian TB, et al. Technical outcomes of sentinel-lymph-node resection and conventional axillary-lymph-node dissection in patients with clinically node-negative breast cancer: results from the NSABP B-32 randomised phase III trial. Lancet Oncol. 2007;8(10):881–8. https://doi.org/10.1016/S1470-2045(07)70278-4.
51. Krag DN, Anderson SJ, Julian TB, et al. Sentinel-lymph-node resection compared with conventional axillary-lymph-node dissection in clinically node-negative patients with breast cancer: overall survival findings from the NSABP B-32 randomised phase 3 trial. Lancet Oncol. 2010;11(10):927–33. https://doi.org/10.1016/S1470-2045(10)70207-2.
52. Kuehn T. Upstage of N-stage by diagnostic axillary lymph node dissection in patients w/ isolated tumor cells or micrometastases in sentinel/target lymph node after neoadjuvant chemotherapy—results from the prospective multicenter AXSANA/EUBREAST 3 study. Clin Cancer Res. 2025;31(12_Supplement):PS6-06. https://doi.org/10.1158/1557-3265.SABCS24-PS6-06.
53. Kuehn T, Bauerfeind I, Fehm T, et al. Sentinel-lymph-node biopsy in patients with breast cancer before and after neoadjuvant chemotherapy (SENTINA): a prospective, multicentre cohort study. Lancet Oncol. 2013;14(7):609–18. https://doi.org/10.1016/S1470-2045(13)70166-9.
54. Lee J, Park S, Bae SJ, et al. Micrometastases in axillary lymph nodes in breast cancer, post-neoadjuvant systemic therapy. Breast Cancer Res. 2024;26(1):120. https://doi.org/10.1186/s13058-024-01874-x.
55. Li J, Cheng J, Liu G, et al. Feasibility of sentinel lymph node biopsy omission after integration of 18F-FDG dedicated lymph node PET in early breast cancer: a prospective phase II trial. Cancer Biol Med. 2022;19(7):1100–8. https://doi.org/10.20892/j.issn.2095-3941.2022.0085.
56. Limberg JN, Jones T, Thomas SM, et al. Omission of axillary lymph node dissection in patients with residual nodal disease after neoadjuvant chemotherapy. Ann Surg Oncol. 2024;31(13):8813–20. https://doi.org/10.1245/s10434-024-16143-6.
57. Lin KM, Patel TH, Ray A, et al. Intradermal radioisotope is superior to peritumoral blue dye or radioisotope in identifying breast cancer sentinel nodes. J Am Coll Surg. 2004;199(4):561–6. https://doi.org/10.1016/j.jamcollsurg.2004.06.018.
58. Lohani KR, Hoskin TL, Yasir S, et al. Clipped axillary node as a potential surrogate for overall axillary nodal status in inflammatory breast cancer patients after neoadjuvant chemotherapy. Ann Surg Oncol. 2024;31(11):7431–40. https://doi.org/10.1245/s10434-024-15796-7.
59. Mamounas EP, Brown A, Anderson S, et al. Sentinel node biopsy after neoadjuvant chemotherapy in breast cancer: results from National Surgical Adjuvant Breast and Bowel Project Protocol B-27. J Clin Oncol. 2005;23(12):2694–702. https://doi.org/10.1200/JCO.2005.05.188.
60. Mamounas E, Bandos H, White J, et al. Omitting Regional Nodal Irradiation after Response to Neoadjuvant Chemotherapy. N Engl J Med 2025;392:2113-2124. https://www.nejm.org/doi/full/10.1056/NEJMoa2414859
61. Mansel RE, Fallowfield L, Kissin M, et al. Randomized multicenter trial of sentinel node biopsy versus standard axillary treatment in operable breast cancer: the ALMANAC trial. J Natl Cancer Inst. 2006;98(9):599–609. https://doi.org/10.1093/jnci/djj158.
62. Martelli G, Boracchi P, De Palo M, et al. A randomized trial comparing axillary dissection to no axillary dissection in older patients with T1N0 breast cancer: results after 5 years of follow-up. Ann Surg. 2005;242(1):1–9. https://doi.org/10.1097/01.sla.0000167759.15670.14.
63. Martelli G, Miceli R, Daidone MG, et al. Axillary dissection versus no axillary dissection in elderly patients with breast cancer and no palpable axillary nodes: results after 15 years of follow-up. Ann Surg Oncol. 2011;18(1):125–33. https://doi.org/10.1245/s10434-010-1217-7.
64. Martelli G, Barretta F, Miceli R, et al. Sentinel node biopsy alone or with axillary dissection in breast cancer patients after primary chemotherapy: long-term results of a pro-

spective interventional study. Ann Surg. 2022;276(5):e544–52. https://doi.org/10.1097/SLA.0000000000004562.
65. Masannat Y, Shenoy H, Speirs V, et al. Properties and characteristics of the dyes injected to assist axillary sentinel node localization in breast surgery. Eur J Surg Oncol. 2006;32(4):381–4. https://doi.org/10.1016/j.ejso.2006.01.010.
66. McMasters KM, Wong SL, Tuttle TM, et al. Preoperative lymphoscintigraphy for breast cancer does not improve the ability to identify axillary sentinel lymph nodes. Ann Surg. 2000;231(5):724–31. https://doi.org/10.1097/00000658-200005000-00013.
67. Montagna G, Laws A, Ferrucci M, et al. Nodal burden and oncologic outcomes in patients with residual isolated tumor cells after neoadjuvant chemotherapy (ypN0i+): the OPBC-05/ICARO study. J Clin Oncol. 2025;43(7):810–20. https://doi.org/10.1200/JCO.24.01052.
68. Montagna G, Mrdutt MM, Sun SX, et al. Omission of axillary dissection following nodal downstaging with neoadjuvant chemotherapy. JAMA Oncol. 2024;10(6):793–8. https://doi.org/10.1001/jamaoncol.2024.0578.
69. Murphy BM, Hoskin TL, Degnim AC, et al. Surgical management of axilla following neoadjuvant endocrine therapy. Ann Surg Oncol. 2021;28(13):8729–39. https://doi.org/10.1245/s10434-021-10385-4.
70. Nguyen TT, Hoskin TL, Day CN, et al. Decreasing use of axillary dissection in node-positive breast cancer patients treated with neoadjuvant chemotherapy. Ann Surg Oncol. 2018;25(9):2596–602. https://doi.org/10.1245/s10434-018-6637-9.
71. Nowikiewicz T, Głowacka-Mrotek I, Tarkowska M, et al. Failure of sentinel lymph node mapping in breast cancer patients qualified for treatment sparing axillary lymph nodes—clinical importance and management strategy—one-center analysis. Breast J. 2020;26(5):873–81. https://doi.org/10.1111/tbj.13769.
72. Park Y, Shin YS, Kim K, et al. Omission of axillary lymph node dissection in patients with ypN+ breast cancer after neoadjuvant chemotherapy: a retrospective multicenter study (KROG 21-06). Eur J Surg Oncol. 2023;49(3):589–96. https://doi.org/10.1016/j.ejso.2022.11.099.
73. Piltin MA, Hoskin TL, Day CN, et al. Oncologic outcomes of sentinel lymph node surgery after neoadjuvant chemotherapy for node-positive breast cancer. Ann Surg Oncol. 2020;27(12):4795–801. https://doi.org/10.1245/s10434-020-08900-0.
74. Povoski SP, Olsen JO, Young DC, et al. Prospective randomized clinical trial comparing intradermal, intraparenchymal, and subareolar injection routes for sentinel lymph node mapping and biopsy in breast cancer. Ann Surg Oncol. 2006;13(11):1412–21. https://doi.org/10.1245/s10434-006-9022-z.
75. Raber BM, Lin H, Shen Y, et al. Trends in regional nodal management of breast cancer patients with low nodal burden. Ann Surg Oncol. 2019;26(13):4346–54. https://doi.org/10.1245/s10434-019-07901-y.
76. Reimer T, Stachs A, Veselinovic K, et al. Axillary surgery in breast cancer—primary results of the INSEMA trial. N Engl J Med. 2024;392(11):1051–64. https://doi.org/10.1056/NEJMoa2412063.
77. Ryu JM, Lee H, Han W, et al. Selective avoidance of sentinel lymph node biopsy after neoadjuvant chemotherapy in human epidermal growth factor 2-positive/triple-negative breast cancer patients with excellent response. J Breast Cancer. 2024;27(2):130–40. https://doi.org/10.4048/jbc.2023.0264.
78. Sakurai T, Endo M, Shimizu K, et al. Axillary reverse mapping using fluorescence imaging is useful for identifying the risk group of postoperative lymphedema in breast cancer patients undergoing sentinel node biopsies. J Surg Oncol. 2014;109(6):612–5. https://doi.org/10.1245/s10434-010-0945-z.
79. Samiei S, Simons JM, Engelen SME, et al. Axillary pathologic complete response after neoadjuvant systemic therapy by breast cancer subtype in patients with initially clinically node-positive disease: a systematic review and meta-analysis. JAMA Surg. 2021;156(6):e210891. https://doi.org/10.1001/jamasurg.2021.0891.

80. Sávolt Á, Péley G, Polgár C, et al. Eight-year follow up result of the OTOASOR trial: the optimal treatment of the axilla—surgery or radiotherapy after positive sentinel lymph node biopsy in early-stage breast cancer: a randomized, single centre, phase III, non-inferiority trial. Eur J Surg Oncol. 2017;43(4):672–9. https://doi.org/10.1016/j.ejso.2016.12.011.
81. Schwieger L, Postlewait LM, Subhedar PD, et al. Patterns of completion axillary dissection for patients with cT1-2N0 breast cancer undergoing total mastectomy with positive sentinel lymph nodes. J Surg Oncol. 2024;129(3):468–80. https://doi.org/10.1002/jso.27503.
82. Simons JM, van Nijnatten TJA, van der Pol CC, et al. Diagnostic accuracy of radioactive iodine seed placement in the axilla with sentinel lymph node biopsy after neoadjuvant chemotherapy in node-positive breast cancer. JAMA Surg. 2022;157(11):991–9. https://doi.org/10.1001/jamasurg.2022.3907.
83. Society of Surgical Oncology. Choosing Wisely. 2016. https://www.choosingwisely.org/clinician-lists/sso-sentinel-node-biopsy-in-node-negative-women-70-and-over/. Published 12 July 2016. Updated 21 July 2021.
84. Sparano JA, Gray RJ, Makower DF, et al. Adjuvant chemotherapy guided by a 21-gene expression assay in breast cancer. N Engl J Med. 2018;379(2):111–21. https://doi.org/10.1056/NEJMoa1804710.
85. Spoto M, Bertolini A, Franceschini D, et al. The radiotherapy omission within the Sinodar one protocol: survival and relapse outcomes and dosimetric analysis. Eur J Cancer. 2024;200:113720.
86. Stafford AP, Hoskin TL, Day CN, et al. Contemporary axillary management in cT1-2N0 breast cancer with one or two positive sentinel lymph nodes: factors associated with completion axillary lymph node dissection within the National Cancer Database. Ann Surg Oncol. 2022;29(8):4740-9.
87. Straver ME, Meijnen P, van Tienhoven G, et al. Sentinel node identification rate and nodal involvement in the EORTC 10981-22023 AMAROS trial. Ann Surg Oncol. 2010;17(7):1854–61. https://doi.org/10.1245/s10434-010-0945-z.
88. Tadros AB, Yang WT, Krishnamurthy S, et al. Identification of patients with documented pathologic complete response in the breast after neoadjuvant chemotherapy for omission of axillary surgery. JAMA Surg. 2017;152(7):665–70.
89. Tasoulis MK, Lee HB, Yang W, et al. Accuracy of post-neoadjuvant chemotherapy image-guided breast biopsy to predict residual cancer. JAMA Surg. 2020;155(12):e204103.
90. Tee SR, Devane LA, Evoy D, et al. Meta-analysis of sentinel lymph node biopsy after neoadjuvant chemotherapy in patients with initial biopsy-proven node-positive breast cancer. Br J Surg. 2018;105(12):1541–52. https://doi.org/10.1002/bjs.10986.
91. Thompson M, Korourian S, Henry-Tillman R, et al. Axillary reverse mapping (ARM): a new concept to identify and enhance lymphatic preservation. Ann Surg Oncol. 2007;14(6):1890–5. https://doi.org/10.1245/s10434-007-9412-x.
92. Tinterri C, Gentile D, Gatzemeier W, et al. Preservation of axillary lymph nodes compared with complete dissection in T1-2 breast cancer patients presenting one or two metastatic sentinel lymph nodes: the SINODAR-ONE multicenter randomized clinical trial. Ann Surg Oncol. 2022;29(9):5732–44. https://doi.org/10.1245/s10434-022-11866-w.
93. Tinterri C, Canavese G, Gatzemeier W, et al. Sentinel lymph node biopsy versus axillary lymph node dissection in breast cancer patients undergoing mastectomy with one to two metastatic sentinel lymph nodes: sub-analysis of the SINODAR-ONE multicentre randomized clinical trial and reopening of enrolment. Br J Surg. 2023;110(9):1143–52. https://doi.org/10.1093/bjs/znad215.
94. van der Noordaa MEM, van Duijnhoven FH, Cuijpers FNE, et al. Toward omitting sentinel lymph node biopsy after neoadjuvant chemotherapy in patients with clinically node-negative breast cancer. Br J Surg. 2021;108(6):667–74. https://doi.org/10.1002/bjs.12026.
95. Verheuvel NC, Voogd AC, Tjan-Heijnen VCG, Roumen RMH. What to do with non-visualized sentinel nodes? A Dutch nationwide survey study. Ann Surg Oncol. 2017;24(8):2155–60. https://doi.org/10.1245/s10434-017-5824-4.

96. Veronesi U, Paganelli G, Giuseppe V, et al. A randomized comparison of sentinel node biopsy with routine axillary dissection in breast cancer. N Engl J Med. 2003;349(6):546–53.
97. Vrancken Peeters MJ, Straver ME, Donker M, et al. Novel surgical technique to selectively remove metastatic axillary lymph nodes in breast cancer patients after neoadjuvant chemotherapy: the MARI procedure—marking of the axilla with radioactive iodine seeds. J Clin Oncol. 2012;30:196. https://doi.org/10.1200/jco.2012.30.27_suppl.196.
98. Weiss A, Lin H, Babiera GV, et al. Evolution in practice patterns of axillary management following mastectomy in patients with 1-2 positive sentinel nodes. Breast Cancer Res Treat. 2019;176(2):435–44. https://doi.org/10.1007/s10549-019-05243-7.
99. Weiss A, Colugnati F, Mitchell M, et al. Contemporary axillary surgical management in patients with pathologically node positive disease after neoadjuvant chemotherapy: a survey of members of the American Society of Breast Surgeons. Ann Surg Oncol. 2024;31(11):7362–71. https://doi.org/10.1245/s10434-024-15705-y.
100. Xing Y, Foy M, Cox DD, et al. Meta-analysis of sentinel lymph node biopsy after preoperative chemotherapy in patients with breast cancer. Br J Surg. 2006;93(5):539–46.
101. Yu M, Liu Y, Huang Z, et al. The feasibility and reliability of sentinel lymph node biopsy after neoadjuvant chemotherapy in breast cancer patients with negative axillary lymph nodes—a meta-analysis. Breast Cancer (Auckl). 2024;18:11782234241255856. https://doi.org/10.1177/11782234241255856.
102. Žatecký J, Coufal O, Zapletal O, et al. Ideal marker for targeted axillary dissection (IMTAD): a prospective multicentre trial. World J Surg Oncol. 2023;21(1):252. https://doi.org/10.1186/s12957-023-03147-x.

Chapter 5
Current Update in Localisation and Management of Breast Cancer in Neoadjuvant Therapy

Jennifer Wang, Simran Malhotra, and Audree B. Tadros

Contents

5.1 Introduction

Neoadjuvant systemic therapy (NST) has been proven to increase rates of breast-conservation surgery (BCS) without compromising disease-free survival or overall survival in operable breast cancers [1, 2]. Among patients who are ineligible for BCS at presentation, NST is given to decrease the size of the residual tumour thereby decreasing the extent of required surgery, improving tumour resectability, and allowing for maximal breast preservation [3]. NST also provides real-time

---

J. Wang
Plastic and Reconstructive Surgery Service, Department of Surgery, Memorial Sloan Kettering Cancer Center, New York, NY, USA
e-mail: wangj24@mskcc.org

S. Malhotra · A. B. Tadros (✉)
Breast Service, Department of Surgery, Memorial Sloan Kettering Cancer Center, New York, NY, USA
e-mail: simran.malhotra@icahn.mssm.edu; tadrosa@mskcc.org

R. Vidya, N. Sharma (eds.), *Breast and Axilla Localisation Techniques*,
https://doi.org/10.1007/978-3-032-17995-1_5

insight on tumour response, which may reveal prognostic information, guide future treatment options, and prevent patients from experiencing side effects of an ineffective therapy [4].

Types of neoadjuvant systemic therapy include neoadjuvant chemotherapy (NAC), immunotherapy, targeted therapy, and hormonal therapy. The type and combination of therapy is dependent on the biologic subtype of breast cancer. Patients with human epidermal growth factor receptor 2 (HER2)-positive breast cancer receiving a combination of NAC and dual HER2-targeted therapy have reported overall pathologic complete response (pCR) rates of 50%–60%, while patients with hormone receptor (HR)-positive/HER2-negative breast cancers undergoing NAC have reported overall pCR rates of 5%–15% [5]. The KEYNOTE-522 Trial, a phase 3 study examining chemotherapy versus chemoimmunotherapy in patients with early-stage triple-negative breast cancer, demonstrated improved rates of pCR with chemoimmunotherapy (64.8%) versus chemotherapy alone (51.2%, $p < 0.01$) [6, 7]. Neoadjuvant endocrine therapy, used in patients with oestrogen receptor (ER)-positive breast cancer who would not benefit from chemotherapy or who would not tolerate chemotherapy, has fewer toxicities compared to chemotherapy and can be used for breast tumour downstaging, with success rates as high as 50% in some studies [8–10].

5.2 Surgical Feasibility of BCS Post-NST

In a recent analysis of the National Surgical Quality Improvement Program (NSQIP) Surveillance, Epidemiology, and End Results (SEER) program, and National Cancer Database (NCDB), rates of BCS are on the rise while rates of mastectomy are declining [11]. This is likely due in part to the increased rates of breast downstaging seen with modern neoadjuvant systemic therapy. Notably, patients do not need to achieve pCR in order to become eligible for BCS. Many patients who achieve a partial response to NST may also be eligible for BCS [12, 13]. Additionally, the entire pre-NAC tumour volume does not need to be resected during surgery [14].

Multiple historic randomized trials have examined the success of NST among patients who were ineligible for BCS at presentation. Published in 1998 and 2001, the National Surgical Adjuvant Breast and Bowel Project (NSABP) B-18 and European Organisation for Research and Treatment of Cancer (EORTC) 10902 trial found increased rates of BCS in patients who received NAC as opposed to adjuvant chemotherapy, with no change in overall survival or locoregional recurrence [2, 15]. In 2005 the European Cooperative Trial in Operable breast cancer (ECTO) found that patients who received a NAC regimen had a BCS rate of 65%, which was significantly greater than the 34% BCS rate in the control arm of patients who underwent surgery first, followed by adjuvant chemotherapy [16]. Rates of conversion from patients who are BCS-ineligible due to large clinical tumour size, to BCS-eligible with NAC are reported to be as high as 75% in some studies [13]. Importantly, these studies included patients regardless of receptor status.

Table 5.1 Response rates to NAC by subtype

	pCR rate (%)	
Subtype	Swisher et al. [12]	Boughey et al. [5]
HR+/HER2+	45.7	45.4
HR−/HER2+	72.4	
HR+/HER2−	16.5	11.4
HR−/HER2−	42	38.2

NAC neoadjuvant chemotherapy, *pCR* pathologic complete response, *HR* hormone receptor, *HER2* human epidermal growth factor receptor 2

However, we know that there are specific subtypes of breast cancer, including triple negative and HER2 positive, that are associated with higher rates of pCR and successful BCS following NAC compared to HR-positive breast cancer (Table 5.1) [5, 12]. More recently, Golshan et al., in two prospective studies, evaluated the effect of differing NAC regimens in patients with triple-negative breast cancer and found conversion rates from BCS ineligibility to BCS eligibility of 42% and 53%, respectively [17, 18]. These results demonstrate the efficacy of NST in downstaging tumours in patients with TNBC. Another prospective study by Golshan et al. demonstrated a conversion rate of 43% in patients with stage II-III HER2-positive breast cancer, confirming that HER2-positive tumours also respond favourably to NST, facilitating BCS in a significant portion of patients [19]. Similarly, Petruolo et al. examined the effect of NST in large tumours precluding BCS and found a conversion rate of 69%. Univariate analysis showed that HER2-positive and triple-negative receptor status independently predicted successful downstaging [13]. These findings highlight that even aggressive breast cancer subtypes are quite suitable for breast downstaging with NAC.

5.3 Review of Short Literature to Date: Local Recurrence Rates and Oncologic Considerations

Downstaging to BCS after NST is oncologically safe and has not been associated with increased risk of locoregional recurrence. In both the NSABP B-18 and EORTC 10902 trials, no significant differences in locoregional recurrence among patients who received NST followed by BCS versus patients who received upfront BCS followed by adjuvant chemotherapy were seen [2, 15, 20]. Similarly, a single-centre experience from The University of Texas MD Anderson Cancer Center (Houston, TX, USA) reported 5-year in-breast tumour recurrence (IBTR)-free and locoregional recurrence-free survival rates of 95% and 91%, respectively, in patients undergoing BCS after NST [21]. In a more contemporary study by Swisher et al., patients receiving NST followed by BCS had a 5-year locoregional recurrence-free survival of 95.4%. Multivariate analysis in this study indicated that patients with HR-negative/HER2-negative receptor status, clinical stage III disease, and lack of pCR had a significantly higher hazard ratio for locoregional recurrence [12]. Huang et al. further highlighted the prognostic role of NST, emphasizing that lack of clinical response to NST is associated with higher locoregional recurrence [4]. Their multivariate regression analysis identified skin/nipple involvement and ER-negative cancer as independent predictors of LRR, with actuarial 5-year and 10-year locoregional recurrence rates of 9% and 11%, respectively. Certain oncologic factors may increase a patient's risk of locoregional recurrence after NST downstaging to BCS, but overall rates of locoregional recurrence are low in this population.

While NST has expanded BCS eligibility, there are some patients who should not be considered for downstaging. Contraindications for downstaging to BCS include patients who have cancer progression or no response to chemotherapy, extensive residual microcalcifications precluding an acceptable cosmetic result, extensive multicentric disease spanning two or more quadrants, and patients with inflammatory breast cancer (IBC). Dawood et al. found that the overall survival and breast cancer-specific survival hazard ratios were significantly higher in patients with inflammatory breast cancer who had a partial mastectomy compared to those who had a mastectomy [22]. Currently, BCS is still considered contraindicated in patients with IBC due to the aggressive nature of this disease and the high probability of uncontrolled locoregional recurrence [23]. Furthermore, non-guideline concordant treatment, including surgery, for patients with IBC has been associated with worse survival outcomes for patients with IBC [24]. While historically, multifocal/multicentric disease was considered contraindications for BCS, recent data have emerged demonstrating the oncologic safety of multiple lumpectomies in this setting. The American College of Surgeons Oncology Group (ACOSOG) Z11102 (Alliance) trial first demonstrated patients with multiple ipsilateral breast cancer have acceptably low 5-year locoregional recurrence rates after BCS followed by adjuvant radiation with lumpectomy site boosts [25]. When comparing patients enrolled in the GeparTrio, GeparQuattro, and GeparQuinto trials with unifocal, multifocal, and multicentric disease who received breast conservation after NAC, Ataseven et al. found no significant difference in disease-free survival between the three groups. Overall survival also did not differ among patients if tumour-free margins were attained during surgery [26]. Therefore, NST is a viable option for patients with multicentric and multifocal disease, presuming negative margins can be achieved with an acceptable cosmetic result.

5.4 Assessing Tumour Response to NST

It is important to assess the extent of breast cancer before and after NST with imaging. Standard preoperative imaging includes breast magnetic resonance imaging (MRI) and mammography. Breast MRI is the most sensitive imaging modality for detecting disease and assessing tumour response [27, 28]. Mammography is not as accurate for assessing tumour response when compared to MRI, but is essential, as it may detect malignant calcifications which may not be evident on MRI. Assessment should also include physical exam in conjunction with imaging for accurate initial tumour staging. Tumours may react to NAC in two ways: pCR or disappearance of all target lesions, and partial response or at least a 30% decrease in the sum of diameters of target lesions. The Response Evaluation Criteria in Solid Tumors (RECIST) guidelines provide criteria used to determine objective tumour response for target lesions and should be used to evaluate tumour response to NST [28].

Common patterns of tumour response to NST include complete or partial response; the latter can be further characterized into a single nidus of residual disease or scattered residual tumour cells (Fig. 5.1) [29]. Regardless of the response

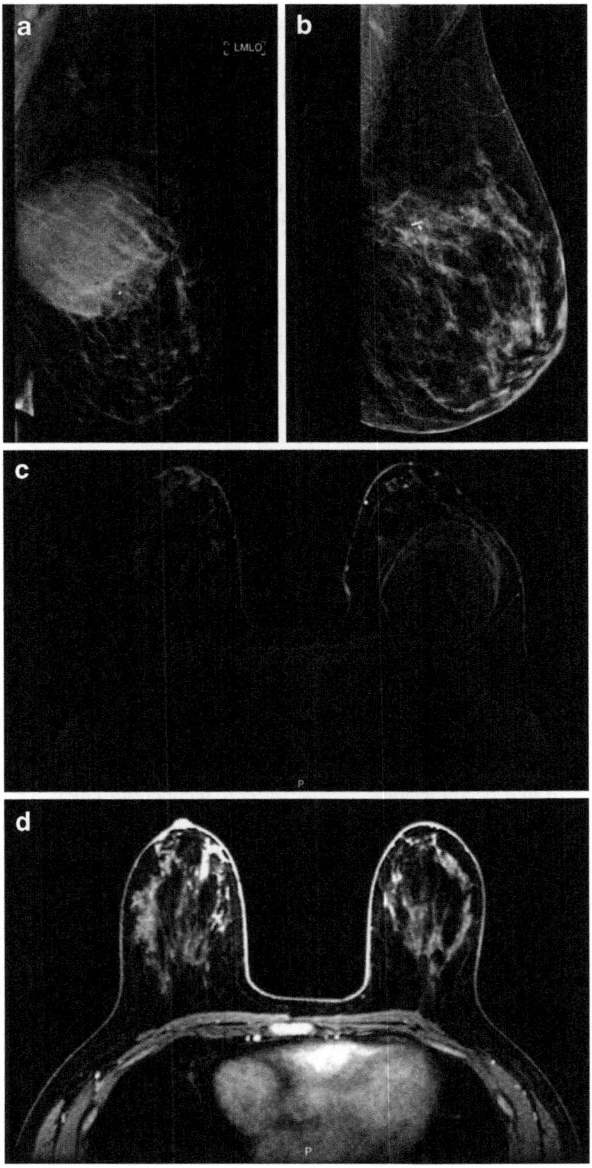

Fig. 5.1 Patterns of tumour response. Patient with a unifocal, TNBC encompassing multiple quadrants of the breast at presentation who underwent NST (KEYNOTE 522) and achieved pCR. (**a**) Pre-NST mammogram with single biopsy clip placed with the tumour; (**b**) post-NAC mammography with a single seed localization at the site of the biopsy clip; (**c**) pre-NAC MRI; (**d**) post-NAC MRI showing a black circle in the area of the biopsy clip with no abnormal findings. Abbreviations: TNBC, triple-negative breast cancer; NST, neoadjuvant systemic therapy; pCR, pathologic complete response; NAC, neoadjuvant chemotherapy

pattern, such downstaging leading to BCS is associated with neither an increased risk of locoregional recurrence nor changes in survival, as shown in both of the landmark EORTC 10902 and NSABP B-18 trials as well as by 12 other worldwide studies reported in a meta-analysis by Mieog et al. [20]. These findings ultimately support the oncologic safety of BCS for operable breast cancer.

5.5 Methods of Tumour Localisation

Accurate localization of the original tumour site is crucial during BCS to ensure tumour removal with negative margins. Standard practice includes placing radiopaque clips at the tumour site following initial diagnostic breast biopsy prior to NST initiation. Among patients undergoing NST, areas of contiguous disease associated with biopsy-proven carcinoma do not require additional biopsy or clip placement prior to NST. If these areas remain following completion of NST, the entire area will require excision. All clips associated with known malignancy prior to NST then require a second localization after NST to target the residual tumour area for surgery. Approaches to this second localization vary immensely. Traditionally, wire-guided localization (WGL) was used to localize tumours. However, there are now numerous options for preoperative tumour localization (Table 5.2) [30].

Table 5.2 Localization techniques

Wire-guided localization	
Wire-guided localization	Insertion of hollow needle through the breast to the lesion under image guidance, wire is threaded through the needle, needle is removed so that the wire remains in place, protruding from the skin
Radioactive localization	
Radioactive seed localization	Placement of 125-iodine seed in the index lesion under image guidance days or weeks prior to surgery; intraoperative detection of seed by handheld gamma probe assists the accurate localization of the lesion
Radio-occult lesion localization	Use of 99 m technetium-labelled radiocolloid to label the index lesion under image guidance, similar intraoperative detection of seed by gamma probe
Magnetic or paramagnetic localization	
Magseed, Sirius Pintuition, MOLLI surgical, TAKUMI/guiding-marker system	Magnetic or paramagnetic (i.e., can be temporarily magnetized by an externally applied field) marker or seed is implanted in index lesion under image guidance days before surgery, intraoperative detection uses a specified compatible probe to accurately locate seed

(continued)

Table 5.2 (continued)

Radar reflector or radiofrequency localization	
SAVI scout	Placement of a passive reflector in index lesion up to 30 days prior to surgery under stereotactic or ultrasound guidance; the reflector is activated intraoperatively by infrared light impulses generated from a compatible probe; two antennas help reflect an electromagnetic wave signal back to the probe for detection
RFID/LOCalizer	Placement of radiofrequency tag with a unique identification number in the index lesion under ultrasound guidance; intraoperative detection uses a specified compatible probe to accurately locate tag; contraindicated in patients with defibrillators and pacemakers

Advantages of WGL are its low cost and availability; however, the main criticisms of this technique include patient discomfort and scheduling difficulties [31, 32]. Hence, the wire has to be placed hours prior to surgery by a breast radiologist, after which the patient must remain still to prevent any wire dislodgement. Other methods including seed localization and commercial products are increasing in popularity, as they allow for better patient comfort and scheduling flexibility with comparable surgical outcomes [33, 34]. However, there is still a lack of adequate data comparing these newer localization techniques and a lack of understanding as to whether WGL is an outdated gold standard. The new MELODY [*Methods for Localization of Different Types of Breast Lesions*] trial is a multinational prospective intergroup cohort study conducted by EUBREAST and iBRA-NET that is currently investigating these very questions [35].

Besides the myriad of localization techniques, different approaches to localization are also available. Single site localization describes a targeted preoperative marking of the residual tumour or area of concern under sonographic or mammographic guidance, followed by same-day surgical removal of the specimen with a localization marker. Bracketed localization, first introduced in 1987 in a study by Silverstein et al., uses two to three wires to 'bracket' large areas (often 3–5 cm in size) of microcalcifications; this allows for a targeted removal of the entire lesion, both permitting BCS and mitigating re-excision risk (Fig. 5.2) [36].

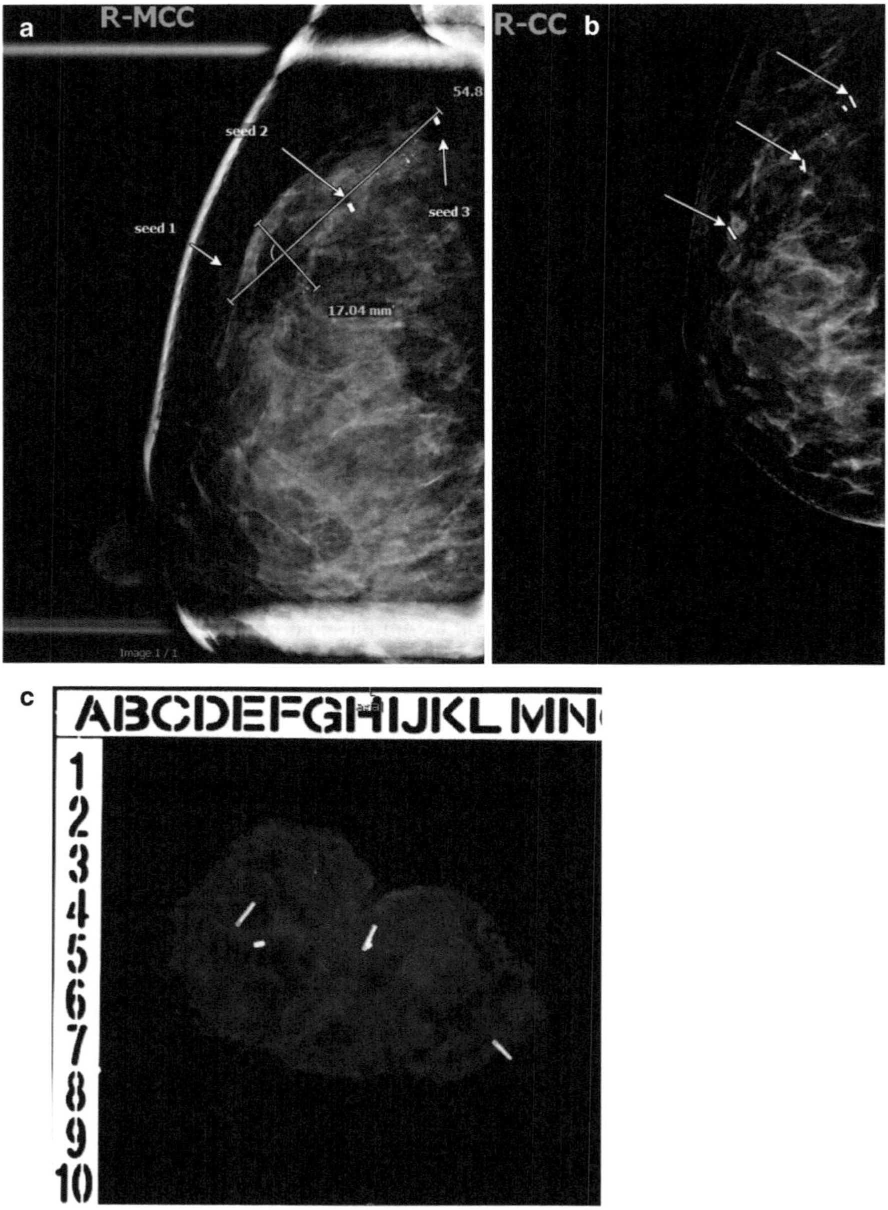

Fig. 5.2 Bracketed localization of multicentric tumour. Patient with extensive multifocal disease who underwent bracketed localization. (**a**) Plan for bracketing to incorporate two biopsy clips and residual calcifications. (**b**) Three-site seed location. (**c**) Lumpectomy specimen containing three radioactive seeds and two biopsy clips

5.6 Surgical Decision Making: What and How Much to Remove in BCS

Decision making in BCS includes determining the extent of volume of breast tissue that requires excision in the context of a patient's breast size and tumour location. A formative study conducted at The University of Texas MD Anderson Cancer Center found lumpectomy patients with a large tumour (2 cm or greater) who received NAC, had significantly smaller volumes of breast tissue excised compared to patients who had adjuvant chemotherapy ($p = 0.004$); but there was *no* difference between these two groups in either the re-excision rate or the total number of breast operations. For those with smaller tumours (2 cm or less), NST receipt had no impact on the volume excised, re-excision rate, or number of operations ($p > 0.05$). This study ultimately showed how BCS can benefit patients with larger tumours post-NST with less-extensive surgeries yet similarly safe oncologic outcomes [14].

While the approach to volume excision is 'less is still good', the approach to residual calcification is more conservative; the removal of all residual calcifications after NST is crucial. An early study reported a 69% positive predictive value for carcinoma in residual calcifications post-BCS [37]. Another study found that removing all suspicious calcifications at the initial surgery using bracketed localization may spare the patient from re-excision, as calcification removal was significantly associated with achieving clear margins *but* did not guarantee it [38]. Most recently, Feliciano et al. found no statistical correlation between changes in calcifications (when comparing pre- and post-NAC changes) and either MRI enhancement resolution or pCR achievement. This study argued that while the residual calcifications seen on post-imaging may be benign, the loss of MRI enhancement does not accurately exclude residual tumour enough to leave calcifications in place; therefore, complete excision is warranted [39]. Hence, this is an important limitation for patients undergoing BCS and should be an active area for future study.

In addition to ensuring adequate residual tumour removal, achieving clear surgical margins is essential to minimize the risk of local recurrence. The Society of Surgical Oncology and the American Society for Radiation Oncology (SSO-ASTRO) guidelines in 2014 recommended that re-excision is indicated for patients with 'tumor on ink' for either the invasive or in situ component, for those treated with BCS and whole-breast irradiation (WBI) [40]. Moreover, another study published in 2018 investigated the optimal margin width for patients who received NAC, BCS, and WBI, and found no association between margin width and local recurrence-free survival, disease-free survival, or overall survival on multivariate analysis. Rather, they found that hormone receptor-negative subtype, breast and/or axillary residual disease, and positive pathologic nodal status were associated with worse disease-free survival [41]. Their study substantiated the earlier 'no ink on tumor' guidelines as sufficient for certain select patients.

For patients with invasive breast cancer who undergo NST followed by BCS, achieving 'no ink on tumor' is considered an acceptable and oncologically safe margin standard. This guideline aligns with the consensus established by SSO-ASTRO, which recommends 'no ink on tumor' as sufficient for patients treated with BCS, regardless of whether NST is given before surgery [40]. A study by Choi et al. examining stage I-III breast cancer patients treated with NAC, BCS, and WBI demonstrated no association between margin width ($\leq$2 mm and $\leq$1 mm) and local recurrence-free survival, disease-free survival, or overall survival on multivariate analysis [41]. Similarly, Mrdutt et al. showed that there was no difference in 4-year IBTR between patients who had a margin width $\leq$2 mm and those who had a margin width >2 mm [42]. Therefore, re-excision is not routinely required if margins are negative, even in the post-NST setting, provided there are no residual extensive intraductal components or other high-risk features that would independently necessitate further surgical intervention.

5.7 Summary with Tips and Pitfalls

Neoadjuvant systemic therapy (NST) allows safe downstaging of breast tumours, enabling breast-conservation surgery (BCS) in patients who were initially ineligible for lumpectomy. This approach does not compromise oncologic outcomes and is supported by data across multiple tumour subtypes. Localization techniques and careful imaging assessment are essential to accurately guide surgery post-NST.

5.7.1 Tips for Clinical Practice

1. *Patient Selection*: Patients do not need to achieve pCR after NST in order to be eligible for BCS.
2. *Clip Placement*: Always place a clip at the tumour site before NST initiation—clips do not migrate and are vital for accurate localization after tumour shrinkage.
3. *Use MRI for Assessment*: MRI is more accurate than mammography or ultrasound for evaluating residual disease and treatment response post-NST.
4. *Localization Technique*: Radioactive and magnetic seed localization is gaining popularity over wire localization for improved patient comfort, flexibility in scheduling, and more precise targeting.
5. *'No Ink on Tumor' Margin Standard*: For patients undergoing BCS post-NST, 'no ink on tumor' remains an acceptable and safe margin standard. The entire pre-NAC tumour volume does not need to be resected.

5.7.2 Common Pitfalls to Avoid

- *Inadequate Pre-NST Imaging*: Failing to fully image extent of disease before NST can lead to incomplete resection.
- *Assuming BCS Is Safe in All*: IBC and extensive multicentric disease remain contraindications for BCS, despite downstaging.

References

1. Rastogi P, Anderson S, Bear H, Geyer C, Kahlenberg M, Robidoux A, Margolese R, Hoehn J, Vogel V, Dakhil S, Tamkus D, King K, Pajon E, Wright M, Robert J, Paik S, Mamounas E, Wolmark N. Preoperative chemotherapy: updates of National Surgical Adjuvant Breast and bowel project protocols B-18 and B-27. J Clin Oncol. 2008;26(5):778–85.
2. Fisher B, Bryant J, Wolmark N, Mamounas E, Brown A, Fisher E, Wickerham D, Begovic M, DeCillis A, Robidoux A, Margolese R, Cruz A, Hoehn J, Lees A, Dimitrov N, Bear H. Effect of preoperative chemotherapy on the outcome of women with operable breast cancer. J Clin Oncol. 1998;16(8):2672–85.
3. Killelea B, Yang V, Mougalian S, Horowitz N, Pusztai L, Chagpar A, Lannin D. Neoadjuvant chemotherapy for breast cancer increases the rate of breast conservation: results from the National Cancer Database. J Am Coll Surg. 2015;220(6):1063–9.
4. Huang E, Tucker S, Strom E, McNeese M, Kuerer H, Hortobagyi G, Buzdar A, Valero V, Perkins G, Schechter N, Hunt K, Sahin A, Buchholz T. Predictors of locoregional recurrence in patients with locally advanced breast cancer treated with neoadjuvant chemotherapy, mastectomy, and radiotherapy. Int J Radiat Oncol Biol Phys. 2005;62(2):351–7.
5. Boughey J, McCall L, Ballman K, Mittendorf E, Ahrendt G, Wilke L, Taback B, Leitch A, Flippo-Morton T, Hunt K. Tumor biology correlates with rates of breast-conserving surgery and pathologic complete response after neoadjuvant chemotherapy for breast cancer: findings from the ACOSOG Z1071 (Alliance) prospective Multicenter clinical trial. Ann Surg. 2014;260(4):608–14.
6. Schmid P, Cortes J, Pusztai L, McArthur H, Kümmel S, Bergh J, Denkert C, Park YH, Hui R, Harbeck N, Takahashi M, Foukakis T, Fasching PA, Cardoso F, Untch M, Jia L, Karantza V, Zhao J, Aktan G, Dent R, O'Shaughnessy J. Pembrolizumab for early triple-negative breast cancer. N Engl J Med. 2020;382(9):810–21.
7. Schmid P, Cortes J, Dent R, McArthur H, Pusztai L, Kümmel S, Denkert C, Park YH, Hui R, Harbeck N, Takahashi M, Im S-A, Untch M, Fasching PA, Mouret-Reynier M-A, Foukakis T, Ferreira M, Cardoso F, Zhou X, Karantza V, Tryfonidis K, Aktan G, O'Shaughnessy J. Overall survival with pembrolizumab in early-stage triple-negative breast cancer. N Engl J Med. 2024;391(21):1981–91.
8. Spring LM, Gupta A, Reynolds KL, Gadd MA, Ellisen LW, Isakoff SJ, Moy B, Bardia A. Neoadjuvant endocrine therapy for Estrogen receptor-positive breast cancer: a systematic review and meta-analysis. JAMA Oncol. 2016;2(11):1477–86.
9. Smith IE, Dowsett M, Ebbs SR, Dixon JM, Skene A, Blohmer J-U, Ashley SE, Francis S, Boeddinghaus I, Walsh G. Neoadjuvant treatment of postmenopausal breast cancer with anastrozole, tamoxifen, or both in combination: the immediate preoperative anastrozole, tamoxifen, or combined with tamoxifen (IMPACT) Multicenter double-blind randomized trial. J Clin Oncol. 2005;23(22):5108–16.
10. Ellis MJ, Suman VJ, Hoog J, Lin L, Snider J, Prat A, Parker JS, Luo J, DeSchryver K, Allred DC, Esserman LJ, Unzeitig GW, Margenthaler J, Babiera GV, Marcom PK, Guenther JM, Watson MA, Leitch M, Hunt K, Olson JA. Randomized phase II neoadjuvant comparison

between letrozole, anastrozole, and exemestane for postmenopausal women with estrogen receptor–rich stage 2 to 3 breast cancer: clinical and biomarker outcomes and predictive value of the baseline PAM50-based intrinsic subtype—ACOSOG Z1031. J Clin Oncol. 2011;29(17):2342–9.
11. Nelson J, Rubenstein R, Haglich K, Chu J, Yin S, Stern C, Morrow M, Mehrara B, Gemignani M, Matros E. Analysis of a trend reversal in US lumpectomy rates from 2005 through 2017 using 3 nationwide data sets. JAMA Surg. 2022;157(8):702–11.
12. Swisher S, Vila J, Tucker S, Bedrosian I, Shaitelman S, Litton J, Smith B, Caudle A, Kuerer H, Mittendorf E. Locoregional control according to breast cancer subtype and response to neoadjuvant chemotherapy in breast cancer patients undergoing breast-conserving therapy. Ann Surg Oncol. 2016;23(3):749–56.
13. Petruolo O, Sevilimedu V, Montagna G, Le T, Morrow M, Barrio A. How often does modern neoadjuvant chemotherapy downstage patients to breast-conserving surgery? Ann Surg Oncol. 2021;28(1):287–94.
14. Boughey JC, Peintinger F, Meric-Bernstam F, Perry AC, Hunt KK, Babiera GV, Singletary SE, Bedrosian I, Lucci A, Buzdar AU, Pusztai L, Kuerer HM. Impact of preoperative versus postoperative chemotherapy on the extent and number of surgical procedures in patients treated in randomized clinical trials for breast cancer. Ann Surg. 2006;244(3):464–70.
15. van der Hage JA, van de Velde CJH, Julien J-P, Tubiana-Hulin M, Vandervelden C, Duchateau L, Investigators C. Preoperative chemotherapy in primary operable breast cancer: results from the European Organization for Research and Treatment of cancer trial 10902. J Clin Oncol. 2001;19(22):4224–37.
16. Gianni L, Baselga J, Eiermann W, Guillem Porta V, Semiglazov V, Lluch A, Zambetti M, Sabadell D, Raab G, Llombart Cussac A, Bozhok A, Martinez-Agulló A, Greco M, Byakhov M, Lopez Lopez J, Mansutti M, Valagussa P, Bonadonna G. Feasibility and tolerability of sequential doxorubicin/paclitaxel followed by cyclophosphamide, methotrexate, and fluorouracil and its effects on tumor response as preoperative therapy. Clin Cancer Res. 2005;11(24 Pt 1):8715–21.
17. Golshan M, Cirrincione C, Sikov W, Berry D, Jasinski S, Weisberg T, Somlo G, Hudis C, Winer E, Ollila D. Impact of neoadjuvant chemotherapy in stage II-III triple negative breast cancer on eligibility for breast-conserving surgery and breast conservation rates: surgical results from CALGB 40603 (Alliance). Ann Surg. 2015;262(3):434–9.
18. Golshan M, Loibl S, Wong S, Houber J, O'Shaughnessy J, Rugo H, Wolmark N, McKee M, Maag D, Sullivan D, Metzger-Filho O, Von Minckwitz G, Geyer C, Sikov W, Untch M. Breast conservation after neoadjuvant chemotherapy for triple-negative breast cancer: surgical results from the BrighTNess randomized clinical trial. JAMA Surg. 2020;155(3):e195410.
19. Golshan M, Cirrincione C, Sikov W, Carey L, Berry D, Overmoyer B, Henry N, Somlo G, Port E, Burstein H, Hudis C, Winer E, Ollila D. Impact of neoadjuvant therapy on eligibility for and frequency of breast conservation in stage II–III HER2-positive breast cancer: surgical results of CALGB 40601 (Alliance). Breast Cancer Res Treat. 2016;160(2):297–304.
20. Mieog J, van der Hage J, van de Velde C. Neoadjuvant chemotherapy for operable breast cancer. Br J Surg. 2007;94(10):1189–200.
21. Chen A, Meric-Bernstam F, Hunt K, Thames H, Oswald M, Outlaw E, Strom E, McNeese M, Kuerer H, Ross M, Singletary S, Ames F, Feig B, Sahin A, Perkins G, Schechter N, Hortobagyi G, Buchholz T. Breast conservation after neoadjuvant chemotherapy: the MD Anderson cancer center experience. J Clin Oncol. 2004;22(12):2302–12.
22. Dawood S, Lei X, Dent R, Gupta S, Sirohi B, Cortes J, Cristofanilli M, Buchholz T, Gonzalez-Angulo AM. Survival of women with inflammatory breast cancer: a large population-based study. Ann Oncol. 2014;25(6):1143–51.
23. Ueno NT, Fernandez JRE, Cristofanilli M, Overmoyer B, Rea D, Berdichevski F, El-Shinawi M, Bellon J, Le-Petross HT, Lucci A, Babiera G, DeSnyder SM, Teshome M, Chang E, Lim B, Krishnamurthy S, Stauder MC, Parmar S, Mohamed MM, Alexander A, Valero V, Woodward WA. International consensus on the clinical management of inflammatory breast cancer

from the Morgan Welch Inflammatory Breast Cancer Research Program 10th Anniversary Conference. J Cancer. 2018;9(8):1437–47.
24. Tadros A, Diskin B, Sevilimedu V, Xu A, Vingan P, Nelson J, Iwai Y, Morrow M, Fayanju OM. Guideline-concordant care for inflammatory breast cancer. JAMA Netw Open. 2025;8(2):e2454506.
25. Boughey J, Rosenkranz K, Ballman K, McCall L, Haffty B, Cuttino L, Kubicky C, Le-Petross H, Giuliano A, Van Zee K, Hunt K, Hahn O, Carey L, Partridge A. Local recurrence after breast-conserving therapy in patients with multiple ipsilateral breast cancer: results from ACOSOG Z11102 (Alliance). J Clin Oncol. 2023;41(17):3184–93.
26. Ataseven B, Lederer B, Blohmer J, Denkert C, Gerber B, Heil J, Kühn T, Kümmel S, Rezai M, Loibl S, von Minckwitz G. Impact of multifocal or multicentric disease on surgery and locoregional, distant and overall survival of 6,134 breast cancer patients treated with neoadjuvant chemotherapy. Ann Surg Oncol. 2015;22(4):1118–27.
27. Reig B, Lewin AA, Du L, Heacock L, Toth HK, Heller SL, Gao Y, Moy L. Breast MRI for evaluation of response to neoadjuvant therapy. Radiographics. 2021;41(3):665–79.
28. Eisenhauer E, Therasse P, Bogaerts J, Schwartz L, Sargent D, Ford R, Dancey J, Arbuck S, Gwyther S, Mooney M, Rubinstein L, Shankar L, Dodd L, Kaplan R, Lacombe D, Verweij J. New response evaluation criteria in solid tumours: revised RECIST guideline (version 1.1). Eur J Cancer. 2009;45(2):228–47.
29. Buchholz TA, Hunt KK, Whitman GJ, Sahin AA, Hortobagyi GN. Neoadjuvant chemotherapy for breast carcinoma. Cancer. 2003;98(6):1150–60.
30. Banys-Paluchowski M, Kühn T, Masannat Y, Rubio I, de Boniface J, Ditsch N, Cakmak GK, Karakatsanis A, Dave R, Hahn M, Potter S, Kothari A, Gentilini OD, Gulluoglu BM, Lux MP, Smidt M, Weber WP, Sezen BA, Krawczyk N, Hartmann S, Micco RD, Nietz S, Malherbe F, Cabioglu N, Canturk NZ, Gasparri ML, Murawa D, Harvey J, Banys-Paluchowski M, Kühn T, Masannat Y, Rubio I, de Boniface J, Ditsch N, Karadeniz Cakmak G, Karakatsanis A, Dave R, Hahn M, Potter S, Kothari A, Gentilini OD, Gulluoglu BM, Lux MP, Smidt M, Weber WP, Aktas Sezen B, Krawczyk N, Hartmann S, Di Micco R, Nietz S, Malherbe F, Cabioglu N, Canturk NZ, Gasparri ML, Murawa D, Harvey J. Localization techniques for non-palpable breast lesions: current status, knowledge gaps, and rationale for the MELODY study (EUBREAST-4/iBRA-NET, NCT 05559411). Cancers. 2023;15(4):1173.
31. Gray RJ, Salud C, Nguyen K, Dauway E, Friedland J, Berman C, Peltz E, Whitehead G, Cox CE, Gray RJ, Salud C, Nguyen K, Dauway E, Friedland J, Berman C, Peltz E, Whitehead G, Cox CE. Randomized prospective evaluation of a novel technique for biopsy or lumpectomy of nonpalpable breast lesions: radioactive seed versus wire localization. Ann Surg Oncol. 2013;8(9):711–5.
32. Moreno-Palacios E, Martí C, Frías L, Meléndez M, Loayza A, Roca MJ, Córdoba V, Oliver JM, Hernández A, Sánchez-Méndez JI, Moreno-Palacios E, Martí C, Frías L, Meléndez M, Loayza A, Roca MJ, Córdoba V, Oliver JM, Hernández A, Sánchez-Méndez JI. Breast-conserving surgery guided with magnetic seeds vs. wires: A single-institution experience. Cancer. 2024;16(3):566.
33. Murphy JO, Moo T-A, King TA, Van Zee KJ, Villegas KA, Stempel M, Eaton A, St. Germain JM, Morris E, Morrow M, Murphy JO, Moo T-A, King TA, Van Zee KJ, Villegas KA, Stempel M, Eaton A, St. Germain JM, Morris E, Morrow M. Radioactive seed localization compared to wire localization in breast-conserving surgery: initial 6-month experience. Ann Surg Oncol. 2013;20(13):4121–7.
34. Pantiora E, Jazrawi A, Hersi A-F, Abdsaleh S, Ahlstedt H, Molnar E, Wärnberg F, Eriksson S, Karakatsanis A. Magnetic seed vs guidewire breast cancer localization with magnetic lymph node detection. JAMA Surg. 2024;159(3):239–46.
35. ClinicalTrials.gov. MEthods for LOcalization of Different Types of Breast Lesions (MELODY) 2023. [updated March 3, 2025]. Available from: https://clinicaltrials.gov/study/NCT05559411?titles=MEthods%20for%20LOcalization%20of%20Different%20Types%20of%20Breast%20Lesions%20(MELODY)&rank=1. Accessed 6 May 2025.

36. Silverstein M, Gamagami P, Rosser R, Gierson E, Colburn W, Handel N, Fingerhut A, Lewinsky B, Hoffman R, Waisman J. Hooked-wire-directed breast biopsy and overpenetrated mammography. Cancer. 1987;59(4):715–22.
37. Gluck B, Dershaw D, Liberman L, Deutch B. Microcalcifications on postoperative mammograms as an indicator of adequacy of tumor excision. Radiology. 1993;188(2):469–72.
38. Liberman L, Kaplan J, Van Zee K, Morris E, LaTrenta L, Abramson A, Dershaw D. Bracketing wires for preoperative breast needle localization. AJR Am J Roentgenol. 2001;177(3):565–72.
39. Feliciano Y, Mamtani A, Morrow M, Stempel MM, Patil S, Jochelson MS, Feliciano Y, Mamtani A, Morrow M, Stempel MM, Patil S, Jochelson MS. Do calcifications seen on mammography after neoadjuvant chemotherapy for breast cancer always need to be excised? Ann Surg Oncol. 2017;24(6):1492–8.
40. Moran MS, Schnitt SJ, Giuliano AE, Harris JR, Khan SA, Horton J, Klimberg S, Chavez-MacGregor M, Freedman G, Houssami N, Johnson PL, Morrow M. Society of Surgical Oncology–American Society for Radiation Oncology consensus guideline on margins for breast-conserving surgery with whole-breast irradiation in stages I and II invasive breast cancer. J Clin Oncol. 2014;32(14):1507–15.
41. Choi J, Laws A, Hu J, Barry W, Golshan M, King T. Margins in breast-conserving surgery after neoadjuvant therapy. Ann Surg Oncol. 2018;25(12):3541–7.
42. Mrdutt M, Heerdt A, Sevilimedu V, Mamtani A, Barrio A, Morrow M, Mrdutt M, Heerdt A, Sevilimedu V, Mamtani A, Barrio A, Morrow M. Margin width and local recurrence in patients undergoing breast conservation after neoadjuvant chemotherapy. Ann Surg Oncol. 2021;29(1):484–92.

Chapter 6
Breast Wire Localisation

Aishwarya Gadwal and Niketa Chotai

Contents

6.1 Introduction

The detection and surgical management of non-palpable breast and axillary lesions have significantly evolved due to widespread adoption of breast cancer screening and rapid advancements in imaging technologies [1, 2]. As a result, the number of such lesions undergoing surgical excision continues to rise. Accurate localisation is essential for complete lesion removal while preserving adjacent healthy tissue—critical not only for oncological control but also for optimal cosmetic outcomes.

Historically, breast lesion excision relied on palpation or rudimentary imaging, often resulting in large tissue resections and suboptimal cosmetic results. The advent of image-guided localisation marked a major shift in surgical planning, enabling more precise targeting and conservative resections. Wire-guided localisation

A. Gadwal
Department of Medical Imaging, University of Toronto, Toronto, Ontario, Canada

N. Chotai (✉)
RadLink Women Imaging Center, Singapore, Singapore

R. Vidya, N. Sharma (eds.), *Breast and Axilla Localisation Techniques*,
https://doi.org/10.1007/978-3-032-17995-1_6

(WGL), introduced in the mid-twentieth century, remains a widely practiced technique and serves as the reference standard, despite increasing interest in wire-free alternatives.

6.2 Historical Background and Evolution

6.2.1 *Early Approaches*

Prior to the availability of modern imaging, surgical excision of breast lesions was based on clinical palpation. This method lacked precision, often resulting in larger resections with negative aesthetic and psychological impact on patients [2].

6.2.2 *Wire-Guided Localisation (WGL)*

WGL was first introduced in 1965 by Dodd et al. as a method to accurately target non-palpable breast lesions under imaging guidance. In this technique, a localisation wire is deployed into the lesion, typically under ultrasound or mammographic guidance. The distal hook anchors the wire within or adjacent to the lesion, serving as a surgical guide. Over the decades, WGL became the gold standard in preoperative localisation for breast-conserving surgery [3].

Despite its efficacy, WGL has known limitations—including risk of wire migration, patient discomfort, and intraoperative challenges—that have spurred the development of alternative localisation technologies [4].

6.3 Procedure

This section outlines a stepwise approach to planning and executing image-guided wire localisation, followed by intraoperative specimen evaluation.

(a) Pre-procedural Planning

Effective pre-procedural planning is essential for successful wire-guided localisation. This process begins with the following:

1. *Review of Prior Imaging*:
    - Assess all available imaging modalities (mammography, ultrasound, and MRI) to determine lesion characteristics such as size, location, morphology, and visibility.

- Identify the most suitable imaging modality for guiding the procedure. The chosen method should allow precise visualisation and access to the lesion while ensuring patient comfort and minimising complications.

2. *Modality Selection*:

- *Ultrasound Guidance*: Most commonly used due to real-time imaging, lack of ionising radiation, better patient tolerance, and cost-effectiveness.
- *Mammographic Guidance*: Essential for localising microcalcifications, architectural distortion, or post-chemotherapy clips not visible on ultrasound.
- *MRI Guidance*: Reserved for lesions visualised exclusively on MRI (the so-called 'MRI-only' lesions).
- *Contrast-Enhanced Mammography* (*CEM*): An emerging modality, useful when lesions are visible only with contrast.

3. *Surgical Coordination*:

- Communicate with the surgical team to understand the planned surgical approach, margin expectations, and timing.
- Consider pathology reports, treatment history (e.g. neoadjuvant therapy), and patient comorbidities to determine if clip localisation, bracketing, or wire-free alternatives may be considered.

(b) Wire Localisation Technique

Wire-guided localisation is typically performed under *local anaesthesia* and with *aseptic precautions*. The procedure varies slightly depending on the guiding modality:

(i) *Ultrasound-Guided Wire Localisation*

- A *needle-wire system* (e.g. Kopans, Hawkins, or Ghiatas wire) is inserted under direct real-time ultrasound guidance.
- The needle is passed through the lesion, and the tip is placed 1 cm beyond the distal margin [5].
- After confirming correct positioning, the wire is deployed by withdrawing the needle while stabilising the wire in situ (Fig. 6.1).
- The final position of the wire hook, the lesion, and its distance from the skin entry site along the wire track are documented.
- Surgeons may prefer:
  - *Central wire passage* through the lesion, or
  - *Anterior placement*, especially if posterior margins will be taken deep up to the chest wall.
- Always align with the surgeon's preference and document the approach clearly.

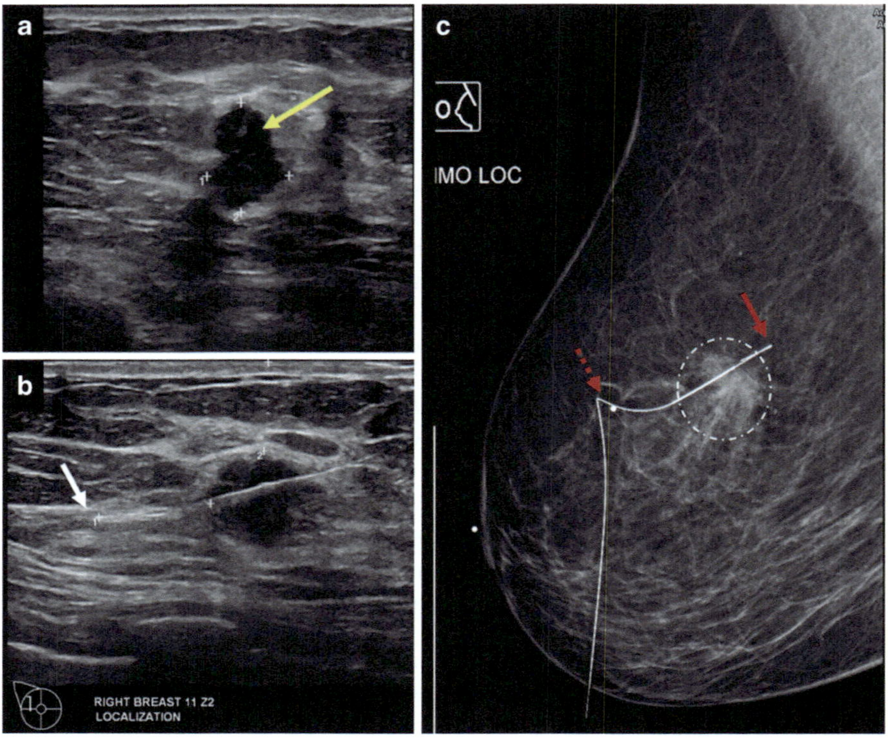

Fig. 6.1 (**a**) Ultrasound image shows a 1.4 cm, biopsy-proven, screen-detected grade 1 invasive ductal carcinoma (yellow arrow) in a 65-year-old woman. (**b**) As the tumour was non-palpable, preoperative localisation was performed using a hook wire. The wire traverses the tumour, with its tip (white arrow) positioned approximately 1 cm beyond the tumour margin. (**c**) Post-localisation mammogram confirms the wire placement, with the targeted tumour located at the thickened portion of the wire (white circle) and the wire tip just beyond the tumour (red arrow). The skin entry site (red dashed arrow) indicates the tumour lies approximately 2.5 cm along the wire path from the skin surface

(ii) *Mammography-Guided Wire Localisation*

- Used for lesions not seen on ultrasound, especially *microcalcifications*, *architectural distortions*, or *post-neoadjuvant therapy clips*.
- The breast is compressed in *stereotactic*, *tomosynthesis*, or *grid-guided* positioning.
- After appropriate *local anaesthesia*, the needle is advanced to the target lesion and *over-inserted by 10 mm* to ensure accurate wire deployment.
- The wire is deployed such that the lesion lies near the *first thick segment* of the wire or at distal thick portion of the wire (Fig. 6.2).
- The external wire is gently secured to prevent migration.
- *Orthogonal mammograms* are obtained post-deployment to:

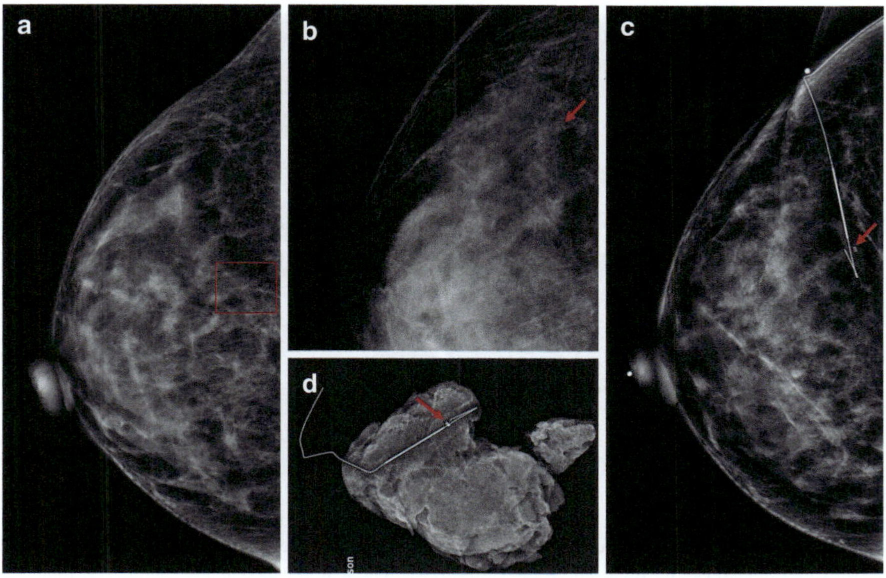

Fig. 6.2 (**a**) A small group of screen-detected amorphous microcalcifications is seen in the outer half of the right breast (red square). (**b**) Magnified view highlights the grouped microcalcifications (red arrow), which were considered indeterminate and biopsied under stereotactic guidance (not shown), yielding a diagnosis of atypical ductal hyperplasia (ADH). (**c**) Mammographic localisation of the marker clip was performed; the clip is visualised at the junction of the hook and the thick portion of the localisation wire (red arrow). (**d**) Specimen radiograph shows the entire wire and the targeted clip (red arrow) clearly within the excised tissue. Final histology revealed no evidence of malignancy

- Confirm correct wire placement relative to the lesion.
- Measure the *skin-to-lesion distance* along the wire path.

In cases where lesion size exceeds *2–2.5 cm*, *bracketing* with multiple wires may be required to mark both ends of the lesion, helping achieve *clear surgical margins*.

(iii) *MRI-Guided Wire Localisation*

- Indicated for lesions visualised exclusively on MRI.
- Requires use of *MRI-compatible wire systems*.
- Performed under standard breast MRI positioning using dedicated breast coils.
- After targeting the lesion, the wire is deployed under imaging guidance.
- A *final confirmatory MRI sequence* with minimal compression is performed to confirm wire location (Fig. 6.3).
- MRI localisation is technically demanding and generally performed in high-volume centres with experienced staff.

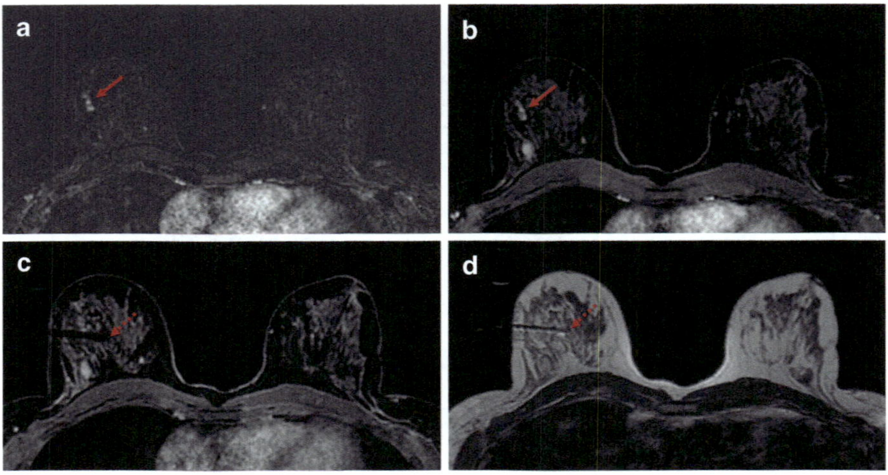

Fig. 6.3 (**a**, **b**) Subtracted and non-subtracted post-contrast MRI images from staging evaluation in a patient with known left breast invasive carcinoma show a linear non-mass enhancement (red arrows) in the lower outer quadrant of the right breast. The lesion was considered indeterminate. A non-enhancing T1 hyperintense lesion posterior to it represents a complicated cyst. (**c**) MRI-guided hook wire localisation and excision biopsy were performed. The needle tip (red arrow) was positioned approximately 1 cm beyond the lesion. (**d**) Following confirmation of appropriate placement, the wire was deployed. A non-fat-saturated T1-weighted MRI confirms the wire tip in a satisfactory position. The target lesion is expected to lie at the level of the second thickened segment of the hook wire. The final histology was reported as intermediate grade DCIS (Ductal carcinoma in situ) with clear margins

(iv) *CEM-Guided Wire Localisation*

- Indicated for lesions visualised exclusively on CEM or MRI.
- Requires use of iodinated intravenous contrast for contrast-enhanced mammogram.
- Performed under standard breast mammographic or stereotactic positioning.
- After confirming the visibility of contrast-enhanced lesion, the wire is deployed under imaging guidance.
- CEM localisation is technically demanding and time-sensitive as contrast would wash out within about 10–12 min and the procedure needs to be completed well within this time.

(v) *Additional Considerations*

- *Clip migration*: If a biopsy clip has migrated, ensure that the original lesion site is targeted—not the migrated clip—to avoid sampling errors.
- *Skin entry point*: Select an entry site that allows a *direct*, *shortest*, *and safe path* to the lesion while *avoiding any other suspicious areas.*
- *Wire choice*: Selection depends on depth, guidance modality, and institutional preference. Common wire types include the following:

  - *Kopans wire.*
  - *Hawkins wire.*
  - *Ghiatas beaded wire.*
  - *Homer wire.*
  - Some wires are repositionable.

(c) Post-Procedural Handling and Surgical Transfer

- The external wire should be *secured to the skin* using adhesive dressings or steri-strips to minimise risk of displacement.
- Patients are advised to avoid *sudden movement* or *arm abduction* on the side of the wire.
- *Prompt transfer* to the operating theatre is crucial, especially since the localisation is often performed on the *same day as surgery*.

(d) Intraoperative Specimen Evaluation

- Once the lesion is excised, the specimen should be imaged using *mammography* or *ultrasound* to:
  - Confirm *presence of the target lesion or marker*.
  - Confirm presence of entire wire in the specimen to rule out fragmentation.
  - Evaluate the *proximity to surgical margins*.
- Typically, *two orthogonal views* of the specimen are obtained for comprehensive margin assessment.
- The radiologist evaluates and documents the findings, advising the surgeon if *further excision* is necessary.
- This step significantly reduces the need for *repeat surgery* due to positive or close margins [3, 6].

6.4 Advantages and Limitations of Wire-Guided Localisation

6.4.1 Advantages

- A well-established and cost-effective technique with consistently high success rates.
- Highly versatile, as it can be performed under various imaging modalities including ultrasound, mammography, MRI, CT, and contrast-enhanced mammography (CEM).
- Widely adopted by radiologists and surgeons, facilitating smooth integration into routine clinical workflows.
- Certain wire systems offer the advantage of being repositionable, allowing for procedural flexibility and improved targeting.

6.4.2 *Limitations*

- Potential risks include wire displacement, fragmentation, or migration.
- Requires meticulous coordination between radiology and the operating room, as localisation must be scheduled precisely on the day of surgery.
- The presence of an external wire can contribute to patient anxiety and physical discomfort.
- The fixed wire trajectory may limit surgical flexibility and could compromise cosmetic outcomes in some cases.

6.5 Future Directions

To address the limitations of wire-guided localisation (WGL), several wire-free alternatives have been developed, including radar reflectors, radioactive seeds, and magnetic seed localisation systems. These innovations aim to enhance patient comfort, offer greater scheduling flexibility, and maintain oncologic efficacy comparable to traditional wire localisation.

Emerging trends in localisation include the following:

- *Hybrid approaches* that combine wire and wire-free technologies for managing complex or multifocal lesions.
- *Biodegradable localisation markers* that eliminate the need for retrieval and reduce long-term foreign body presence.
- *Artificial intelligence (AI)* applications for automated lesion detection, procedural planning, and workflow optimisation.

These advancements are poised to support more personalised, precise, and patient-centred surgical care.

6.6 Conclusion

Wire-guided localisation remains a foundational technique in the surgical management of non-palpable breast lesions. While newer technologies continue to evolve, WGL offers the enduring advantages of high accuracy, cost-effectiveness, and widespread clinical familiarity. As breast-conserving surgery advances, the integration of innovative localisation methods, advanced imaging, and multidisciplinary collaboration will shape the next era of precision breast surgery. Until then, WGL remains a reliable, accessible, and evidence-based solution in daily practice.

References

1. Banys-Paluchowski M, Kühn T, Masannat Y, Rubio I, De Boniface J, Ditsch N, et al. Localization techniques for non-palpable breast lesions: current status, knowledge gaps, and rationale for the MELODY study (EUBREAST-4/iBRA-NET, NCT 05559411). Cancer. 2023;15(4):1173. Available from: https://www.mdpi.com/2072-6694/15/4/1173.
2. Cheung BHH, Co M, Lui TTN, Kwong A. Evolution of localization methods for non-palpable breast lesions: a literature review from a translational medicine perspective. Transl Breast Cancer Res. 2024;5:12. Available from: https://tbcr.amegroups.com/article/view/85225/html.
3. Kalambo M, Dogan BE, Whitman GJ. Step by step: planning a needle localization procedure. Clin Imaging. 2020;60(1):100–8. Available from: https://linkinghub.elsevier.com/retrieve/pii/S0899707119302633.
4. Shirazi S, Hajiesmaeili H, Khosla M, Taj S, Sircar T, Vidya R. Comparison of wire and non-wire localisation techniques in breast cancer surgery: a review of the literature with pooled analysis. Medicina (Mex). 2023;59(7):1297. Available from: https://www.mdpi.com/1648-9144/59/7/1297.
5. Khare S, Singh T, Santosh I, Laroiya I, Singh G. Wire- and ultrasound-guided localization: a novel technique for excision of nonpalpable breast tumors. Breast Cancer Basic Clin Res. 2020;14:1178223420938068. Available from: https://journals.sagepub.com/doi/10.1177/1178223420938068.
6. Cheang E, Ha R, Thornton CM, Mango VL. Innovations in image-guided preoperative breast lesion localization. Br J Radiol. 2018;91(1085):20170740. Available from: https://academic.oup.com/bjr/article/doi/10.1259/bjr.20170740/7449417.

Chapter 7
Localisation Using Scout

Raghavan Vidya, Saima Taj, and Sheetal Sharma

Contents

R. Vidya · S. Taj
Department of Breast Surgery, The Royal Wolverhampton NHS Trust, Wolverhampton, UK
e-mail: Raghavan.Vidya@nhs.net; S.Taj1@nhs.net

S. Sharma (✉)
Department of Breast Radiology, NHS University Hospitals of Liverpool Group, Liverpool, UK
e-mail: Sheetal.Sharma@liverpoolft.nhs.uk

R. Vidya, N. Sharma (eds.), *Breast and Axilla Localisation Techniques*,
https://doi.org/10.1007/978-3-032-17995-1_7

7.1 Introduction

7.1.1 Background

Breast cancer is the commonest malignancy in the UK with 55,500 new cases diagnosed annually, and surgery remains an important component of treatment. Breast screening and advances in imaging modalities have led to an increase in identification of non-palpable breast lesions that need preoperative localisation prior to surgery [1].

Historically, excision of impalpable breast lesions was usually directed by preoperative wire placement into, or adjacent to, the target lesion [2]. Wire localisation has several disadvantages; most notably, displacement of the wire and difficulty in the surgeon accurately discerning the position of the tip of the wire intraoperatively [3]. The entry point of the wire may be some distance from the wire tip, which can make it difficult to place the surgical incision optimally; this can lead to a larger area of dissection than is necessary to remove the target lesion. Additionally, wire placement occurs on the day of surgery, which removes flexibility for scheduling in both radiology and surgery and can lead to delays in the operating theatre. While wire-guided localisation was the gold standard for more than a decade, it is now being replaced by new wire-free techniques which offer a greater degree of both accuracy and flexibility [4, 5].

Introduction of a new non-wire system can be challenging as it requires investment and staff training. Additionally, in the initial stages, scheduling and coordination of care are needed to allow extra time for reflector localisation.

The Scout® surgical guidance system offers a non-radioactive, FDA-approved alternative for the localisation and excision of nonpalpable breast lesions. Utilising electromagnetic wave technology, the system enables real-time intraoperative guidance for both breast and axillary procedures [6–8]. Unlike traditional wire localisation methods, Scout® employs a small, implantable reflector that is inserted into the target tissue prior to the day of surgery. The Scout® system detects the reflector using a unique radar signal, allowing for precise and efficient lesion localisation.

7.2 Indications for Scout® Localisation

Scout® is indicated for patients undergoing breast-conserving surgery (BCS) where the target lesion is non-palpable. It may also be used for axillary lymph node localisation (Table 7.1).

An alternative localisation method should be planned in case of technical failure, and early implementation should focus on lesions ≤6 cm deep to ensure familiarity with the system.

Table 7.1 Indications and contraindications for Scout®

Category	Details
Breast lesions	Non-palpable invasive carcinoma or DCIS
	Lesions pre- and post-neoadjuvant therapy
Lymph node localisation	Biopsy-proven malignant axillary lymph node to guide axillary surgery
Bracketing use	Large lesions or multifocal disease requiring multiple reflectors
Contraindications	Nickel/titanium allergy, lesions >6 cm deep, obscured targets

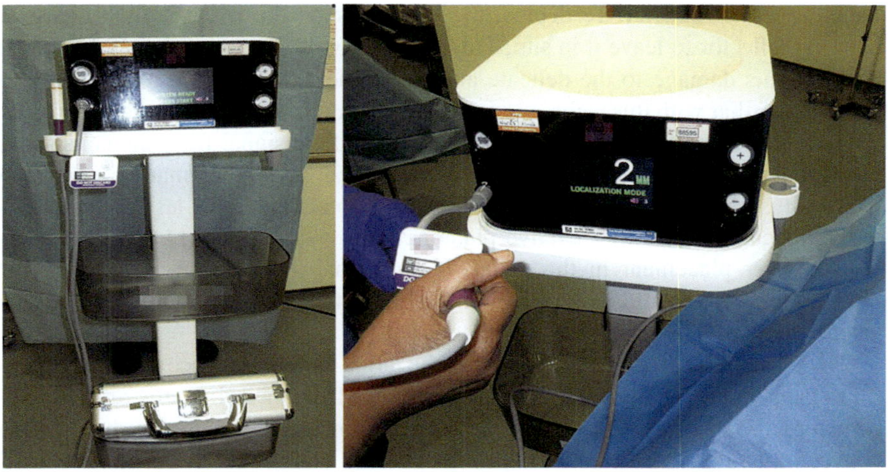

Fig. 7.1 The Scout® system including the console, hand piece, and reflector

7.3 Principles of Scout Localisation

A Scout® reflector is placed within the breast tissue under either mammographic or sonographic guidance. The reflector comprises an infrared (IR) light receptor, a resistor, and two antennae. Detection of the reflector is performed transcutaneously, using a handpiece that emits both IR light and electromagnetic waves [4] (see Fig. 7.1). The system transmission is mediated by the IR receptor, which facilitates an electrical connection between the antennae, mediated by the resistor, and this enables the handpiece to detect the reflector via reflected electromagnetic signals. Additionally, an integrated electrostatic discharge (ESD) component protects and safeguards the reflector from damage during surgery in the event of electrocautery transmission from instruments. The antennae are made from nitinol, a durable shape-memory alloy known for its strength, flexibility, and resistance to fracture. It is similar to materials used in coronary stents and cardiac valves.

7.4 Technique: Insertion

This system uses a radar reflector activated with infrared light. The reflector is passive until activated from the console by a hand piece. The Scout® reflects the radar signal, which is then detected by the hand piece and console (Cox CE).

The reflector is 12 mm in length, with a 4 mm body and two antennae, each 4 mm in length. The reflector can be inserted with either ultrasound or mammographic guidance through a preloaded 16-gauge introducer needle (see Fig. 7.2). The tip of the needle should be positioned approximately 1 mm distal to the intended location of the reflector. To deploy, the introducer needle is carefully withdrawn over the reflector to leave it in situ. This contrasts with, for example, marker clips, and prevents damage to the delicate antennae. There is a short learning curve to become familiar with this technique (see Fig. 7.3). Following Scout® placement, the reflector can be activated and detected with an audible signal from the console. If the Scout® has been placed in the breast the patient undergoes mammography to document and check the reflector position in relation to the target lesion. The mammograms can assist with operative planning. Mammography is not typically performed after placement in the axilla. If more than one Scout® is required for bracketing, there should be a minimum of 15–20 mm between the two devices to ensure that they can be detected separately.

The distance between the reflector and the target and the distance from the reflector to the skin are measured. The shortest distance from the skin to the reflector can be recorded. For cases with more than one reflector in the same breast, the distance between the reflectors on both images is measured and the greater distance should

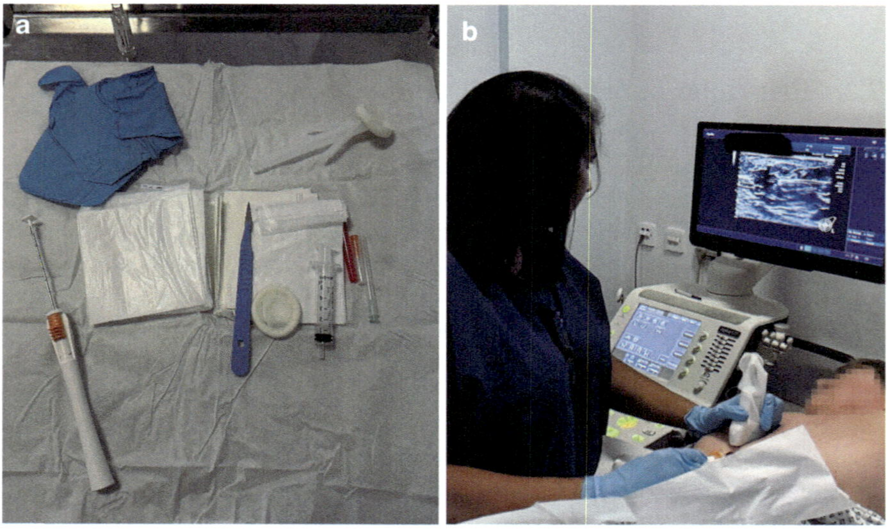

Fig. 7.2 (**a**) The trolley set up for Scout® insertion. (**b**) Performing ultrasound-guided Scout® insertion

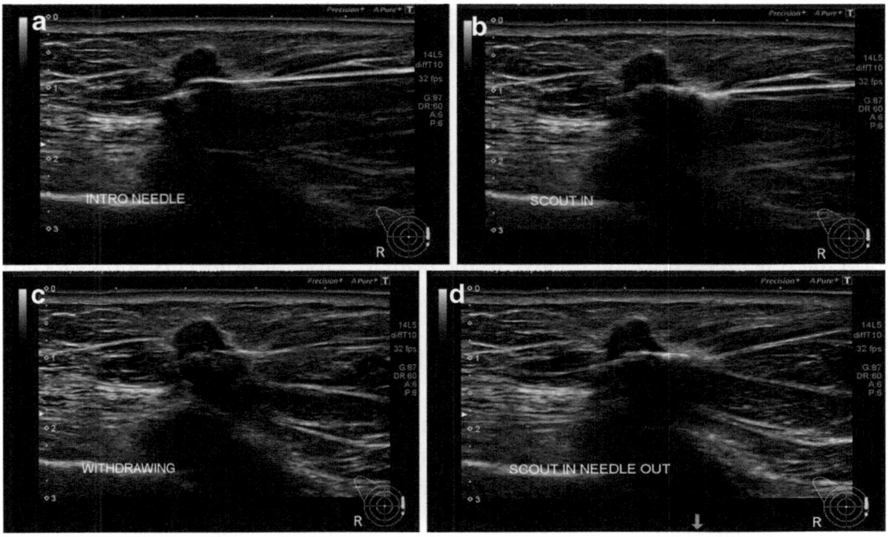

Fig. 7.3 Scout® insertion (**a**) needle visible within lesion during ultrasound-guided localisation (**b**) Scout® within lesion. (**c**) Withdrawing needle over the Scout® (**d**) Scout® within lesion and needle being withdrawn from patient

Table 7.2 Summary of technical execution of Scout® insertion and precautions to be taken

Step	Action
1. Planning	Confirm imaging visibility Determine number and position of reflectors
2. Placement	Use ultrasound or stereotactic guidance Insert 16G needle ~1 mm past target
	Deploy reflector by withdrawing needle over it (do not push)
	For bracketing: keep ≥15–20 mm between reflectors
3. Confirmation	Detect reflector with console and handpiece (optional) Confirm with mammography
	Record device identifiers, reflector depth, and position
4. Documentation	Record LOT number, placement success, signal quality Include in patient's report
5. Surgery	Check for signal in theatre before anaesthesia Intraoperative—use sterile handpiece to locate reflector Follow signal to guide dissection
	Confirm retrieval of reflector in specimen

be recorded. Immediately after placement, the reflector can be activated and detected while the patient is still in the breast imaging department to verify detection from the skin surface.

All device identifiers, including the LOT number, should be documented in the radiology report (Table 7.2). The reflector is approved by the US Food and Drug Administration (FDA) for placement more than 30 days prior to surgery both between reflector placement and removal, which allows for maximum scheduling flexibility for the radiologists and surgeons resulting in an improved patient pathway.

7.5 Mammographic Evaluation

Mammographic imaging is performed post-reflector insertion, to identify and confirm the reflector's position relative to the primary target lesion. This allows localisation when bracketing lesions with multiple reflectors or when placing reflectors in anatomically challenging or deep locations. The radiological images help to document accurate placement, guide surgical planning, and serve as a reference for intra-operative navigation (Fig. 7.4).

If reflectors are placed in the axilla, mammograms are generally not performed. Distance measurements from skin to reflector and between reflectors (if applicable) are recorded and included in the radiology report to assist the surgical team.

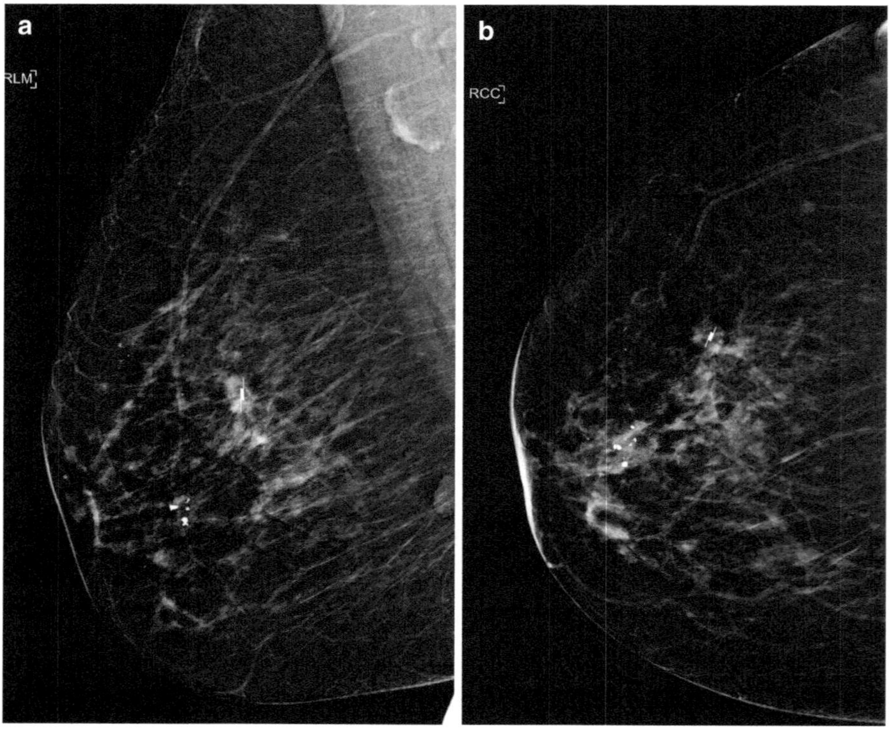

Fig. 7.4 (**a**) Right lateral and (**b**) CC views following Scout® localisation of cancer

7.6 Technique: Excision

In the theatre, prior to anaesthesia, the surgeon checks the precise site of the Scout® reflector and marks the site (Fig. 7.4). This ensures the signal and position of reflector is checked prior to surgery. Incision is planned depending on the tumour location. Dissection is performed using diathermy and care is taken not to apply diathermy close to the reflector. During surgery, the Scout® system is activated with a sterile handheld probe that emits infrared light and electromagnetic signals. These signals interact with the reflector, which then emits a return signal detected by the probe. The console provides both audible tones and a digital readout in millimetres, guiding the surgeon in real time towards the target. The console reader provides the distance in millimetres indicating the distance between the reflector and probe and emits more audible sound as the distance decreases (Fig. 7.5). This live navigation allows for accurate excision with minimal disruption to surrounding tissue, ultimately allowing the surgeon to remove the abnormal tissue accurately (Fig. 7.6a). The surgeon can also place a single suture close to the reflector to aid in the dissection (Fig. 7.6b). The wide local excision is performed with the aim of removing a minimum 1 mm margin of normal tissue around the tumour (Fig. 7.7a).

The specimen is orientated, marked with sutures or clips as per local protocol. Intraoperative specimen X-ray is carried out to confirm removal of lesion with adequate margins (Fig. 7.7b). Local anaesthesia is given, and a layered closure is performed.

The specimen is sent to Histopathology for evaluation, including surgical pathology and margin status. Clear margin includes tumour ≤1–2 mm from ink, for invasive and in situ pathology and positive margin is defined as tumour on ink.

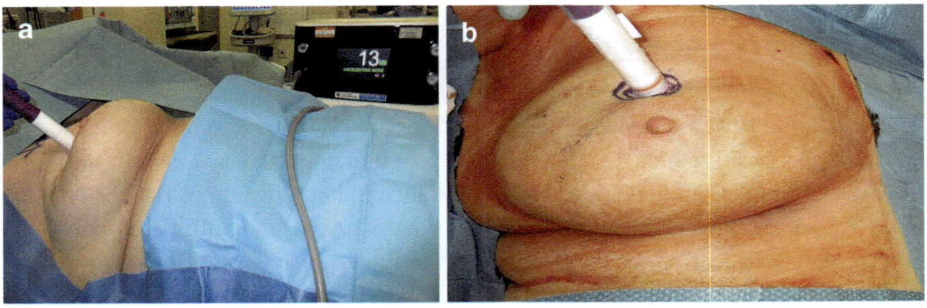

Fig. 7.5 (**a**, **b**) Scout® localisation in theatre

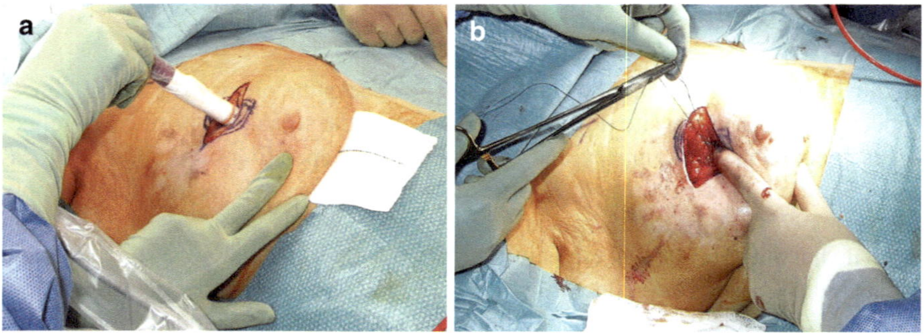

Fig. 7.6 (**a**) Intraoperative Scout® localisation. (**b**) Localisation of the reflector guided by application of suture Scout® to guide dissection

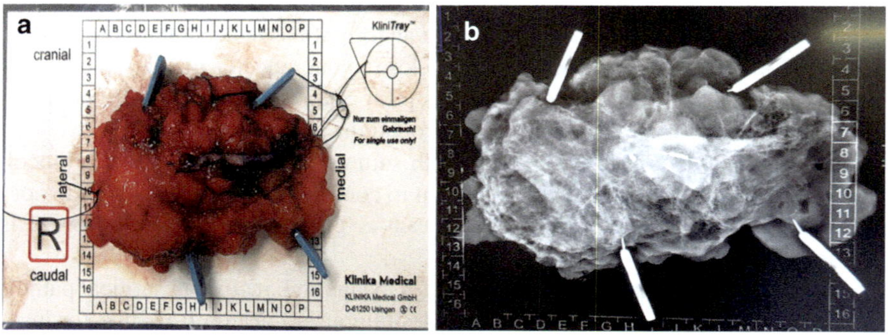

Fig. 7.7 (**a**) Surgical specimen of wide local excision. (**b**) X-ray showing Scout® and clip in centre with good margins

7.7 Axillary Localisation

The combination of marked lymph node and sentinel lymph node biopsy for biopsy-proven node-positive breast cancer is known as targeted axillary dissection (TAD). Scout® can be inserted under ultrasound guidance to mark the abnormal lymph node (Fig. 7.8). This can be carried out prior to neoadjuvant chemotherapy, known as single stage localisation, or at a later stage of a previously marked node known as secondary localisation. Scout® reflectors have FDA approval for soft tissue implantation for an unlimited preoperative period. A Scout® reflector can be inserted at the time of biopsy under ultrasound guidance to mark the lymph node.

The position and signal of Scout® is checked under ultrasound guidance and using the handheld console unit.

At surgery, the reflector is identified using the detection probe. The continuous feedback provides the exact depth and location of the lesion and the continuous audio signal guides the surgical excision. The specimen is X-rayed intraoperatively to confirm the removal of the marked lymph node (Fig. 7.9).

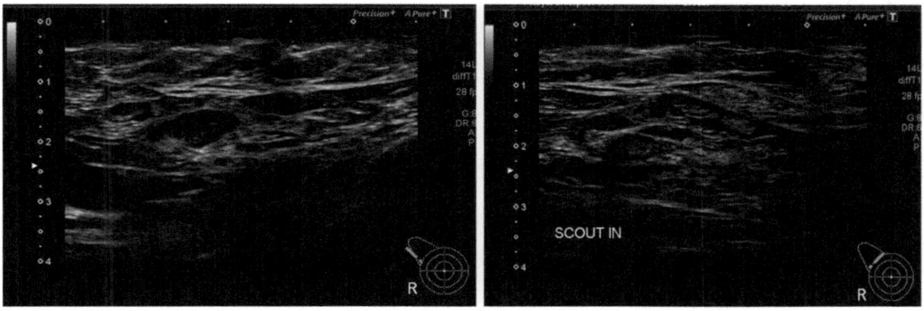

Fig. 7.8 Scout® localisation in lymph node

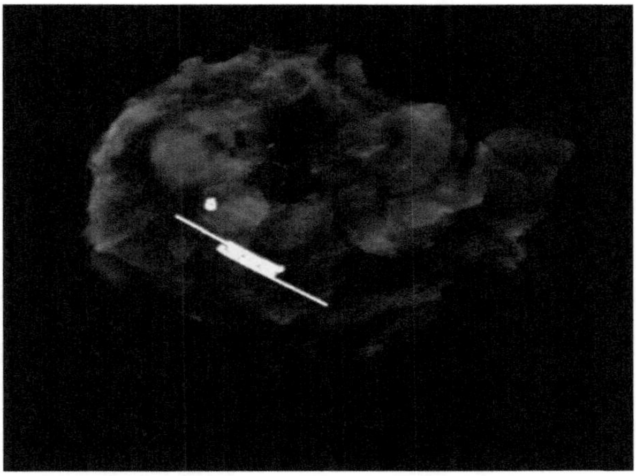

Fig. 7.9 X-ray showing excised lymph node with Scout® and clip

7.8 Advantages and Limitations

The Scout® system demonstrates an accurate detection capacity of up to 6 cm in depth. Notable limitations include the inability to reposition the reflector post-deployment, the absence of a delivery system that is compatible with MRI, contra-indication in patients with nickel allergies, and the risk of intraoperative detection failure attributable to the presence of haematoma [5, 8]. It is acknowledged that electrocautery can inactivate the reflector if it is brought into close proximity. Instances of reflector deactivation through electrocautery via short-circuiting have been documented. Nevertheless, this phenomenon is unlikely to impede surgical excision as, under such circumstances, the marker is likely to become visible to the operating surgeon. A summary of advantages and limitations is seen in Table 7.3.

Table 7.3 Advantages and limitations of Scout®

Advantages	Limitations
No external component	Cost
No radioactive component	Difficulty with detection if placed >6 cm deep from the skin surface
Reduced chance of displacement	Difficulty with detection in the presence of a haematoma
Live localisation during surgery	Potential difficulty with detection if deep to dense breast parenchyma
Good patient/clinician acceptance	Signal detection may be absent:
Minimal MRI artifact compared with other non-wire alternatives (see Fig. 7.10)	If the reflector is contacted directly with the intraoperative electrocautery device
Licensed for use in the axilla	If the reflector is exposed to older halogen operating room lights
No time limit once inserted (can be placed at the time of biopsy)	

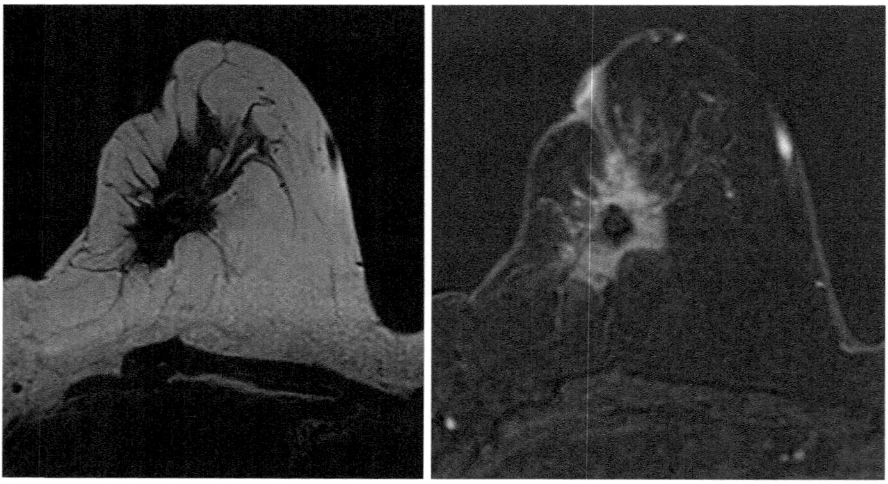

Fig. 7.10 MRI breast with signal dropout from Scout®

7.9 Literature Review

The Scout® surgical guidance system has become a reliable, non-radioactive alternative to traditional wire-guided and radioactive seed localisation methods for non-palpable breast lesions [9]. By employing a radar-reflective implant combined with electromagnetic wave detection, Scout® provides real-time intraoperative localisation that enhances surgical accuracy, workflow efficiency, and patient comfort. The initial clinical evaluation was performed by Cox et al. in 2016 in a prospective feasibility study involving 15 patients with non-palpable breast lesions. The results were very encouraging with a 100% success rate in reflector placement, lesion retrieval, decoupling of radiology and surgery and improved patient experience compared to wire localisation [10]. Subsequent prospective multicentre study by Mango et al. involving 154 patients confirmed 100% success rates for reflector placement, localisation, and lesion excision. The study also reported no device-related complications further validating the system's safety and efficacy in a wider clinical context [11].

The first systematic review of 842 Scout® cases, reported a 99.6% deployment success rate with a significant lower re-excision rate of 12.9% compared to traditional wire localisation of 21.1% ($p < 0.01$), thereby demonstrating improved outcomes with greater surgical precision [12]. A recent study by Sharma et al. (senior author), using Scout localisation system in both breast and axilla, reported high success rates with no device-related adverse events ascertaining the safety and reliability across varied surgical settings [13]. A more recent large-scale pooled analysis by Morrow et al. reported a similar 99.6% success rate with low re-excision rate, thereby supporting its adoption as a standard localisation technique [14].

The feasibility and effectiveness of radar reflector localisation (Scout®) to guide excision of axillary lymph nodes in patients with node-positive breast cancer has been well demonstrated [15, 16]. Scout® application has also been extended to axillary surgery, particularly in targeted axillary dissection (TAD) following neoadjuvant chemotherapy. A systematic review by West et al., analysing 252 TAD procedures, observed a 99.6% success rate in lymph node localisation and a 100% retrieval rate, demonstrating high concordance between marked and sentinel lymph nodes with no significant device migration or complications [17]. Weiss et al. observed in a sample of 172 patients that there was a 100% reflector localisation rate with high surgeon satisfaction emphasizing Scout® clinical reliability and ease of use [18]. Subsequent report by the RADIOSO Milan Trial confirmed high tumour-free margins (95.5%) with no re-excision portraying the clinical benefits of this wireless technology [19].

Targeted axillary dissection in breast cancer patients using Scout radar reflector localisation after neoadjuvant systemic therapy observed 92% clinical axillary downstaging, 44% pathological complete response, and a complete 100% reflector retrieval in all patients [20]. A recent systematic review demonstrated the Scout® radar reflectors are reliable and accurate in localisation of lymph nodes in targeted axillary dissection [21]. The review demonstrated a 99.6% successful localisation rate, (95% confidence [CI]: 98.9–100), 100% retrieval rate, and 81% (95% CI: 76–86) concordance rate between sentinel node biopsy and marked lymph node biopsy. Interestingly no major complications or reflector migrations was observed in the study. We need to add the R in a circle after the word Scout in a few places where it is absent.

In summary, novel Scout radar localisation system has significant benefits in comparison to wire localisation with high lesion detection rate and favourable advantages in the combined radiological-surgical pathway. Its combination of technical precision, safety, logistical flexibility, and positive impact on patient and surgeon experience supports its increasing adoption in breast and axillary cancer surgery.

7.10 Tips to Help with Scout® Usage

- In the initial stages of introducing Scout® localisation to a unit we would recommend starting with lesions less than 6 cm in depth to build experience.
- There is a learning curve with image-guided insertion. The tip of the introducer needle should be approximately 1 mm distal to the intended position of the distal end of the reflector. The introducer needle is withdrawn over the reflector to leave it in place; this is a different skill to 'pushing out' a device into the breast tissue.
- Record the device LOT number in the radiology report for the procedure. In the case of any problems with the device, this assists the manufacturer in investigating the issue.
- Check the console is correctly plugged in, turned on, and in the 'ready' state.
- The probe should be covered with a sterile probe cover (not a sterile glove as this reduces sensitivity of signal detection).
- Check in anaesthetic room prior to anaesthetic induction that Scout® can be located and if bracketing that both devices can be differentiated.
- Be aware of the risk of signal loss after an electrocautery device comes into close contact with the reflector. However, in practice, this means the surgeon has reached the lesion and may be able to visualise the reflector at this stage allowing accurate removal.
- There is a risk of antenna transection during surgical dissection, so caution is advised.
- Have a plan in place for an alternative method of localisation in case of Scout® failure.

7.11 Summary

- Scout® can be placed in advance of operation date with no time limit between insertion and removal.
- Scout® is licensed for use in axillary nodes.
- Patients should receive an information leaflet about Scout® prior to insertion.
- Prospective outcomes of Scout® localisation should be audited.
- Exclusion criteria for using Scout® are patients who are allergic to Nickel and/or Titanium.
- Caution when using Scout® for bracketing lesions that are close together.
- Wire localisation can continue to be available when clinicians feel that this would be preferable for an individual patient or in case of Scout® failure.

References

1. Cheang E, Ha R, Thornton CM, Mango VL. Innovations in image-guided preoperative breast lesion localisation. Br J Radiol. 2018;91(1085):1–2.
2. Hall FM, Kopans DB, Sadowsky NL, Homer MJ. Development of wire localisation for occult breast lesions: Boston remembrances. Radiology. 2013;268(3):622–7.
3. Kapoor MM, Patel MM, Scoggins ME. The wire and beyond: recent advances in breast imaging preoperative needle localisation. Radiographics. 2019;39(7):1886–906.
4. Mango V, Ha R, Gomberawalla A, Wynn R, Feldman S. Evaluation of the SCOUT surgical guidance system for localisation and excision of nonpalpable breast lesions: a feasibility study. AJR Am J Roentgenol. 2016;207(4):W69–72.
5. Mango VL, Wynn RT, Feldman S, Friedlander L, Desperito E, Patel SN, Gomberawalla A, Ha R. Beyond wires and seeds: reflector-guided breast lesion localisation and excision. Radiology. 2017;284(2):365–71.
6. Falcon S, Weinfurtner RJ, Mooney B, Niell BL. SAVI SCOUT® localisation of breast lesions as a practical alternative to wires: outcomes and suggestions for trouble-shooting. Clin Imaging. 2018;52:280–6.
7. Cornella KN, Palafox BA, Razavi MK, Loh CT, Markle KM, Openshaw LE. SCOUT as a novel localisation and surgical navigation system for more accurate localisation and resection of pulmonary nodules. Surg Innov. 2019;26(4):469–72.
8. Cox CE, Garcia-Henriquez N, Glancy MJ, Whitworth P, Cox JM, Themar-Geck M, Prati R, Jung M, Russell S, Appleton K, King J, Shivers SC. Pilot study of a new nonradioactive surgical guidance technology for locating nonpalpable breast lesions. Ann Surg Oncol. 2016;23(6):1824–30.
9. Shirazi S, Hajiesmaeili H, Khosla M, Taj S, Sircar T, Vidya R. Comparison of wire and non-wire localisation techniques in breast cancer surgery: a review of the literature with pooled analysis. Medicina (Kaunas). 2023;59(7):1297. https://doi.org/10.3390/medicina59071297. PMID: 37512107; PMCID: PMC10383802.
10. Cox CE, Garcia-Henriquez N, Glancy MJ, Whitworth PW. A prospective feasibility study of the SAVI SCOUT® surgical guidance system for localisation of nonpalpable breast lesions. AJR Am J Roentgenol. 2016;207(2):W69–75. https://doi.org/10.2214/AJR.15.15962.
11. Mango VL, Wynn RT, Feldman S, Friedlander L, Falzon L, Zhang Z, et al. Beyond wires and seeds: reflector-guided breast lesion localisation and excision in a multicenter trial. Breast J. 2016;22(2):151–6. https://doi.org/10.1111/tbj.12565.
12. Kasem I, Mokbel K. Savi SCOUT® radar localisation of non-palpable breast lesions: systematic review and pooled analysis of 842 cases. Breast Cancer. 2020;27(4):1–9. https://doi.org/10.3390/cancers16071345.
13. Sharma S, Siddiqui S, Henderson J, et al. Clinical experience with SAVI SCOUT® radar reflector localisation: safety and efficacy in breast and axillary procedures. Breast Cancer Res Treat. 2021;188(3):601–7. https://doi.org/10.1007/s10549-021-06257-x.
14. Morrow M, Tamkus D, Abu-Khalaf M, et al. Pooled analysis of SCOUT® radar reflector localisation in breast surgery: clinical outcomes and re-excision rates. Ann Surg Oncol. 2024;31(2):480–8. https://doi.org/10.1245/s10434-023-13257-0.
15. Feinberg JA, Axelrod D, Guth A, Maldonado L, Darvishian F, Pourkey N, Goodgal J, Schnabel F. Radar reflector guided axillary surgery in node positive breast cancer patients. Expert Rev Med Devices. 2022;19(10):791–5. https://doi.org/10.1080/17434440.2022.2139177. Epub 2022 Nov 8. PMID: 36345879.
16. Weinfurtner RJ, Leon A, Calvert A, Lee MC. Ultrasound-guided radar reflector localisation of axillary lymph nodes facilitates targeted axillary dissection. Clin Imaging. 2022;90:19–25. https://doi.org/10.1016/j.clinimag.2022.07.007. Epub 2022 July 25. PMID: 35908456.
17. West NP, Goyal A, Guidroz J, Pilewskie M, Boughey JC. Evaluating radar reflector localisation in targeted axillary dissection in patients undergoing neoadjuvant systemic therapy for

node-positive early breast cancer: a systematic review and pooled analysis. Cancers (Basel). 2024;16(7):1345. https://doi.org/10.3390/cancers16071345.
18. Weiss A, Ramey L, Wilson T, Etikan T, May J, Silverstein M. Radar localisation of breast and axillary lesions with SCOUT: a prospective single-institution pilot study. ANZ J Surg. 2024;94(5):E1–6. https://pubmed.ncbi.nlm.nih.gov/38741456.
19. Bianchi S, Maisonneuve P, Ghidini A, et al. The RADIOSO Milan Trial: impact of SCOUT radar localisation on surgical margins and re-excision rates in breast conserving surgery. Eur J Cancer. 2024;175:12–9. https://doi.org/10.1016/j.ejca.2023.12.005.
20. Caudle AS, Yang WT, Krishnamurthy S, et al. Targeted axillary dissection in breast cancer patients using SCOUT radar reflector localisation after neoadjuvant systemic therapy. Ann Surg Oncol. 2021;28(8):4211–8. https://doi.org/10.1245/s10434-021-09714-8.
21. Varghese J, Patani N, Wazir U, Novintan S, Michell MJ, Malhotra A, Mokbel K, Mokbel K. Wire-free targeted axillary dissection: a pooled analysis of 1300+ cases post-neoadjuvant systemic therapy in node-positive early breast cancer. Cancers (Basel). 2024;16(12):2172. https://doi.org/10.3390/cancers16122172. PMID: 38927878; PMCID: PMC11201777.

Chapter 8
Localisation Using Magnetic Magseed

Julie Simpson and Emma MacInnes

Contents

J. Simpson
Department of Radiology, St James University Hospital, Leeds, UK
e-mail: julie.simpson14@nhs.net

E. MacInnes (✉)
Department of Breast Surgery, St James University Hospital, Leeds, UK
e-mail: emma.macinnes1@nhs.net

R. Vidya, N. Sharma (eds.), *Breast and Axilla Localisation Techniques*,
https://doi.org/10.1007/978-3-032-17995-1_8

8.1 Introduction

Over the past decade, there has been widespread, rapid adoption of a variety of devices for localising impalpable areas within the breast to guide surgical excision. Wires have largely been replaced by a series of implantable devices that allow surgeons to use paired probes to detect the device intraoperatively. Magseed® is the most widely used of all the implantable devices. Its worldwide adoption has provided greater data demonstrating safety and efficacy than are available for the less widely adopted devices. It is specifically recommended by NICE.

As Magseeds® are inert, there are no requirements for radioactive licensing or for additional precautions at insertion or in the operating theatre. The seed does not degrade, and the risks associated with insertion are minimal. Magseeds® are very simple devices, made of stainless steel and that introduces issues that are not seen with some other localisation devices. The use of an electromagnetic probe to detect the seed means that any other ferrous item, for example, a stainless steel surgical instrument, will also cause the probe to register proximity. Like most other localiser seeds, they do also introduce artefact on MRI scans meaning, for centres using MRI to monitor response to neoadjuvant systemic therapies, a standard radiological marker clip would be required for the duration of anticipated MRI surveillance. They can, in centres using imaging modalities other than MRI, be inserted at the start of NACT and the same clip used to guide surgery.

Magseed® is well supported by industry with a helpful range of educational resources and widespread mentorship available. Radiological insertion is very similar to that of any other marker device. The cost of a seed is covered by the NHS tariff for localisation insertion (at time of print). The development of the next-generation seed and probe, whilst not yet widely available or with the same quality of evidence to support, would seem to address the limitations of the current device.

This chapter provides information about the technology and the specifics of the device and the probe, provides a summary of evidence relating to Magseed® localisation, provides instruction on techniques for both insertion and Magseed®-guided breast excision, and details tips and tricks based on extensive first-hand experience. Advantages and pitfalls are also explored and in the context of this book, providing a helpful overview for those unfamiliar with this localisation device. As with all new approaches, there is a learning curve to using Magseed® for breast localisation. Our hope is that by sharing our experience, we can accelerate others in theirs.

8.2 Device Description

Magseeds® are inert, metallic markers used to localise impalpable breast lesions for surgical excision. They are classed as IIb and are CE-approved medical devices. The seed itself is made of surgical grade, stainless steel, with a fine thread running around the length, aiding secure tissue placement. The seed measures 5 mm × 1 mm and is the smallest of the implantable breast localisation devices. Magseeds® are not magnetic but due to the ferrous component of steel, create a graded change relative to the seed's proximity to the electromagnetic Sentimag® probe. Magseeds® are single use and have a long-term soft tissue licence, meaning there is no time-frame requirement between insertion and removal, and they can be left in situ if plans change subsequent to insertion. Magseeds® are not radioactive.

Magseeds® are introduced via an 18G needle, the slimmest of all non-wire introducers. They can be inserted either under ultrasound guidance or stereotactically. They are visible on all breast imaging modalities and although MRI is conditionally compatible, they do create a 2–4 cm void artefact, so are recommended only for localisation to guide surgery. Magseeds® can be placed in breast tissue, within areas of calcification, within lesions and within lymph nodes in either breast or axilla.

The method of localisation requires use of the Sentimag® probe. This is a small, portable unit with a probe on a cable that plugs into the unit base. The probe is placed into a disposable plastic wrap, similar to those used for laparoscopy or sentinel node probes. Placing the probe near to a metallic, ferrous object, will result in a change in the electromagnetic field, with a graded 'signal' to demonstrate proximity of the probe to the metallic object. The distance from the probe to the seed (or other ferrous object) is accessible both with a visual display unit, giving a numerical indication of proximity, and with an audible 'woo' noise, which shifts in tone, according to proximity. Most surgical instruments are made from stainless steel, and so the operating field needs to be free from any other metallic source of interference for the Sentimag® probe to accurately detect the signal from the Magseed®. Reusable plastic instruments are provided to facilitate surgery with Magseeds®. These include Langenbeck retractors, Babcock's forceps, and Allis forceps.

The Sentimag® unit has the option to select from 3 settings, changing the signal tone and indication of distance according to different preset levels of signal shift: 1 is the least sensitive, 2 moderate (and mostly commonly used for detecting Magseeds®), and 3 the most sensitive, and more appropriate for Magtrace®-guided procedures.

Magseed® Pro is the next iteration of the Magseed® and expected to become available in 2026. This seed is very different in appearance to the original Magseed®. It is self-expanding and anchors in tissues once deployed. It claims to create 96% less MRI artefact compared with the original Magseeds®. In addition to an upgrade to the Magseed® design, a next-generation Sentimag® Unit will also become available in 2026. This upgraded unit allows surgeons to distinguish between the signal derived from a Magseed® and the signal derived from Magtrace®, which are currently indistinguishable using the original Magseed® and Sentimag® unit. This upgrade will facilitate MagTotal localisation, combining Magseeds® with Magtrace®, with the ability to discern between the two signals even in overlapping areas of the breast. Magseed® Pro provides better bracketing options than the original Magseeds®, with seeds being used closer together without compromise. Of note, the upgraded Sentimag® Smart probes do not register a signal from standard metallic surgical instruments. The improved technology finally allows surgeons to choose between two display options: the measured distance between the seed and the probe, and the signal count, to guide the procedure.

8.3 Technique

Magseed® localised breast surgery requires the seed to be inserted under radiological guidance, and then located within the operating theatre. This section covers the basics of these techniques, sharing tips and tricks to cover more challenging scenarios.

Through MDT discussion, it is important to select cases appropriate for Magseed® localisation and to plan the appropriate timing of Magseed® insertion. Points to consider are as follows:

- Multifocality. At least 2 cm separation are recommended between Magseeds® to allow confident localisation of the two separate signals. This is an issue where two separate excisions are planned, although less of an issue if the Magseeds® are being used to bracket a wider area for excision.
- Planned management pathway. Magseed® cannot be inserted if breast MRI is planned due to the significant artefact. Patients undergoing neoadjuvant chemotherapy prior to breast-conserving surgery should have their Magseed® inserted after the end-of-treatment MRI.

Once all diagnostic work-up is complete, unless the patient is undergoing neoadjuvant chemotherapy, Magseeds® can be inserted at any time prior to surgery. This allows the procedure to be planned at a time that is suitable for the breast imaging department whilst also providing flexibility to the patient when booking appointments.

Consent for Magseed® insertion is discussed at the time of surgical planning, or by the radiologist, if more appropriate. As with any localisation, to facilitate workflow in the department, each case is reviewed prior to booking to determine the likely imaging modality. However, flexibility is necessary as lesions biopsied under ultrasound guidance may no longer be amenable to ultrasound-guided localisation following neoadjuvant treatment or where disease was very subtle prior to biopsy.

As with all localisation procedures, insertion is undertaken using a non-touch aseptic technique and local anaesthetic. Magseeds® are pre-loaded within a wax plug in an 18G needle, along with a steel obturator for deployment. To prevent accidental deployment, there is a white plastic clip (*) on the obturator lying between its blue plastic end and the hub of the needle. This must be removed before the Magseed® can be deployed (Fig. 8.1).

Whether using ultrasound or X-ray, the approach is planned to achieve accurate targeting and planned localisation. Unlike with wires, the surgical approach does not need to be considered. Once the needle tip is accurately positioned, the obturator is pushed up to the hub of the needle to deploy the Magseed®. The Magseed® can usually be easily seen on ultrasound (Fig. 8.2) and when inserted stereotactically, a stereo pair is obtained to confirm deployment (Fig. 8.3). As with marker clip insertion, rotation of the needle is recommended prior to removal of the needle to minimize the chances of the seed being dislodged back along the needle track.

A post-procedure ipsilateral mammogram is undertaken to confirm accuracy of position of the Magseed®(s) and to provide further guidance to the surgeon at the time of excision. The patient returns home with the Magseed® in situ. If the

Fig. 8.1 Magseed® needle delivery system showing clip (*) to prevent accidental deployment

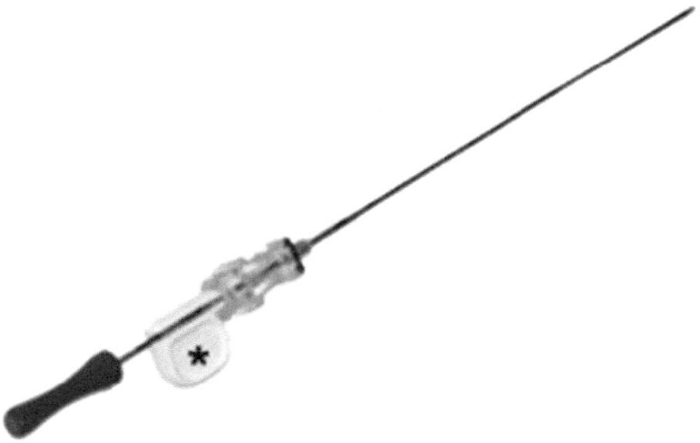

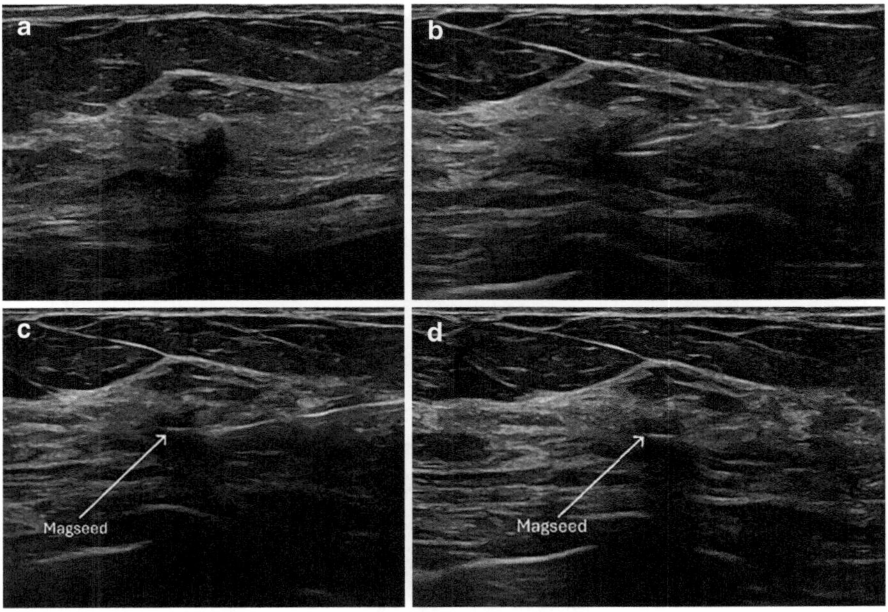

Fig. 8.2 Ultrasound-guided Magseed® localisation of a small carcinoma

position is unsatisfactory, the surgical team is alerted and alternative localisation planned on the day of surgery.

Correlating with the design and the fine thread running around the stainless-steel seed, Magseeds® have a serrated appearance on specimen X-rays allowing them to be distinguished from smooth edged surgical clips (see Figs. 8.4 and 8.5).

The Sentimag® probe requires a power supply and sterile probe cover, which is applied to the probe by the scrub team once the patient is anaesthetised and prepared for surgery. This will be familiar to any team that have used laparoscopic probe covers. The surgeon has access to recalibrate the probe by using a foot pedal that is readily distinguishable from a diathermy pedal due to the texture of the device.

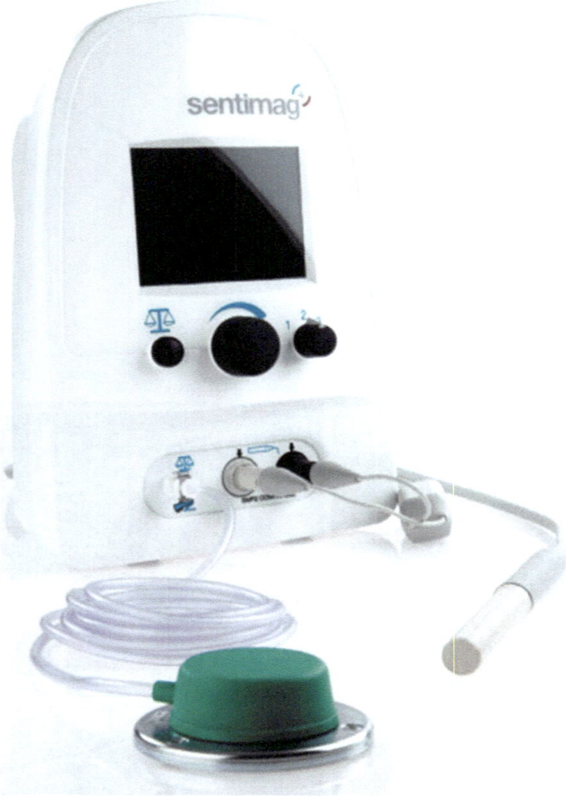

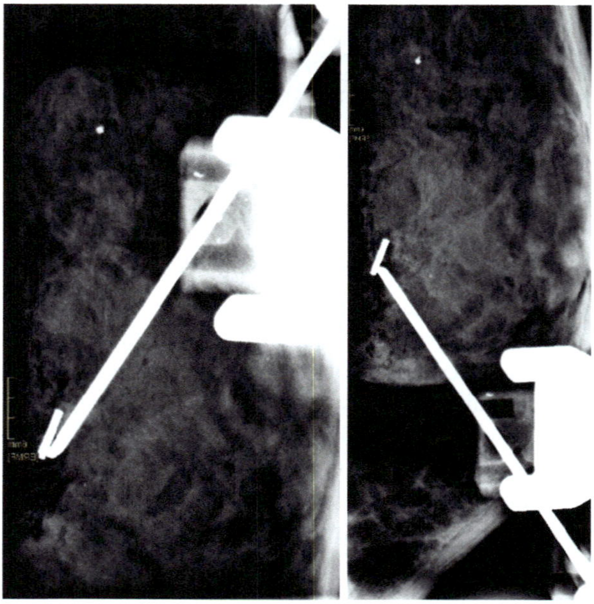

Fig. 8.3 Stereo pair confirming Magseed® deployment

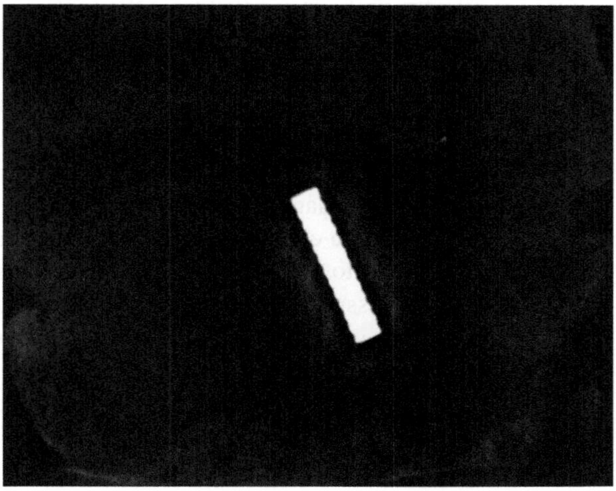

Fig. 8.4 Magnified specimen X-ray containing a Magseed® showing the serrated edge

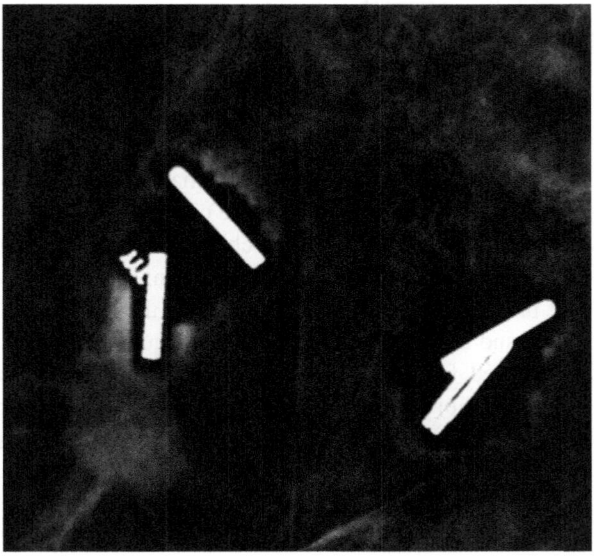

Fig. 8.5 Magnified specimen X-ray showing the difference in appearance between a Magseed® and surgical clips

Once sterile, the probe is handled from the cable side of the black band that runs around the middle of the probe. This avoids any conflicting signal from the surgeon's hands whilst sensing. The probe should be recalibrated whenever it is used, usually holding the probe near to but not in contact with the patient. In some cases, performing a 'skin balance', with the probe in contact with the patient, but away from an area of anticipated signal, may be more appropriate than 'air balance', for example use of the Sentimag® probe in the axilla.

The Sentimag® probe can detect a Magseed® from a distance of around 4 cm. This can be increased to allow detection of deeper lesions by using the probe to compress the breast tissue between the skin and the seed. Once the Magseed® has been inserted, it can be detected using the probe at any point in time. Some surgeons choose to check the seed position prior to anaesthesia, although this is not recommended as a necessary step. Due to the seed design with screw-type threads, once sited, it is very unlikely that a seed will dislodge prior to surgery, and there are no documented cases of seed migration. As long as it can be seen on mammogram, it should be possible to find the seed once the patient is asleep. A disadvantage of exploring whilst the patient is awake is that in women with larger or denser breasts, it may be necessary to push the probe into the breast sufficiently firmly that the assessment can become uncomfortable and equally risks being disconcerting to the patient, if a strong signal is not immediately found. Some surgeons may request an alternative localisation technique be performed if they are unable to find a signal prior to surgery; however evidence has shown, once a seed is in place, surgery can proceed and in all cases where there has been limited or no signal preoperatively, a good signal has become accessible once through skin.

As with any image-guided technique, the use of two-view mammography is beneficial in providing an estimated location, beyond knowing simply the breast quadrant in which to explore. In most cases, the probe can be held perpendicular to the breast and lifted on and off to assess sequential areas. This is different to the technique used for Geiger counter type probes used in radioisotope-guided sentinel lymph node biopsy, where either sweeping the probe across the breast into the axilla or employing a 'joystick' type movement is often appropriate. By sweeping the Sentimag® probe, the signal begins to deteriorate requiring more frequent recalibration. It is sometimes helpful to 'lift' the breast and to use the probe from the inframammary fold or lateral breast crease, essentially probing along the chest wall plane, to access the deeper tissues. It is worth remembering that the probe is designed to receive signal from directly in front of the tip as well as circumferentially around the tip, which is particularly beneficial in larger, more ptotic breasts.

In cases where Magtrace® is being injected intraoperatively to guide sentinel lymph node biopsy, it is recommended that the seed position is clarified first. In many centres, Magtrace® is injected preoperatively and in these cases, the injection point must be selected in light of the known position of the Magseed®, to avoid one overlying the other.

More than one Magseed® can be utilised to 'bracket' a larger lesion. At least 2 cm separation is recommended between Magseeds® to allow for greater confidence in localisation of the two separate signals. In most cases, overlap would rarely

Table 8.1 Distance from probe to seed

Signal	Minimum distance from probe
>9999	In contact
2500	1 cm
500	1.5 cm

be a significant issue as the tissue between Magseeds® would often form part of the area being excised, meaning the peripheral signal, which should not overlap, would be more important and should not be compromised by use of bracketing Magseeds®. In cases where lesions are targeted under stereotactic guidance, the potential for seeds to move when the breast compression is released should be taken into account, and, in these cases, a separation distance greater than 2 cm should be considered.

Once a signal has been identified, the breast can be marked using ink, and a skin incision made. The author advocates the use of a silk suture to mark the anterior aspect of the specimen early in the procedure, essentially marking the breast tissue site of maximal signal in that plane. Once dissection moves into the radial margins, use of plastic reusable retractors allows for use of the probe intermittently without needing to change instruments. This allows the surgeon to check that the signal strength is appropriate for the area of breast being targeted for excision. On setting 2 on the Sentimag® probe, Table 8.1 shows the minimum distances between the probe and the seed.

A signal of 500 suggests the seed is around 1.5cm away from the probe tip. A signal of 9999 means the probe is immediately adjacent. It is clearly necessary to appreciate the individual localisation details for each case to know what margin around a seed is desirable, for example if a seed sits a few millimetres medial to the target lesion, it may be that a stronger signal is appropriate for the medial margin and a correspondingly weaker signal for the opposing lateral margin. Once the specimen has been excised, the probe can be used to assess the margins around the seed ex vivo, which can guide the need for any re-excision requirements.

Magseed® allows for supervision of trainees with transparency of the intraoperative process of seed localisation to both the trainee and trainer. The learning curve for Magseed®-guided breast surgery is quick, and the technique is easy to teach. That the trainer is able to observe the signal strength allows for greater confidence than was feasible with wire-guided excisions, which required more 'feel' and which was harder to teach without being scrubbed and having 'hands on'.

8.4 Case Study 1

Magseeds® are mostly used for localising small impalpable masses, clusters of calcifications, stromal deformities, or marker clips following response to neoadjuvant chemotherapy. This case illustrates how Magseed® has been used to guide

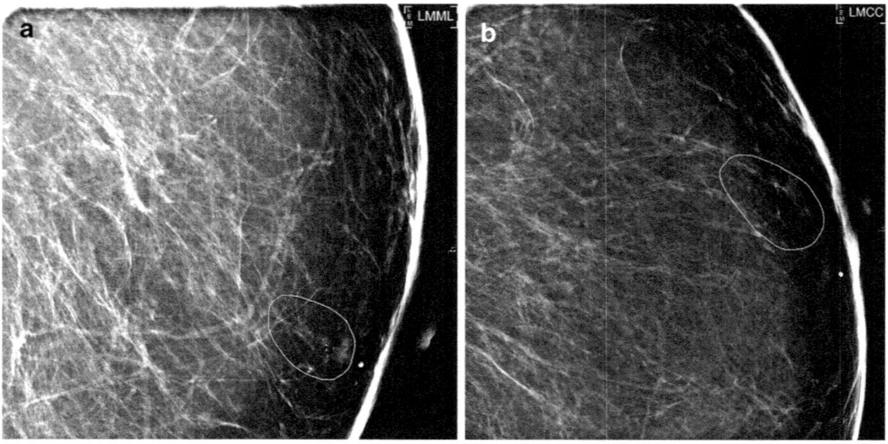

Fig. 8.6 (**a**) Left lateral and (**b**) CC magnification views showing subareolar calcification

wide local excision of calcification detected on a prevalent screening mammogram. Calcification is sparse and in a ductal distribution extending radially in the left 3 o'clock subareolar region (Fig. 8.6a, b).

Stereotactic vacuum-assisted 9G biopsy confirmed a grade 2 carcinoma with ductal and lobular morphology with intermediate grade DCIS. The marker clip deployed via a lateromedial approach was positioned medial to residual calcification. Following MDT discussion, surgery was planned without further imaging in view of the low breast density. The initial surgical plan was to localise the residual calcification and include the nipple. However, the patient wished to preserve the nipple. Calcification extended close to but not up to the nipple, so with appropriate consent the plan was revised to undertake wide local excision including areolar skin en bloc, preserving the nipple. Given the radial distribution of sparse calcification, Magseed® localisation was planned to localise the peripheral aspect of the area of calcification.

Following consent, the peripheral aspect of the calcification was targeted for localisation via a lateromedial approach. A Magseed® was successfully deployed and confirmed to be in a satisfactory position on post-procedure mammography (Fig. 8.7a, b).

Surgery was undertaken uneventfully with a good Magseed® signal over the lateral areola and specimen X-rays confirming excision of the Magseed®, the marker clip, and residual calcification (Fig. 8.8a, b).

Pathology showed a 7 mm grade 2 NST with high-grade solid DCIS, total extent 20 mm with good circumferential margins including 5 mm superficially.

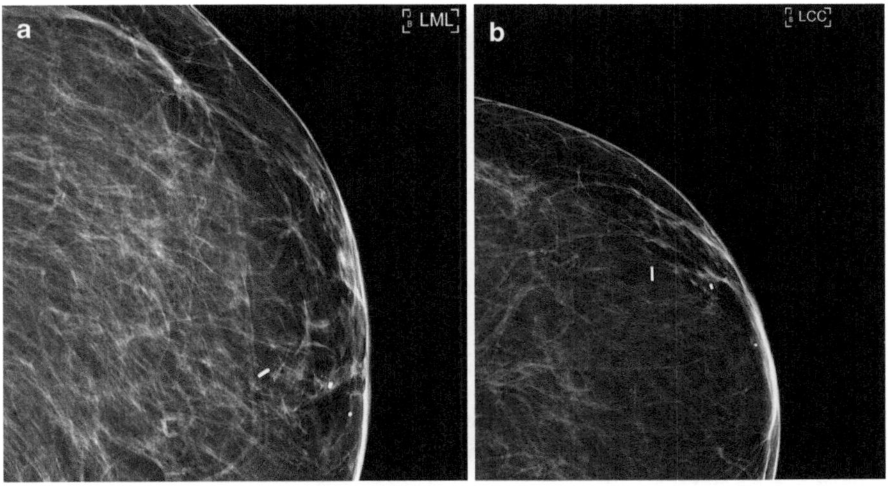

Fig. 8.7 (**a**) Left lateral and (**b**) CC views following Magseed® localisation of the peripheral aspect of subareolar calcification

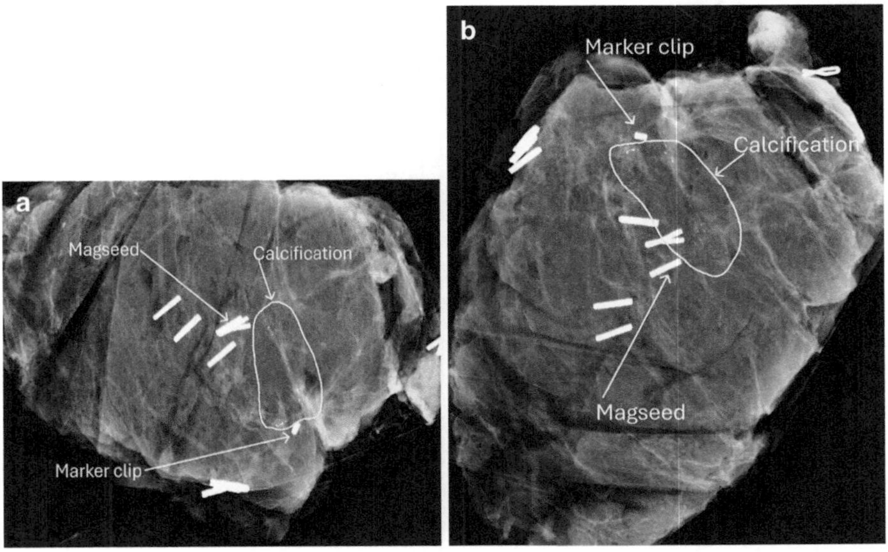

Fig. 8.8 (**a**, **b**) WLE specimen X-rays

8.5 Case Study 2

This case illustrates the use of Magseed® in a small, screen detected breast cancer. The diagnosis was made on an incident screen, with an 11 mm spiculate mass associated with microcalcification sitting in the upper outer quadrant of the right breast (Fig. 8.9a–d).

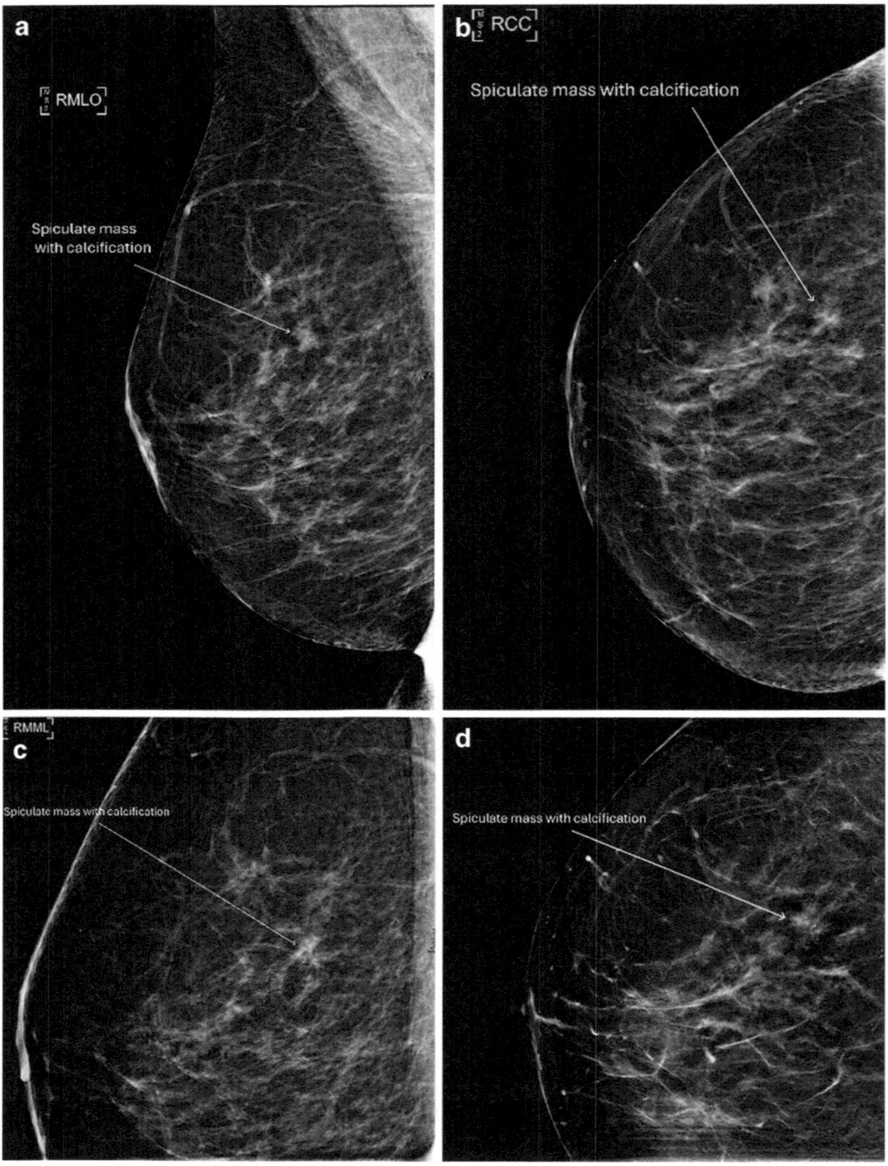

Fig. 8.9 (**a**) Right MLO and (**b**) CC screening mammogram with (**c**) lateral and (**d**) CC magnification views

Pathology demonstrated a grade 2 cancer of no special type, with associated ductal carcinoma in situ. The breast volume, determined mammographically, was 576cm^3 and the density 21% (BIRADS B). The post-biopsy mammogram showed that the clip position was medial to the lesion and that post-biopsy haematoma

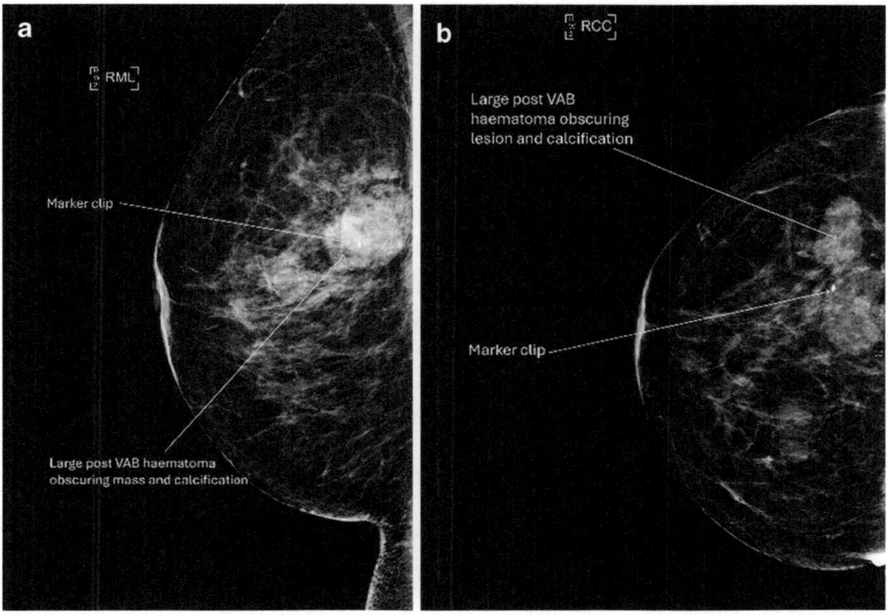

Fig. 8.10 (**a**) Right lateral and (**b**) CC mammogram following diagnostic vacuum biopsy showing medially sited marker clip and large haematoma obscuring lesion

obscured the residual lesion (Fig. 8.10a, b). Residual-associated calcification was visible on a further delayed right mammogram following resolution of the haematoma.

In this case, a Magseed® was used to localise the area of impalpable disease, initially aiming to target the residual microcalcification, which sat distant to the biopsy placed clip; however the calcification was not appreciable at the time of localisation and so the clip was targeted instead. The Magseed® was inserted under stereotactic guidance. It was noted that the seed position was 10 mm medial to the residual calcification, and 6 mm medial and 3 mm inferior to the radiological clip (Fig. 8.11a, b). This phenomenon is common for areas that have been both sampled and localised using stereotactic guidance.

The degree of separation tolerable between the seed and the area being targeted for excision will depend on the size of the target lesion, the size of the breast, and the planned excision size, along with the views of the radiologist and operating surgeon. In this case, it was felt acceptably close to proceed without further localisation. The seed was sited deep in the upper outer quadrant of the breast, and, in theatre, the probe was used in a lateral-to-medial orientation, from the lateral breast fold, to locate the signal.

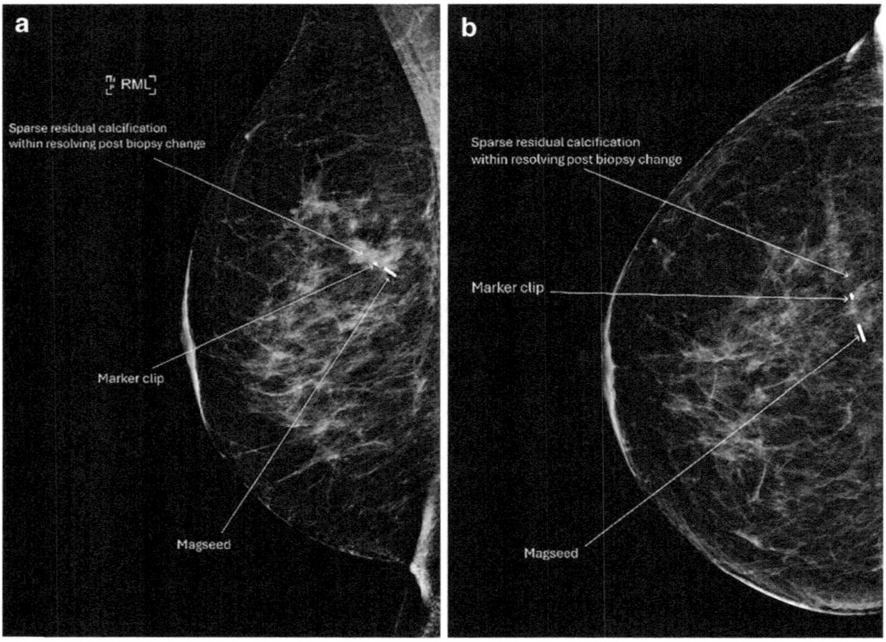

Fig. 8.11 (**a**) Right lateral and (**b**) CC mammogram following stereotactic Magseed® localisation

DIAGRAM of the planned excision from the surgeon's point of view (i.e. schematic of breast with probe pointing to position of Magseed® and different colour markings to show the anticipated position of the clip and lesion).

The operation proceeded uneventfully, and the specimen was excised (Fig. 8.12a, b) with greater signal strength at the medial margin and lesser laterally, in accordance with the anticipated location of the seed to the lesion.

Pathology showed adequate margins circumferentially and the patient ultimately proceeded on to radiotherapy and endocrine treatment.

8.6 Advantages and Pitfalls

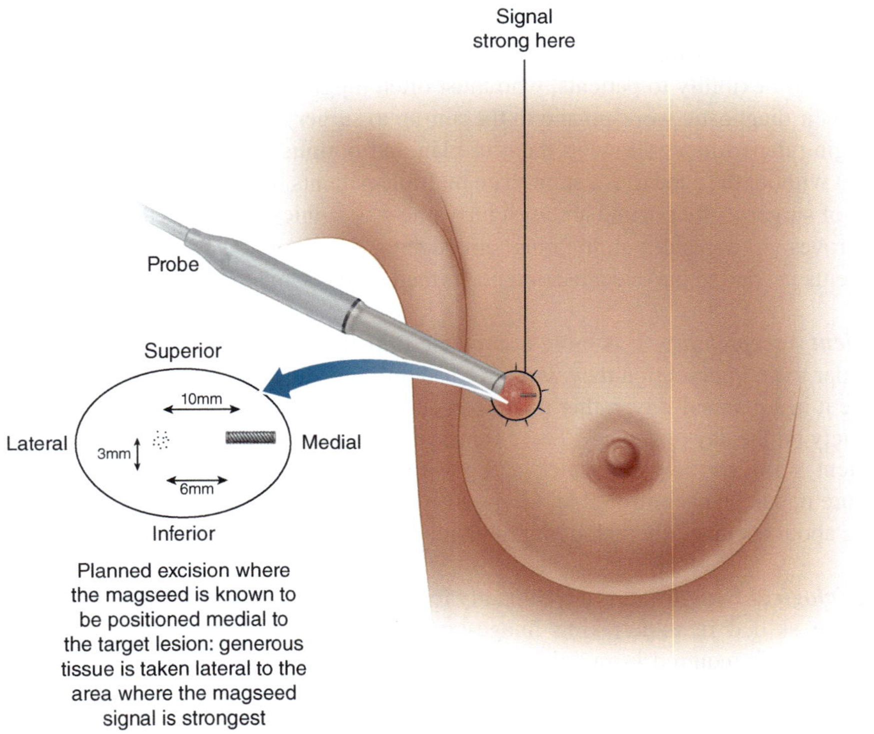

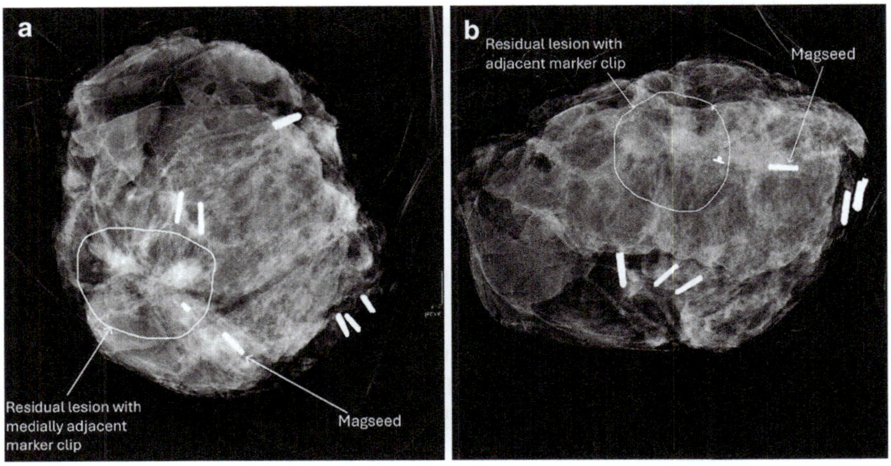

Fig. 8.12 (**a**, **b**) Specimen X-rays following excision showing the residual lesion, marker clip, and Magseed® relative to the margins

There are several advantages of Magseed® localisation over wire localisation from an imaging, surgical, and patient perspective.

Timing Magseeds® are inert, do not degrade over time, and have a long-term soft tissue licence, so they can be inserted at any time prior to surgery. This gives increased flexibility to patients, who must often juggle multiple appointments during their diagnostic work-up and in the run-up to surgery. It is also beneficial to the imaging department, allowing them to plan and optimise workflow in the department without the need to accommodate multiple patients for wire localisation on the day of surgery, often in and amongst busy one-stop clinics. The workflow in theatre improves as a result, eliminating any delays that would have happened, had patients needed to have localisation performed on the same day.

Patient Acceptability It is more acceptable to patients to have a procedure that is similar to an intervention they will have had during their diagnostic work-up and to have it in a planned way, rather than as an additional procedure adding to stress and anxiety on the day of surgery. There is no wire protruding from the breast whilst the patient waits for surgery, which along with the large dressing needed to safely secure it, can be uncomfortable. Magseed® localisation eliminates any patient concern about accidentally dislodging the wire whilst they wait to go to theatre.

Radiological Benefits It is a technically reliable and straightforward procedure for anyone skilled in undertaking image-guided breast intervention. No additional equipment is required in radiology. The needle is easy to visualise on ultrasound with smooth deployment of the seed at the needle tip. The seed is usually clearly seen as an echogenic linear artefact giving confidence in accurate positioning. The post-procedure mammogram is quicker and easier to perform, without a wire protruding from the skin.

Surgical Benefits Magseed® localisation eliminates the risk of wire dislodgement and wire transection and there is no interference with the surgical approach. Implantation into the breast tissue is secure with no evidence of seed migration. Magseeds® are widely used with good data and training pathways.

8.7 Disadvantages of Magseed® Localisation

MRI Artefact* Magseed® is MRI conditional. Patients can safely have an MRI in a 1.5 or 3 T scanner without risk of the Magseed® moving or of significant heating but the Magseed® will create a signal void of 2–4 cm. As such, Magseed® cannot be deployed until after the completion of neoadjuvant chemotherapy when MRI is being used to monitor response. All diagnostic imaging with MRI should be undertaken before Magseed® localisation.

Multiple Magseeds® * Signals can overlap and the Sentimag® probe is unable to distinguish between the two seeds. This must be considered when more than one seed is deployed, particularly when undertaking multiple separate excisions, as the separation distance of lesions, and hence Magseeds®, can be less in the non-compressed breast in the surgical position than it appears on mammography. This is less of an issue when multiple seeds are used for bracketing excision of a large area and in this case, some centres use multiple seeds to create a single area of high signal to map the area for localisation purposes.

Intraoperative Probe Recalibration* The need to pause to recalibrate over several seconds can introduce time to surgery but is unlikely to significantly impact on overall operating time. This has been addressed to allow much quicker recalibration in the new probe.

Need for Non-metallic Instruments* To avoid interference with the Sentimag® probe and reliable detection of the Magseed®, there should be no metallic instruments in the surgical field.

Probe Display Limitations* The probe provides a logarithmic indication of seed proximity but does not display distance directly. This has been addressed in the new probe, which is not available at time of print but is anticipated to become available in 2026.

Cost The cost of a Magseed® (£250) is approximately sevenfold that of a wire (£35).

Allergy According to the manufacturer's product specifications, Magseed® is not indicated for use in Nickel-allergic patients; however it contains much less Nickel than a guidewire.

Pacemakers The Sentimag® probe should not be placed within 15 mm of any part of an operational pacemaker. Pacemakers are not an absolute contraindication to the use of Magseed®, but care must be taken both with the case selection and with the intraoperative instrument handling and position.

* These issues have been addressed and improved upon in the next generation of Magseed® and probe.

8.8 Short Literature Review

8.8.1 Magseed® Localisation in Breast Cancer Surgery: A Review of the Literature for Efficacy, Clinical Workflow, Benefits, and Patient Experience

Magseed® has over 13,000 patients published in the peer-reviewed literature at the time of writing and has emerged as a viable alternative to wire-guided localisation. Magseed® reported benefits including scheduling flexibility and efficiencies [1, 12], reduced migration [5], shorter operating and localisation procedures[4,] and reduced operating room delays [2, 16], alongside a potentially better patient experience [12]. The addition of Magtrace®, on the single 'Sentimag®' platform, for axillary staging has the potential to amplify many of these benefits, particularly when used with the 'MagTotal' technique [4, 11]. Unlike radioactive seeds, Magseed® is non-radioactive, eliminating regulatory and safety concerns related to radiation exposure.

8.8.2 Surgical Outcomes, Clinical Workflow and Scheduling Flexibility

Magseed® has been demonstrated to be non-inferior to wire-guided localisation. An iBRA-NET multidisciplinary group, prospective cohort study of 2300 patients across 35 UK centres, found no difference in re-excision rates compared to a wire-guided arm of the study. However, statistically significant improvements were noted with Magseed® in the primary endpoint of successful index lesion localisation. A failed localisation was also a statistically more common occurrence in the wire-guided arm [1].

Magseed® has significantly reshaped the workflow for breast cancer surgeries. Unlike traditional wire-guided localisation (WGL), which requires same-day placement due to wire protrusion and patient discomfort, Magseed® allows for flexible, preoperative placement [14]. The Magseed® marker is small, measuring only 5 mm, and is easily visualized with ultrasound [5, 13, 15] or mammography [13, 15], ensuring precise placement [12, 16].

Radiologists can place the magnetic seed any time before surgery, freeing up critical operating room time and reducing coordination challenges [2]. Shorter localisation times are also reported [3, 18], which may correlate to lower morbidity. Using the sharp 18 g needle to place the 5 × 0.9 mm seed results in high satisfaction scores for radiologists [4, 5, 12, 16]. Its small size may reduce the likelihood of complications such as pneumothorax,

From a surgeon's perspective, Magseed® enables predictable and streamlined localisation [4]. The absence of a percutaneous wire reduces the risk of migration

[5], minimizes logistical concerns [1, 4, 6, 16], and allows the surgeon to make incisions based on optimal surgical access [7–9]. Consequently, this provides surgeons with more control, potentially leading to more successful resections [8, 10–12, 14] and the possibility of better cosmetic outcomes [11, 12].

The clinical effectiveness of Magseed® is closely tied to its radiological properties and ease of intraoperative detection. The Magseed device, when paired with the Sentimag® magnetic sensing probe, allows precise localisation within the breast, offering reliable navigation during surgery. Importantly, Magseed® can be placed either centrally within the lesion or at its margins, providing flexibility depending on lesion type and location.

8.8.3 Health Economics

The potential economic advantages of Magseed® are shorter localisation procedures and reduced times for excision [4]. The ability to decouple localisation from surgery offers the potential for cost benefits by improving scheduling efficiencies and reducing logistical complexities [2, 12, 16–18] and, possibly, re-operations [7, 8, 16, 18–21]. Magseed® potentially reduces operating room delays and decreases operating room overruns or cancellations due to late localisation procedures [2, 4, 16].

The elimination of radiotracers in favour of the MagTotal approach presents clear cost advantages, including savings on radioactive materials, compliance-related costs, and additional staff training for handling radiological substances. This is particularly important for hospitals and health systems seeking cost-effective alternatives that do not compromise quality of care [22].

8.8.4 Patient Experience

Magseed® improves patient comfort and reduces anxiety [12]; as well as accommodates the patient through scheduling flexibility [2, 12, 16–18]. The ability to schedule Magseed® placement at any convenient time, rather than on the day of surgery, significantly alleviates patient stress. Patients report a greater sense of autonomy in their treatment process, as the more flexible scheduling allows them to attend the localisation procedure at a time that suits their personal commitments. Additionally, the MagTotal technique, which streamlines both tumour localisation and sentinel node detection, further reduces procedural burdens on patients, requiring fewer hospital visits and fewer invasive procedures [2, 4, 11, 12, 16–18].

Magseed® eliminates the need for an external wire protruding from the breast. Preoperative placement is minimally invasive and well-tolerated by patients [12], with fewer complications, such as displacement or wire-associated trauma [12].

The integration of Magseed® for lesion localisation with Magtrace® for axillary staging on the Sentimag® platform has the important benefit of potentially improving surgical outcomes [4, 11] whilst minimizing the risks of MRI artefact and skin staining [23–25] during long-term post-procedure follow-up. It further reduces procedural burden on patients, allowing for fewer hospital visits and fewer invasive procedures [4, 11].

8.8.5 Magseed® in the Axilla, Targeted Axillary Dissection

In a prospective registry study of 50 post-neoadjuvant chemotherapy (NAC) patients by Simons et al. [27], 17 radiologists placed 50 Magseeds® in sentinel nodes at the first attempt, with a 100% successful retrieval rate at surgery [27]. Similar results were found in a study by Reitsamer et al. [26], who found a 100% identification rate for targeted lymph nodes marked with Magseed®. The study highlights that Magseed® deployment is straightforward to perform under ultrasound, with no reported complications such as haematoma or bleeding [26]. Barry et al. [28], also found Magseed® to be a highly effective tool for accurately marking axillary lymph nodes and facilitating precise localisation and removal during surgery. Of note, the authors found that Magseed® placement is particularly accurate when placed prior to the NAC cycle [28]. However, Bravo et al. [29], in a multicentre prospective observational study, found no influence on outcomes of timing of placement; with a false negative rate for targeted axillary dissection of 0%. All magnetic seeds were identified and removed in just over 10 min during surgery. They concluded that Magseed® could be used for long-term marking of axillary lymph nodes [29].

8.8.6 Conclusion

Magseed® localisation leads to improvements in clinical workflow and scheduling flexibility resulting in a more efficient process for both surgeons and radiologists, with fewer logistical challenges and improved operating room efficiency. The health economics of Magseed® also suggest direct cost reductions associated with optimized resource utilization and reduced operating delays.

Clinical outcomes with Magseed® are consistent, with reduced re-excision rates and effective localisation. Importantly, the radiological ease of placement, combined with the absence of radiation safety concerns, enhances the preoperative experience for radiologists and patients alike.

Finally, the MagTotal® procedure, utilizing a totally magnetic technique, integrates the benefits of tumour localisation and sentinel node detection into a streamlined workflow and is reported in the MagTotal® randomized control trial, which is the highest level of evidence (Oxford scale 1b) currently published for any non-radioactive localisation device.

8.9 Summary

Magseed® localisation of impalpable breast lesions is a safe, reliable, and straightforward procedure which offers many benefits over wire localisation for patients, radiologists, and surgeons. Despite the greater cost of a Magseed® compared to wire localisation, it has become widely adopted.

References

1. Dave RV, et al. Wire- and magnetic-seed-guided localisation of impalpable breast lesions: iBRA-NET localisation study. Br J Surg. 2022;109(3):274–82. https://doi.org/10.1093/bjs/znab443.
2. Chacko SM, Marshall HN. Implementation of preoperative magnetic seed localisation for breast and axillary lesions: an alternative to wires and radioactive seeds. J Radiol Nurs. 2018;37(3):154–7. https://doi.org/10.1016/j.jradnu.2018.03.015.
3. Tayeh S, et al. The use of magnetic seeds and radiofrequency identifier tags in breast surgery for non-palpable lesions. Anticancer Research, 2020, 1 January, pp. 315–322. Available at: https://research.ebsco.com/linkprocessor/plink?id=2c208c5b-4246-3225-8adb-5d506f3d6ff2. Accessed 31 Jan 2024.
4. Pantiora E, et al. Magnetic seed vs guidewire breast cancer localisation with magnetic lymph node detection: a randomized clinical trial. JAMA Surg [Preprint]. 2023; https://doi.org/10.1001/jamasurg.2023.6520.
5. Harvey JR, et al. Safety and feasibility of breast lesion localization using magnetic seeds (Magseed): a multi-centre, open-label cohort study. Breast Cancer Res Treat. 2018;169(3):531–6.; ISSN 0167-6806 1573-7217 [Preprint]. https://doi.org/10.1007/s10549-018-4709-y.
6. Ross FA, et al. Magseed localisation of non-palpable breast lesions: experience from a single centre. Clin Radiol. 2022;77(4):291–8. https://doi.org/10.1016/j.crad.2022.01.034.
7. Bravo EI, et al. Reliability of Magseed ® marking before neoadjuvant systemic therapy with subsequent contrast-enhanced mammography in patients with non-palpable breast cancer lesions after treatment: the MAGMA study. Breast Cancer Res Treat. 2024:1–11. https://doi.org/10.1007/s10549-024-07407-6.
8. D'Angelo A, et al. Magnetic seed versus skin tattoo localization of non-palpable breast lesions: a single institution cohort study. Eur Radiol [Preprint]. 2023; https://doi.org/10.1007/s00330-023-10008-4.
9. Bell E, Gray K, Lang A, Lannigan A, MacPherson B, Murphy D, McIlhenny J. Oncoplastic surgery and Magseed ® markers: a five-year snapshot of ambition and evolution in breast conserving surgery [poster], Presented at: 22nd QI and audit symposium 2024, 12 April 2024. Edinburgh, UK; 2024.
10. Cieciorowski M, et al. Assessment of the use of the Magseed marker in the localization of non-palpable lesions in the mammary gland. Pol Przegl Chir. 2022;95(4):1–5. https://doi.org/10.5604/01.3001.0016.0664.
11. Hersi A-F, et al. A combined, totally magnetic technique with a magnetic marker for non-palpable tumour localization and superparamagnetic iron oxide nanoparticles for sentinel lymph node detection in breast cancer surgery. Eur J Surg Oncol. 2019;45(4):544–9. https://doi.org/10.1016/j.ejso.2018.10.064.
12. Micha AE, Sinnett V, Downey K, Allen S, Bishop B, Hector LR, Patrick EP, Edmonds R, Barry PA, Krupa KDC, Rusby JE. Patient and clinician satisfaction and clinical outcomes of Magseed compared with wire-guided localisation for impalpable breast lesions. Breast Cancer.

2021;28(1):196–205. https://doi.org/10.1007/s12282-020-01149-1. Epub 2020 Sep 24. PMID: 32974810; PMCID: PMC7796883
13. Murphy E, Quinn E, Stokes M, Kell M, Barry M, Flanagan F, Walsh SM. Initial experience of magnetic seed localization for impalpable breast lesion excision: first 100 cases performed in a single Irish tertiary referral centre. Surgeon. 2022;20(3):e36–42. https://doi.org/10.1016/j.surge.2021.02.010. Epub 2021 Apr 8. PMID: 33840595
14. Redfern RE, Shermis RB. Initial experience using Magseed for breast lesion localization compared with wire-guided localization: analysis of volume and margin clearance rates. Ann Surg Oncol. 2022;29(6):3776–83. https://doi.org/10.1245/s10434-022-11327-4.
15. Liang DH, et al. Clinical outcomes using magnetic seeds as a non-wire, non-radioactive alternative for localization of non-palpable breast lesions. Ann Surg Oncol. 2022;29(6):3822–8. https://doi.org/10.1245/s10434-022-11443-1.
16. Singh P, et al. Effectiveness and safety of Magseed -localization for excision of breast lesions: a prospective, phase IV trial. Ann Surg Open. 2020;1(2) https://doi.org/10.1097/as9.0000000000000008.
17. Constantinidis F, Sakellariou S, Chang SL, Linder S, MacPherson B, Seth S, Gill N, Seth A. Wireless localisation of breast lesions with Magseed. A radiological perspective of 300 cases. Br J Radiol. 2022;95(1133):20211241. https://doi.org/10.1259/bjr.20211241. Epub 2022 Feb 24. PMID: 35201906; PMCID: PMC10993964
18. Lake B, et al. The magnetic effect: sustainability of patient centric outcomes, time and cost saving following 5 years of Magseed experience. The Shrewsbury and Telford Hospital NHS Trust; 2023. ESSO 2023 poster presentation
19. Crèvecoeur J, Jossa V, Di Bella J, Coibion M, Crèvecoeur A. Clinical experience of the Magseed ® magnetic marker to localize non-palpable breast lesions: a cohort study of 100 consecutive cases. Gland Surg. 2023;12(5):566–76. https://doi.org/10.21037/gs-22-552. Epub 2023 Apr 11. PMID: 37284712; PMCID: PMC10240439
20. Clement C, Schops L, Nevelsteen I, Thijssen S, Van Ongeval C, Keupers M, Prevos R, Celis V, Neven P, Han S, Laenen A, Smeets A. Retrospective cohort study of practical applications of paramagnetic seed localisation in breast carcinoma and other malignancies. Cancers (Basel). 2022;14(24):6215. https://doi.org/10.3390/cancers14246215. PMID: 36551700; PMCID: PMC9777317
21. Depretto C, Della Pepa G, De Berardinis C, Suman L, Ferranti C, Marchesini M, Maugeri I, Martelli G, Gennaro M, Folli S, Pruneri G, Scaperrotta GP. Magnetic localization of breast lesions: a large-scale European evaluation in a National Cancer Institute. Clin Breast Cancer. 2023;23(8):e491–8. https://doi.org/10.1016/j.clbc.2023.08.004. Epub 2023 Aug 22. PMID: 37704563
22. Menen. 2024. Magnetic Tracer Aids in Commission on Cancer Compliance Reducing Time to Surgery and Increasing Surgical Volumes. Miami Breast 2024 poster presentation.
23. Pantiora E, Tasoulis MK, Valachis A, Eriksson S, Kühn T, Karakatsanis A, Rubio IT. Evolution and refinement of magnetically guided sentinel lymph node detection in breast cancer: meta-analysis. Br J Surg. 2023;110(4):410–9. https://doi.org/10.1093/bjs/znac426. PMID: 36560842; PMCID: PMC10364535
24. Jazrawi A, Pantiora E, Abdsaleh S, et al. Prospective evaluation of MRI artefacts following breast conserving surgery and sentinel lymph node dissection with the magnetic technique. Eur J Surg Oncol. 2024; https://doi.org/10.1016/j.ejso.2024.109368.
25. Jazrawi A, Wärnberg M, Hersi AF, Obondo C, Pistioli L, Eriksson S, Karakatsanis A, Wärnberg F. A comparison of skin staining after sentinel lymph node biopsy in women undergoing breast cancer surgery using blue dye and Superparamagnetic Iron Oxide Nanoparticle (SPIO) tracers. Cancers (Basel). 2022;14(23):6017. https://doi.org/10.3390/cancers14236017. PMID: 36497498; PMCID: PMC9741074
26. Reitsamer R, Peintinger F, Forsthuber E, Sir A. The applicability of Magseed ® for targeted axillary dissection in breast cancer patients treated with neoadjuvant chemotherapy. Breast.

2021;57:113–7. https://doi.org/10.1016/j.breast.2021.03.008. Epub 2021 Mar 25. PMID: 33813230; PMCID: PMC8050798
27. Simons JM, Scoggins ME, Kuerer HM, Krishnamurthy S, Yang WT, Sahin AA, Shen Y, Lin H, Bedrosian I, Mittendorf EA, Thompson A, Lane DL, Hunt KK, Caudle AS. Prospective registry trial assessing the use of magnetic seeds to locate clipped nodes after Neoadjuvant chemotherapy for breast cancer patients. Ann Surg Oncol. 2021;28(8):4277–83. https://doi.org/10.1245/s10434-020-09542-y. Epub 2021 Jan 8. PMID: 33417121
28. Barry PA, Harborough K, Sinnett V, Heeney A, St John ER, Gagliardi T, Bhaludin BN, Downey K, Pope R, O'Connell RL, Tasoulis MK, MacNeill F, Rusby JE, Gui G, Micha A, Chen S, Claudia Krupa KD. Clinical utility of axillary nodal markers in breast cancer. Eur J Surg Oncol. 2023;49(4):709–15. https://doi.org/10.1016/j.ejso.2022.12.019. Epub 2023 Feb 1. PMID: 36764880
29. Martínez M, Jiménez S, Guzmán F, Fernández M, Arizaga E, Sanz C. Evaluation of axillary lymph node marking with Magseed ® before and after Neoadjuvant systemic therapy in breast cancer patients: MAGNET study. Breast J. 2022;2022:6111907. https://doi.org/10.1155/2022/6111907. PMID: 35855102; PMCID: PMC9288346

Chapter 9
Localisation Using Radio-Guided Occult Lesion Localisation (ROLL)

Germana Lissidini, Elisa Ileana Bottazzoli, Luca Nicosia, and Paolo Veronesi

Contents

G. Lissidini (✉) · E. I. Bottazzoli
Breast Surgery Division, European Institute of Oncology, IRCCS, Milan, Italy
e-mail: germana.lissidini@ieo.it; ElisaIleana.Bottazzoli@ieo.it; http://www.ieo.it/

L. Nicosia
Breast Imaging Division, Radiology Department, IEO European Institute of Oncology IRCCS, Milan, Italy
e-mail: luca.nicosia@ieo.it

P. Veronesi
Breast Surgery Division, European Institute of Oncology, IRCCS, Milan, Italy

Breast Imaging Division, Radiology Department, IEO European Institute of Oncology IRCCS, Milan, Italy

Department of Oncology and Hemato-Oncology, University of Milan, Milan, Italy
e-mail: paolo.veronesi@ieo.it; http://www.ieo.it/

R. Vidya, N. Sharma (eds.), *Breast and Axilla Localisation Techniques*,
https://doi.org/10.1007/978-3-032-17995-1_9

9.1 Introduction

The global expansion of screening programmes, primarily employing bilateral mammography and breast ultrasound, has significantly increased the early detection of breast cancer in clinical practice [1]. As a result, breast surgeons frequently encounter non-palpable in situ or invasive lesions requiring surgical excision [2]. In such cases, precise localization techniques are essential to facilitate breast-conserving surgery (BCS), which aims to excise the tumour with sufficient margins of healthy tissue while preserving as much of the breast as possible. Accurate localization is pivotal in achieving oncological safety, maintaining favourable cosmetic outcomes, and minimizing the removal of healthy tissue. Over time, several preoperative localization techniques have been employed [2], including carbon particle injections and the placement of anchoring or guiding wires within the lesion. Despite their utility, these methods present notable drawbacks, such as challenges in the histological assessment of carbon-marked specimens and complications associated with hook-wire placement, including bleeding, infection, pneumothorax, and wire displacement [2–4].

To address these limitations, a novel approach known as Radio-Guided Occult Lesion Localization (ROLL) was developed in 1997 at the European Institute of Oncology in Milan [5]. This technique involves the injection of colloidal human serum albumin particles (10–150 μm in diameter), labelled with approximately 3.7 MBq of technetium-99 m (99mTc), directly into the lesion under mammographic or ultrasonographic guidance [5]. ROLL has since gained widespread acceptance and remains one of the most effective options for localizing non-palpable lesions [6–9]. Beyond its accuracy, the technique offers significant intraoperative advantages. By utilizing a gamma-detection probe, the surgeon can assess the extent of resection in real time, ensuring the radicality of the procedure. This capability not only distinguishes ROLL from conventional localization methods but also streamlines surgical procedures, reducing operative time and enhancing overall efficiency.

9.2 Indications

ROLL is currently recommended for the localization of non-palpable breast lesions detectable through ultrasound or mammographic imaging. These include clusters of microcalcifications, small spiculated opacities, irregular masses, or parenchymal distortions. The technique is particularly applicable in cases where a metallic marker has been placed in the lesion following biopsy or after neoadjuvant therapy when breast-conserving surgery is planned.

However, ROLL is not suitable for certain conditions. Its application is contraindicated in the presence of multicentric or multifocal lesions, diffuse microcalcifications, or retroareolar lesions. In the latter case, the risk of radioactive contamination of the mammary ducts precludes its use.

9.3 Technical Execution

The radio-guided localization and subsequent removal of non-palpable breast lesions certainly represent a multidisciplinary procedure and involves multiple specialists including a breast surgeon, a breast radiologist, a pathologist, and a nuclear medicine doctor. It requires an optimal organization within the centre and the presence of a nuclear medicine department in order to be performed.

Along the following chapter, we will evaluate in detail the main passages required to localize and subsequently remove a non-palpable lesion of the breast:

- Intralesional inoculation of the radioactive tracer.
- Mammographic/ultrasound-guided verification of centring.
- Acquisition of the scintigraphic image.
- Surgical excision.
- Intraoperative radiograph of the removed surgical piece.
- Histological examination.

9.3.1 Tracer Inoculation

Tracer inoculation for ROLL is typically performed either on the day of the planned breast-conserving surgery or a few hours prior [6]. The process begins with the localization of the non-palpable lesion using ultrasound or mammography, with the latter being the preferred method in cases involving microcalcifications or the presence of a metallic marker.

Subsequently, a saline solution (approximately 0.2 mL) containing a small amount of radiopharmaceutical is injected directly into the lesion (Fig. 9.1). This radiopharmaceutical consists of approximately 0.05 mg of macroaggregates of human serum albumin, with particle diameters ranging from 10 to 150 μm, labelled with 3–10 MBq of technetium-99 m (99mTc).

The macroaggregates used in ROLL differ from the colloidal particles employed in sentinel lymph node identification. Their larger size prevents migration through lymphatic channels, ensuring that the radiopharmaceutical remains localized at the injection site. This characteristic necessitates precise intralesional injection to achieve accurate localization.

An accurate evaluation of the protectionist parameters has demonstrated a very high safety profile for this method, due to the extremely low quantity of injected radioactivity which will be completely removed during surgery; the patient will, however, be advised to avoid direct contact with subjects under the age of 16 and with pregnant women for a brief period after the procedure.

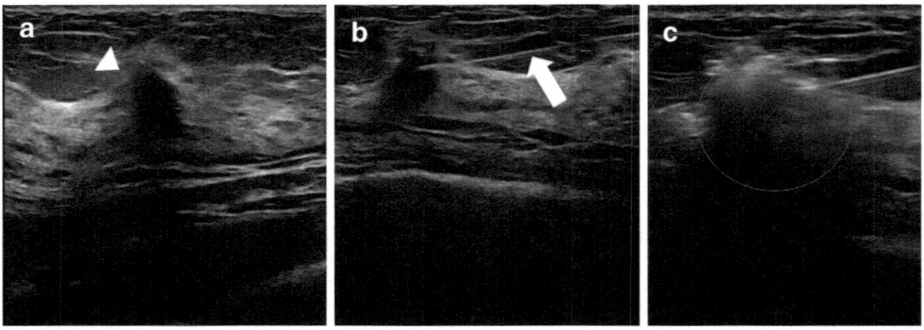

Fig. 9.1 Injection of the tracer in a non-palpable lesion using echographic guidance [7, 8]: The needle reaches the small non-palpable lesion, seen as a ipoechogenic nodule with a rear shadow cone. In (**a**), the pathological nodule (arrowhead) is shown. In (**b**), the needle (elongated arrow) is visible within the lesion during ultrasound-guided localization. In (**c**), the spread of the tracer within the area of the nodule (circular area) is evident

9.3.2 Mammographic Evaluation

When the non-palpable lesion is represented by a cluster of microcalcification, a metallic landmark, or other findings visible only at mammography, it is preferable to perform a 2-projections stereotactic mammography. In these cases, following the injection of the radioactive tracer, a 0.2–0.3 ml of water-soluble, radiopaque solution is injected into the same site to verify the correct centring (Fig. 9.2).

9.3.3 Acquisition of the Scintigraphic Image

Breast scintigraphy in antero-posterior projections and lateral-lateral, performed after inoculation of the radioactive tracer, compared with the radiological image, allows to verify not only the correct centring of the lesion (Fig. 9.3), but also check for the tracer spreading status or see if there are multiple areas of radioisotope activity of the mammary gland, as well as contamination of the skin. These are all conditions that would make it difficult to identify and surgically remove the non-palpable lesion itself.

In these first three phases of the ROLL (the inoculation of the tracer, mammography when necessary, and scintigraphy), the close collaboration between the nuclear medicine doctor and the radiologist is essential to the success of the method.

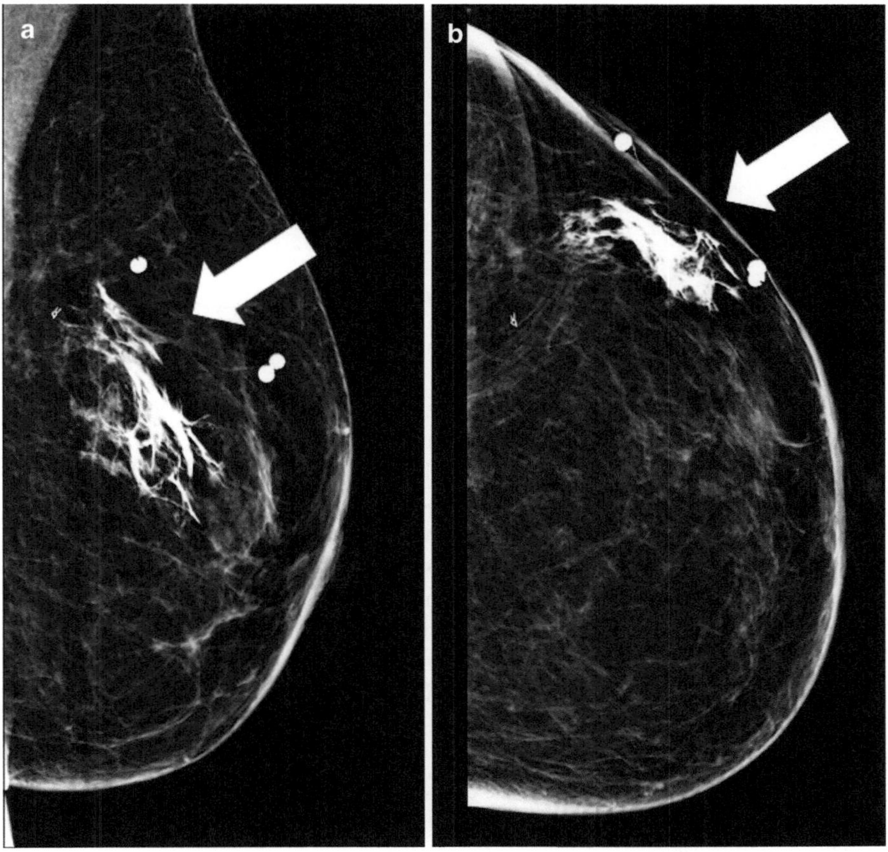

Fig. 9.2 Injection of a radiopaque solution to verify the correct localization of a non-palpable lesion after a mammographically guided insertion of the tracer [6]. In (**a**, **b**), we see the radiotracer (arrow) injected with stereotactic guidance, respectively, in the medio-lateral (**a**) and cranio-caudal (**b**) projections

9.3.4 Surgical Resection

The ROLL technique is closely associated with subsequent breast-conserving surgery, aiming to achieve complete resection of the target lesion while optimizing cosmetic outcomes. A critical aspect of performing this type of surgery is the use of a specialized wireless gamma probe [10, 11]. This probe is indispensable in three key phases of the procedure. First, prior to the initiation of surgery, it is used to accurately locate the lesion that has been pre-marked with technetium. This enables the surgeon to select the most appropriate incision, balancing both oncological efficacy and aesthetic considerations. During the surgery, the same probe, enclosed in sterile covers, is employed continuously to assist in the localization of the lesion throughout the resection process. This approach ensures maximal conservation of

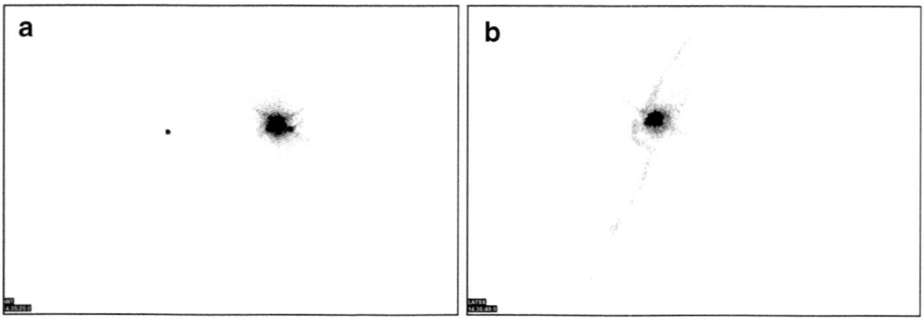

Fig. 9.3 Scintigraphical evaluation after the inoculation of radioactive tracer in antero-posterior (**a**) and latero-lateral (**b**) projections [9]

healthy tissue. When the probe is directed towards the area where the radiotracer is injected, it emits a distinct, rhythmic audible signal, and the screen displays high radiotracer counts (Fig. 9.4).

A key objective of this surgical approach is achieving complete excision, particularly in the case of B4 and B5 lesions. To achieve this, it is crucial to extend the resection deep into the pectoralis fascia, maintaining a margin of at least 10 mm around the lesion, particularly for infiltrating tumours. At our centre, we routinely assess the adequacy of resection not only by using the gamma probe but also through macroscopic examination of the excised tissue, confirming that the lesion is centrally located within the specimen.

Finally, once the resection is complete, the probe is again utilized to verify that the lesion is fully contained within the excised specimen and to rule out any residual radiotracer uptake in the remaining breast tissue.

The primary objective of breast-conserving surgery, as previously discussed, is the complete excision of the index lesion. The breast surgeon plays a pivotal role in achieving this goal, not only through the execution of the surgical procedure but also by providing the pathologist with detailed information to aid in the precise localization of the lesion within the excised tissue. To facilitate this process, it is crucial to 'orient' the excised specimen by placing a distinct number of sutures along each margin. This technique allows the pathologist to accurately describe the lesion's distance from the specimen's margins and, subsequently, assess whether the resection is adequate. This information is essential for determining the adequacy of the surgical margins and for planning the appropriate adjuvant therapy.

9.3.5 *Intraoperative X-Ray of the Removed Sample*

In certain cases, particularly when the index lesion consists of a cluster of microcalcifications, a radial scar, or when it is marked with a metallic landmark—either due to complete excision during a VABB biopsy or because the landmark was placed

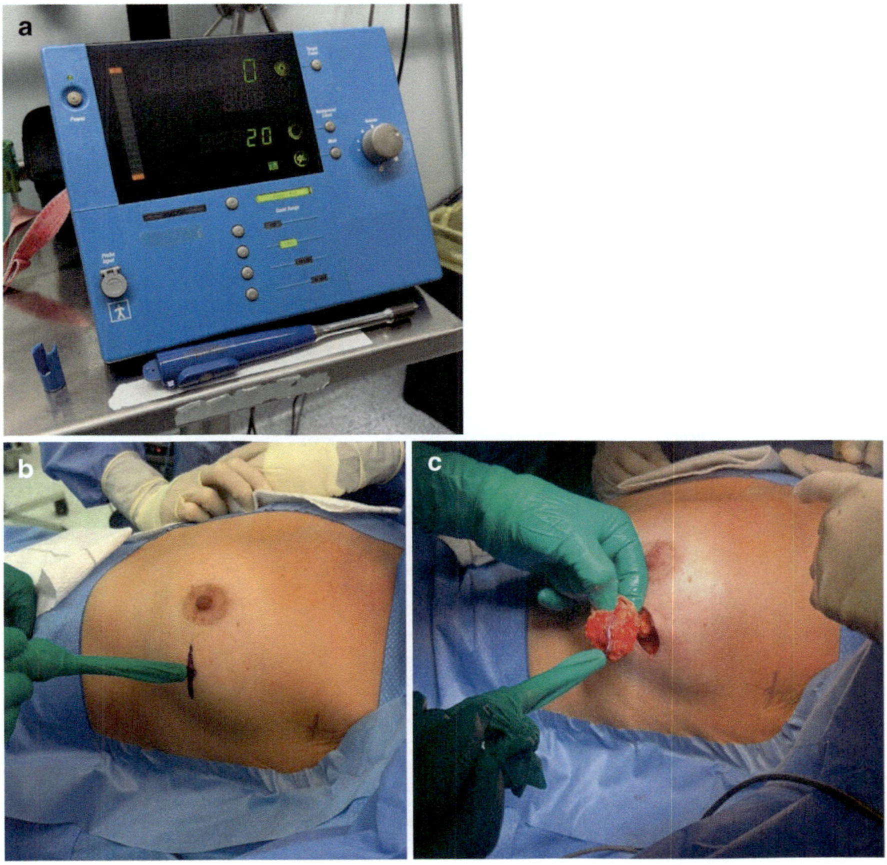

Fig. 9.4 Intraoperative evaluation of the non-palpable lesion marked with radiotracer, using wireless probe. In (**a**), the wireless gamma probe is shown, ready to be used during surgery. In (**b**), the gamma probe is used by the surgeon to localize the non-palpable lesion in order to choose the correct site for the incision; during surgery it is constantly used to manage the complete resection of the sample (**c**)

prior to neoadjuvant therapy—an intraoperative X-ray of the excised specimen is typically performed. This allows for immediate verification of the complete removal of the marked, non-palpable lesion during surgery and facilitates margin re-excision when necessary.

When this procedure is conducted, it is essential to mark the sutures used for orienting the specimen with radiopaque clips, ensuring the number of clips corresponds to the number of sutures (Fig. 9.5).

In most institutions, the X-ray is performed by sending the specimen to the radiology department; however, in a few centres, such as ours, a portable X-ray device is available in the operating room, enabling quicker and more efficient imaging during the procedure.

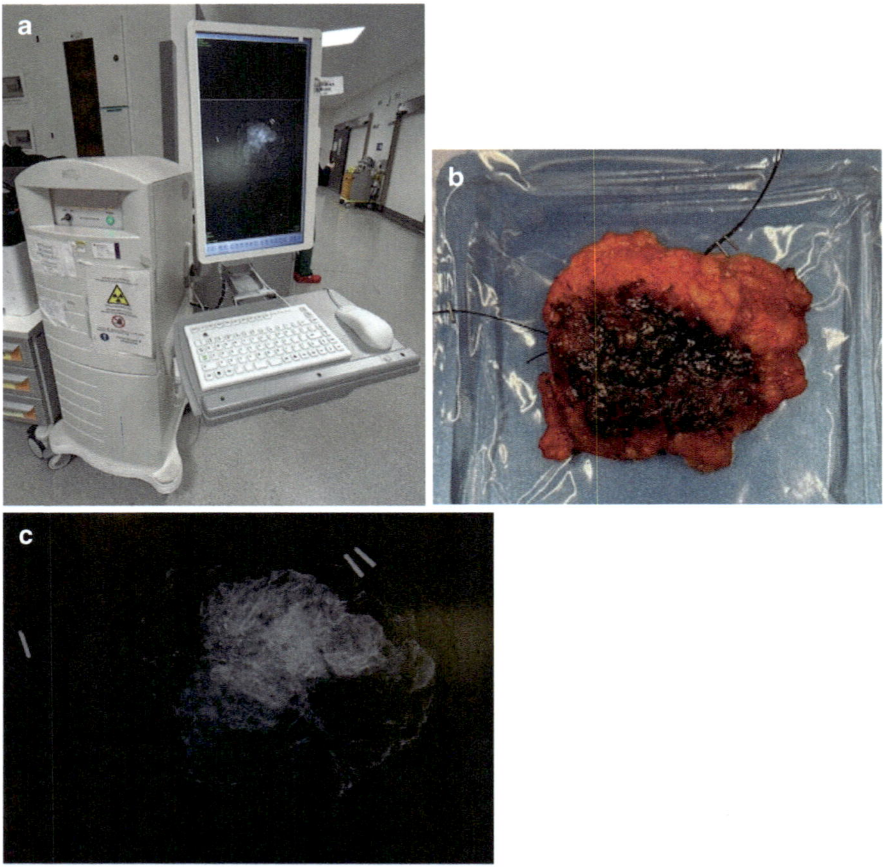

Fig. 9.5 Resected sample and its x-ray evaluation. In (**a**), the portable X-ray device in shown in the surgical block. In (**b**), after the excision of the sample, it is fundamental to orientate it with stitches and, when an X-ray has to be performed, clips. The intraoperative X-ray allows the surgeon to see the lesion in the sample and to verify the radicality of surgery, as shown in (**c**)

9.3.6 Histological Examination

The histological examination of the excised specimen is crucial for determining the histological and molecular characteristics of the target lesion, verifying whether the lesion has been entirely removed during surgery, and assessing whether the resection margins are adequate to consider the procedure oncologically safe and radical.

A comprehensive histological report must be available post-surgery, detailing all relevant features of the lesion necessary for selecting the appropriate adjuvant therapy. These include size, margin status, histological classification, grading, biological markers, growth index, and evidence of vascular or lymphatic invasion. In fact, adjuvant radiotherapy is generally recommended following breast-conserving surgery. However, additional therapies such as hormonal treatment or chemotherapy are determined based on the findings of the histological analysis. For this reason, it is imperative that the histological evaluation be conducted by a pathologist with expertise in breast tissue analysis.

9.3.7 Sentinel Node Identification

Similar to the evolution of surgery for primary breast lesions, axillary surgery has also undergone significant changes over time, progressively becoming more conservative. When clinically indicated, sentinel lymph node biopsy is now considered the preferred surgical approach.

In cases where breast surgery involves a radio-guided quadrantectomy with sentinel lymph node biopsy, the ROLL technique must be employed. Simultaneously, it is crucial to identify the sentinel lymph node using lymphoscintigraphy.

To achieve this, two distinct radiotracers are used: one for localizing the non-palpable breast lesion (macroaggregated albumin injected intralesionally) and another for identifying the sentinel lymph node (microaggregated albumin injected subdermally or perilesionally).

This combined technique is referred to as SNOLL: Sentinel Node and Occult Lesion Localization.

9.4 Results

Over the past decade, the ROLL technique has demonstrated several advantages, including higher rates of clear margins, reduced excision volume, improved cosmetic outcomes, better lesion centricity in the surgical specimen, and the ability to simultaneously localize the sentinel lymph node. These benefits are particularly evident when compared to other techniques for non-palpable lesion localization, such as Wire-Guided Localization (WGL). Furthermore, ROLL is associated with a low incidence of serious complications, although operator experience is crucial to avoid failures in lesion identification [10].

It is important to note that, even in cases where mammographic control and/or post-inoculation scintigraphy reveal imperfect centring of the lesion, a larger resection around the marked area can still result in complete excision of the lesion. The procedure becomes more challenging if there is leakage of the radiopharmaceutical within the breast tissue, which can create additional radioactive areas, or if radioactive contamination of the skin occurs.

One of the key advantages of ROLL is the reduced localization time compared to WGL, which also contributes to a shorter overall surgical duration [10, 11]. This could be explained by the relative simplicity of radiotracer injection in ROLL compared to the more complex wire placement required for WGL. Additionally, the gamma probe used in ROLL allows the surgeon to more precisely direct the incision and dissection, with the added benefit of real-time feedback on the lesion's location throughout the surgery, as previously discussed.

Literature data indicate that ROLL significantly reduces the likelihood of involved resection margins when compared to WGL [11]. This could be due to the improved lesion centricity achieved with ROLL, which allows the surgeon to confidently excise the tissue of interest while being guided by the frequency and intensity of the radioactivity. As the signal diminishes, the surgeon is alerted to the proximity of the lesion's centre. The gamma probe also provides a pseudo-3D image of the lesion, a feature absent in WGL, which relies more on the surgeon's experience and judgement. Furthermore, residual radioactivity can be easily checked from the wound, ensuring that the tumour has been radically excised [12].

Another notable advantage of ROLL is the feasibility of performing it simultaneously with sentinel node biopsy, which is particularly beneficial in the management of early-stage breast cancer [12].

The incidence of occult, non-palpable breast carcinomas is steadily increasing, and it is expected that in the future, a significant proportion of breast cancers will fall into this category [13]. The high curability rates of patients with non-palpable breast carcinomas, identified through mammography, ultrasound, and MRI, highlight the critical role of surgical techniques like ROLL that allow for immediate resection of the breast with clear and safe margins surrounding the primary lesion.

9.5 Advantages and Limitations

Over the years, the ROLL technique has demonstrated numerous advantages, establishing itself as a safe and effective method that does not require external devices. Its primary benefit is the ability to localize both the target lesion and the sentinel lymph node using the same radiotracer. Other advantages include reduced localization and surgery times, a lower incidence of positive margins, a decreased reoperation rate, and improved patient comfort compared to alternative localization techniques, such as WGL [2, 14]. Additionally, ROLL offers superior cosmetic outcomes, particularly when compared to WGL, as it allows the surgeon greater flexibility in making an incision that ensures radical resection while preserving as much healthy breast tissue as possible.

However, ROLL also has certain limitations. It necessitates close multidisciplinary collaboration between nuclear medicine and surgical departments and requires specific equipment and training due to the radioactive nature of the materials involved. Another potential drawback is the limited surgical flexibility, as the radiotracer must be injected hours before the procedure. Any delay in surgery could compromise the localization of the marked lesion, as the radiotracer may lose efficacy over time. Furthermore, the high cost of the procedure remains a notable disadvantage [2].

9.6 Conclusions

The ROLL technique for preoperative localization of non-palpable lesions has become widely adopted and offers several improvements in breast cancer surgery. It facilitates more efficient and faster conservative surgeries with improved outcomes, both in terms of oncological radicality and aesthetic results. The surgeon can select an incision that ensures complete excision of the index lesion with clear margins, while preserving as much healthy breast tissue as possible.

A successful implementation of ROLL requires a multidisciplinary approach and strong collaboration between specialists dedicated to breast pathology, making this cooperation essential for achieving optimal results.

References

1. Nicosia L, Gnocchi G, Gorini I, et al. History of mammography: analysis of breast imaging diagnostic achievements over the last century. Healthcare. 2023;11(11):1596. https://doi.org/10.3390/healthcare11111596.
2. Cheung BHH, Co M, Lui TTN, Kwong A. Evolution of localization methods for non-palpable breast lesions: a literature review from a translational medicine perspective. Transl Breast Cancer Res. 2024;5:12. https://doi.org/10.21037/tbcr-23-49.
3. De Cicco C, Pizzamiglio M, Trifirò G, et al. Radioguided occult lesion localisation (ROLL) and surgical biopsy in breast cancer. Technical aspects. Q J Nucl Med Off Publ Ital Assoc Nucl Med AIMN Int Assoc Radiopharmacol IAR. 2002;46(2):145–51.
4. Postma EL, Witkamp AJ, Van Den Bosch MA, Verkooijen HM, Van Hillegersberg R. Localization of nonpalpable breast lesions. Expert Rev Anticancer Ther. 2011;11(8):1295–302. https://doi.org/10.1586/era.11.116.
5. Luini A, Zurrida S, Galimberti V, Paganelli G. Radioguided surgery of occult breast lesions. Eur J Cancer Oxf Engl 1990. 1998;34(1):204–5. https://doi.org/10.1016/s0959-8049(97)00376-6.
6. Aydogan F, Ozben V, Celik V, et al. Radioguided occult lesion localization (ROLL) for non-palpable breast cancer: a comparison between day-before and same-day protocols. Breast. 2010;19(3):226–30. https://doi.org/10.1016/j.breast.2010.01.017.
7. Follacchio GA, Monteleone F, Anibaldi P, et al. A modified sentinel node and occult lesion localization (SNOLL) technique in non-palpable breast cancer: a pilot study. J Exp Clin Cancer Res. 2015;34(1):113. https://doi.org/10.1186/s13046-015-0230-x.
8. Barros A, Cardoso M, Sheng P, Costa P, Pelizon C. Radioguided localisation of non-palpable breast lesions and simultaneous sentinel lymph node mapping. Eur J Nucl Med Mol Imaging. 2002;29(12):1561–5. https://doi.org/10.1007/s00259-002-0936-9.
9. De Cicco C, Trifirò G, Intra M, et al. Optimised nuclear medicine method for tumour marking and sentinel node detection in occult primary breast lesions. Eur J Nucl Med Mol Imaging. 2004;31(3):349–54. https://doi.org/10.1007/s00259-003-1390-z.
10. Elzohery YH, Gomaa MM, Mohamed G, Fadlalla WM, Taha SN, Ibraheem MH. Comparison of wire-guided localization (WGL) and radio-guided occult lesion localization (ROLL) in localization of non-palpable breast lesions. World J Surg Oncol. 2023;21(1):266. https://doi.org/10.1186/s12957-023-03152-0.
11. Kiruparan N, Kiruparan P, Debnath D. Use of wire-guided and radio-guided occult lesion localization for non-palpable breast lesions: a systematic literature review and meta-analysis of current evidence. Asian J Surg. 2022;45(1):79–88. https://doi.org/10.1016/j.asjsur.2021.06.055.

12. Rönkä R, Krogerus L, Leppänen E, Von Smitten K, Leidenius M. Radio-guided occult lesion localization in patients undergoing breast-conserving surgery and sentinel node biopsy. Am J Surg. 2004;187(4):491–6. https://doi.org/10.1016/j.amjsurg.2003.12.040.
13. Veronesi U, Luini A, Botteri E, et al. Nonpalpable breast carcinomas: long-term evaluation of 1,258 cases. Oncologist. 2010;15(12):1248–52. https://doi.org/10.1634/theoncologist.2010-0123.
14. Chan BK, Wiseberg-Firtell JA, Jois RH, Jensen K, Audisio RA. Localization techniques for guided surgical excision of non-palpable breast lesions. Cochrane Breast Cancer Group, ed. Cochrane Database Syst Rev. 2015;2016(3) https://doi.org/10.1002/14651858.CD009206.pub2.

Chapter 10
Localisation Using Iodine Seeds

Emilie Fentener van Vlissingen, Iris van der Ploeg, and Marie-Jeanne T.F.D. Vrancken Peeters

Contents

10.1 Introduction

Radioactive seed localization (RSL) is a localization technique in which surgical resection is guided by the radioactivity emitted by an Iodine-125 (^{125}I) seed. Originally the seeds were developed for brachytherapy, a form of radiation treatment in which a sealed radioactive source is placed directly in or near the tumour. In 2001, Gray et al. first described the application of ^{125}I-seeds for RSL, introducing

E. F. van Vlissingen · I. van der Ploeg
Department of Surgical Oncology, Netherlands Cancer Institute Antoni van Leeuwenhoek, Amsterdam, The Netherlands
e-mail: e.fv.vlissingen@nki.nl; i.vd.ploeg@nki.nl

M.-J. T. F. D. Vrancken Peeters (✉)
Department of Surgical Oncology, Netherlands Cancer Institute Antoni van Leeuwenhoek, Amsterdam, The Netherlands

Department of Surgical Oncology, Amsterdam University Medical Center, Amsterdam, The Netherlands
e-mail: m.vrancken@nki.nl

R. Vidya, N. Sharma (eds.), *Breast and Axilla Localisation Techniques*,
https://doi.org/10.1007/978-3-032-17995-1_10

Table 10.1 Current clinical applications of radioactive seed localization for breast cancer treatment

	Breast-conserving surgery	Axillary-preserving surgery
Diagnostics	Diagnostic excision of breast lesion [1]	Diagnostic excision of lymph node [2]
Primary breast-conserving surgery	Non-palpable breast cancer [3] Non-palpable multifocal breast cancer [4] Non-palpable DCIS [5] Extensive DCIS [6]	
Breast-conserving surgery after PST	cT1–2-3 breast cancer patients [7]	
Axillary staging after PST		cN+ breast cancer patients MARI procedure [8]. TAD procedure [9]. RISAS procedure [10].

PST primary systemic treatment, *DCIS* ductal carcinoma in situ, *MARI* marking axillary lymph nodes with radioactive iodine seeds, *TAD* targeted axillary dissection, *RISAS* radioactive iodine seed and sentinel node biopsy

an alternative to conventional localization techniques in breast-conserving surgery (BCS) [1]. Since then, ^{125}I-seed localization has been introduced in various stages of the breast cancer treatment pathway, including both breast-conserving and axillary-preserving surgery (Table 10.1).

10.2 Development Towards Radioactive Seed Localisation (RSL)

The global incidence of breast cancer continues to rise, making it the most common malignancy among women worldwide [11–13]. Management of breast cancer consists of a multidisciplinary treatment strategy, involving systemic therapy, surgery, and radiotherapy. Over the past decades, advantages across these fields have led to de-escalated treatment options, enabling tailoring therapy based on tumour biology and individual patient characteristics, while maintaining oncologic safety.

This shift towards de-escalation started when prospective randomized clinical trials demonstrated comparable overall survival outcomes between patients undergoing breast-conserving surgery (BCS) followed by radiotherapy (RT), and those treated with mastectomy [14–16]. Furthermore, the implementation of population-based screening programs, and the improvements in imaging techniques, have led to the detection of more early-stage and non-palpable tumours, including both ductal carcinoma in situ (DCIS) and invasive breast cancer (iBC) [17]. In parallel, the increasing use and effectiveness of neoadjuvant systemic treatment (NST) result in substantial tumour downstaging. As a result, many tumours initially large and palpable at diagnosis now achieve a pathological complete or near complete response, allowing for BCS instead of mastectomy [18, 19]. As a result of these developments, over 60% of breast cancer patients currently undergo BCS.

The main surgical challenge in BCS is to achieve complete tumour excision with negative margins, while preserving enough healthy breast tissue to maintain favourable cosmetic outcome. As argued before, the population of breast cancer patients with small or non-palpable tumours is increasing. For these patients, accurate intraoperative localization is technically challenging. Therefore, several tumour localization techniques have been developed to guide resection and improve margin control.

The most longstanding method is *wire-guided localization (WGL).* With this technique, preoperatively a wire is inserted under ultrasound or stereotactic guidance into the centre of the tumour. Intraoperatively the location of the wire is used to determine tumour location and estimate its margins. Despite widespread adoption and longtime use, WGL is associated with high rates of positive resection margins, ranging between 13% and 58% [1, 18–23]. Together with the risk of wire displacement, patient discomfort, and suboptimal cosmetic outcomes [23–25] this makes the WGL technique a less favorable technique compared to the more recently explored localization techniques.

Another technique developed is *intraoperative ultrasound-guided localization.* Intraoperatively, the ultrasound provides a real-time visualization of the tumour margins. This technique leads to fewer positive resection margins compared to WGL. However, its applicability is limited because certain lesions, including DCIS and tumours with near or complete pathological response (pCR), are not sonographically visible [26–28]. These limitations make it an unreliable technique, and therefore it is not used often.

Eventually, *radio-guided localization techniques* were introduced to overcome the limitations of earlier mentioned approaches. One of these methods is called *radioactive occult lesion localization (ROLL).* In ROLL, a technetium-labelled radiotracer is injected intratumourally prior to surgery. Intraoperatively, a gamma probe is used to identify the location with the highest signal intensity, which is then removed by the surgeon. However, diffuse uptake of the technetium tracer into the surrounding tissue complicates precise excision [26, 29–34].

To address this limitation, *Radioactive Seed Localization (RSL)* was developed. Instead of a liquid radiotracer, a sealed ^{125}I-seed is implanted directly into the lesion preoperatively. The gamma probe detects the seed with accurate localization, enabling targeted resection [26, 29–34]. Multiple randomized trials and large cohort studies have demonstrated that both ROLL and RSL have superior outcomes compared to WGL, with respect to re-excision rates due to positive resection margins and improved cosmetic outcomes [2, 35–38].

10.3 Radioactive Seed Localisation (RSL)

With the Radioactive Seed Localization (RSL) technique, an ^{125}I-seed is implanted in target tumour preoperatively. Under ultrasound or stereotactic guidance, the ^{125}I-seed is accurately placed in the centre of the tumour (Fig. 10.1). Prior to first incision, the surgeon uses a gamma-probe for transcutaneous identification of the location with maximal ^{125}I activity. This location can be externally marked to guide optimal entry site of the first incision. Intraoperatively, the gamma probe is used for accurate localization of the ^{125}I-seed and the surrounding pathological tissue in the breast (Fig. 10.1), or in the axillary (Fig. 10.2). After excision, ^{125}I activity is measured within the surgical cavity to confirm complete removal, and the excised tissue is verified to contain the ^{125}I-seed. This confirms that the target lesion has been removed, which minimizes the risk of residual tumour tissue [3, 29–34].

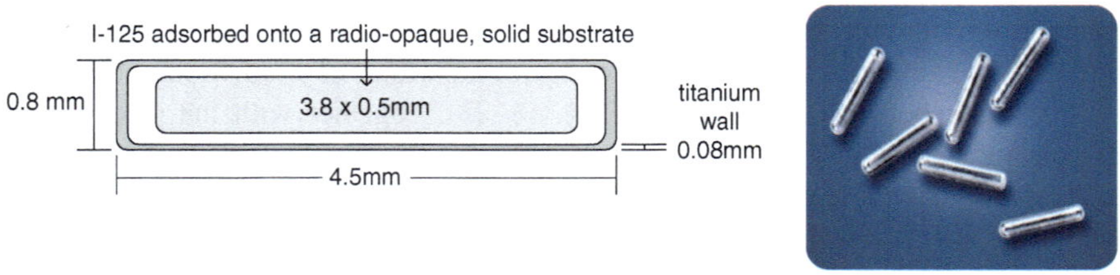

Fig. 10.1 (**a**) Implantation of an ^{125}I-seed by US guidance. (**b**) Post-implantation mammography to validate the implantation location. (**c**) Intraoperative ^{125}I-seed localization while using a gamma probe

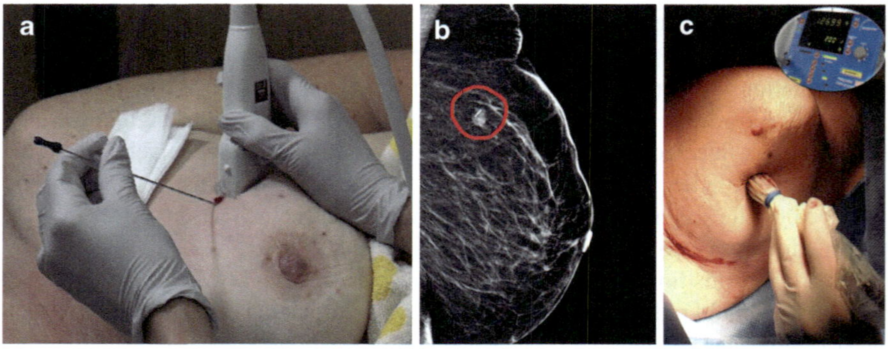

Fig. 10.2 (**a**) Implantation of an ^{125}I-seed by US guidance in a pathologic lymph node. (**b**) Post-implantation ultrasound to validate the implantation location. (**c**) Intraoperative ^{125}I-seed marked lymph node localization while using a gamma probe

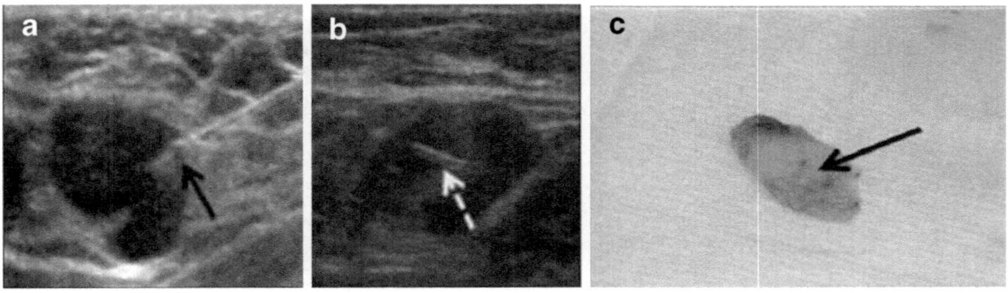

Fig. 10.3 ^{125}I-seed

10.4 Technical Aspects of the ^{125}I-Seed

Understanding the technical aspects of the ^{125}I-seed is essential, as precise placement, timing of the placement, accurate intraoperative localization, and reliable verification of excision directly impact surgical outcomes, patient safety, and oncological outcome.

An ^{125}I-seed consist of a small, welded titanium capsule containing radioactive Iodine-125 absorbed onto a nickel/copper coated, gold cored aluminium wire, measuring approximately 4 mm × 0.8 mm in size (Fig. 10.3) [3, 39]. While several manufacturers produce these seeds, the available models differ only minimally in design and radiation characteristics [1, 3, 16, 21–23, 40–43].

During the early implementation of RSL, high-activity ^{125}I-seeds developed for brachytherapy were used, containing a radiation dose ranging 10–30 MBq. With the recognition of the suitability of ^{125}I-seeds as a localization technique, efforts have been made to standardize the procedure using low-activity ^{125}I-seeds specifically designed for RSL. Nowadays, the radiation activity of the ^{125}I-seeds used in RSL varies slightly between institutions, typically ranging 3–13 MBq, with a half-life of 59.6 days [3, 44].

10.5 Advantages of Radioactive Seed Localisation (RSL)

Radioactive seed localization (RSL) offers several important advantages over both radioactive occult lesion localization (ROLL) and wire-guided localization (WGL). A key benefit lies in the precise and stable localization provided by the ^{125}I-seed, which facilitates optimal incision planning and allows precise lesion excision with negative excision margins and minimal removal of healthy tissue. This is in contrast to the diffuse signal produced by technetium-based injections in ROLL and the less precise guidance offered by WGL [45–47].

In addition, RSL provides flexibility for treating more complex disease presentation. Multiple ^{125}I-seeds can be placed to bracket edges of extensive DCIS (Fig. 10.4a) or to localize multiple tumour foci in multifocal breast cancer

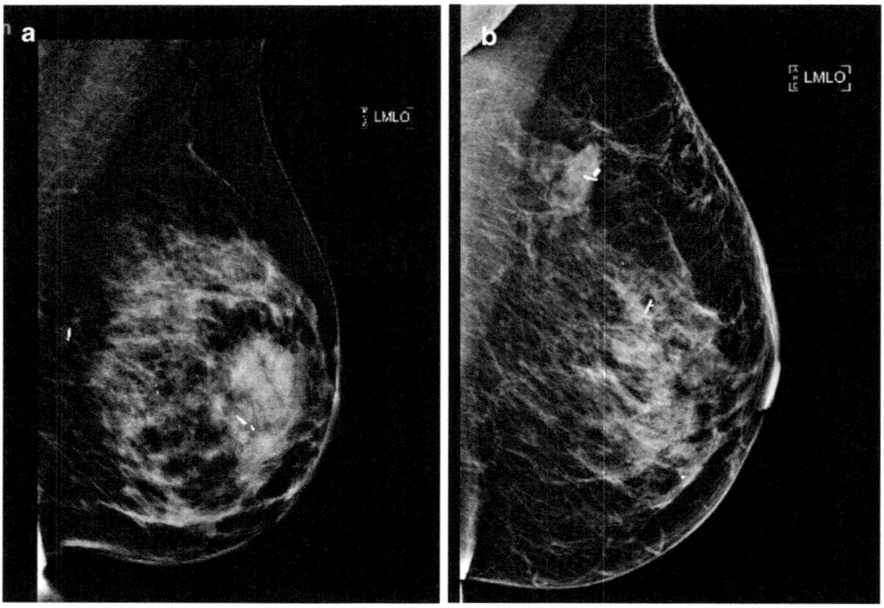

Fig. 10.4 (**a**) Extensive DCIS with multiple seeds, (**b**) Multifocal BC with multiple seeds

(Fig. 10.4b). Although the use of multiple wires is technically possible with WGL, using multiple ^{125}I-seeds is technically simpler and better tolerated by patients, as it has less discomfort and avoids restricted mobility associated with preventing wire displacement [7, 45, 48, 49].

Another major advantage lies in the radioisotope characteristics of Iodine-125. The ^{125}I-seed has a half-life of approximately 59.6 days, which allows the seed to be implanted up to 12 months before surgery. This characteristic makes RSL particularly valuable for patients undergoing neoadjuvant systemic treatment (NST). In these patients, placement of the seed prior to the treatment ensures that the lesion remains clearly identifiable throughout therapy and at the time of surgery. Even when the tumour reaches near or pathological complete response, becoming non-palpable and/or nearly invisible on conventional imaging, the seed provides reliable intraoperative guidance [29, 40, 41].

This extended half-life also improves logistical flexibility in surgical scheduling, unlike technetium-based localization. This requires same-day or near same-day procedural scheduling due to the short half-life of 6 h of technetium (Tc-99 m) [44].

A general technical challenge when using radionuclides is the ability to differentiate between different radioactive signals, when multiple types of radionuclides are used. This situation frequently occurs during BCS, as most patients eligible for BCS also receive a sentinel lymph node biopsy (SLNB). In such cases, the gamma probe must be able to differentiate the signal originating from the radioactive source in the breast and the Tc-99 m in the axilla used for SLNB.

Fortunately, differentiation between Iodium-125 and Tc-99 m is technically achievable. ^{125}I-seeds emit low-energy photons at approximately 35.5 keV, whereas Tc-99 m emits gamma photons at 140 keV [47, 50]. This difference allows reliable signal discrimination using dual-window gamma probes with appropriately calibrated thresholds. Clinical studies have demonstrated that dual-tracer use is both safe and effective when certain technical conditions are met, including correct energy-window configuration, the use of high-resolution gamma probes, and appropriate activity ratios [44, 47, 50]. These findings support the routine use of dual-tracer techniques in BCS when both tumour localization and sentinel node mapping are indicated.

Beyond localization of the primary breast lesion, RSL has also contributed to advances in axillary management. The ability to accurately mark and later retrieve a previously biopsy-proven metastatic axillary lymph node after NST has played an important role in the development of targeted axillary approaches, which support selective de-escalation of axillary surgery.

10.6 Radioactive Seed Localisation (RSL) in Axillary Nodes

Beyond its established role in breast-conserving surgery (BCS), ^{125}I-seeds have been increasingly applied to guide tailored axillary treatment following neoadjuvant systemic treatment (NST). With the ongoing improvement of NST efficacy, the number of patients achieving a pathological complete response (pCR) is rising, not only in the breast but also in the axilla. Following the shift from mastectomy to BCS, less invasive axillary techniques have been developed to assess nodal response after NST. This includes Marking the Axilla with Radioactive Iodine seeds (MARI) and the Targeted Axillary Dissection (TAD) [51, 52].

Within the MARI protocol, an ^{125}I seed with an activity typically ranging from 0.2 to 1.0 MBq is used. This activity is intentionally lower than the activity of seeds commonly applied for breast tumour localization (1.0–7.6 MBq), to limit radiation exposure to the more fragile axillary tissue. Prior to the start of NST in cN+ patients, the ^{125}I-seed is placed in the largest pathological proven tumour-positive axillary lymph node, classified as the MARI-node [9].

A treatment algorithm was developed to personalize axillary therapy based on the MARI procedure. Pre-NST staging with FDG-PET/CT stratifies patients according to the number of tumour-positive axillary lymph nodes (cALN<4 or cALN≥4). This is combined with the pathological status of the MARI node (ypMARI-negative or ypMARI-positve) (Fig. 10.5) [9]. Following these combined factors, patients with cALN<4 and a ypMARI-negative result receive no further axillary treatment. Those with cALN<4 and ypMARI-positive disease, as well as patients with cALN≥4 but ypMARI-negative disease, are treated with axillary radiotherapy (ART). Patients classified as cALN≥4 and ypMARI-positive undergo axillary lymph node dissection (ALND) followed by ART [9, 53, 54].

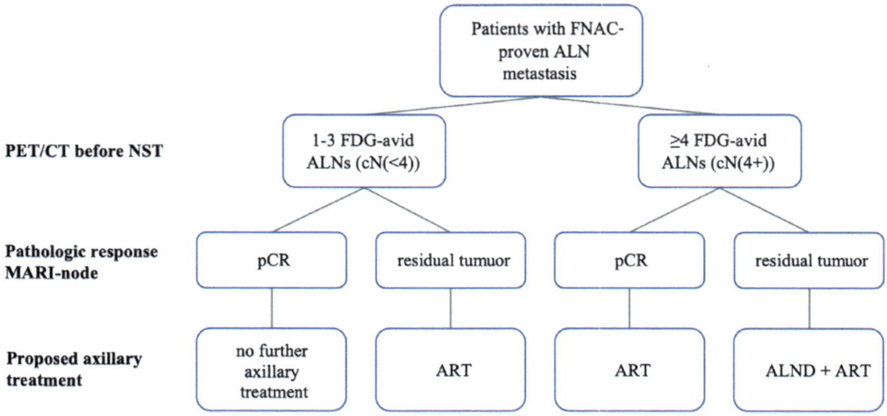

Fig. 10.5 MARI protocol treatment algorithm at the Netherlands Cancer Institute. FNAC, fine-needle aspiration cytology; ALN, axillary lymph node; PET/CT, positron emission tomography combined with computed tomography; MARI, marking axillary lymph nodes with radioactive iodine seeds; pCR, pathologic complete response; ALND, axillary lymph node dissection; ART, axillary radiotherapy

The MARI technique was first implemented in 2008 in the Netherlands Cancer Institute (NCI). Initial findings demonstrated that the procedure has a false negative rate (FNR) of 7% for predicting pCR in additional axillary nodes. When isolated tumour cells were classified as negative, consistent with definitions used in major sentinel lymph node trials, the FNR decreases to 4% [55]. Recent studies demonstrated that the MARI protocol is an effective staging and treatment algorithm, resulting in the omission of ALND in 80% of cN+ patients undergoing NST, while maintaining excellent 5-year invasive disease-free survival and overall survival in limited as well as extensive nodal disease [56–58].

An alternative approach involving marking an axillary node with an ^{125}I-seed is Targeted Axillary Dissection (TAD). In this technique, the biopsy-proven positive axillary node is marked with a conventional marker pre-NST, followed by placement of an ^{125}I-seed just prior to surgery. During surgery, the marked axillary node is removed, alongside a sentinel lymph node biopsy (SLNB). TAD shows a false negative rate of 4% [10]. This combined approach has also been validated in the Dutch RISAS trial, which demonstrated improved diagnostic accuracy after NST and supports the clinical application of TAD to reduce false-negative rates [59].

10.7 Radiation Risks

The ^{125}I-seed is a low-energy radioactive source. Its clinical application versus radiation toxicity has been extensively evaluated, demonstrating minimal radiation exposure to both patients and healthcare providers, while providing sufficient signal strength for accurate intraoperative detection [26, 46, 57]. A large retrospective cohort study involving 25.000 patients confirmed that radiation dose rates from RSL are low and do not pose a significant risk to patients or close contacts post-implantation [19, 46].

In pregnancy-related breast cancer, which has an increasing incidence of approximately 1 in 3.000 pregnancies [58, 60, 61], representing a relevant subgroup of BC patients, the use of ^{125}I-seeds for tumour localization remains controversial due to potential foetal radiation exposure.

Heeling et al. estimated foetal radiation exposure from ^{125}I-seeds, reporting a maximum dose of 11.6 mSv, which is well below 100 mSv set by the International Commission on Radiological Protection (ICRP) but exceeding the often clinically used 1 mSv. To keep foetal exposure below 1 mSv, they recommend removing the seed within 2 weeks of implantation after 26 weeks gestational age (GA), and within 1 week after 32 weeks GA [62]. A recent updated model shows substantially lower foetal doses, with a worst-case maximum of 1.6 mSv. This further supports the safe use of ^{125}I-seeds during pregnancy [63].

Postpartum, ^{125}I-seeds are often avoided due to concerns about infant exposure during breastfeeding or close contact. However, a recent study found that seed implantation allows for safe breastfeeding and close contact on the contralateral breast, regardless of the duration of implantation but with strict rules [64, 65]. When the ipsilateral breast is used, contact should be limited to a maximum of 5 h a day to keep radiation exposure below 1 mSv when the ^{125}I-seed will be removed within 14 days of implantation. For longer implantation periods, for example during NST, prolonged ipsilateral contact is not recommended [65]. Importantly, ^{125}I-seeds do not affect breast milk, and therefore pumped milk can be safely used throughout the implantation period [65, 66].

Continued efforts to minimize radiation exposure remain essential. Reducing seed activity in accordance with the ALARA (As Low As Reasonably Achievable) principle is a key strategy [19, 57]. While earlier studies reported activity levels of 3–12 MBq, a recent study reduced seed activity to 2.8 MBq without compromising detectability, enabled by improved knowledge of seed visibility and probe sensitivity [19]. Strict procedural safety is also critical. This includes accurate documentation at implantation, intraoperative verification of seed removal, and careful handling to prevent seed damage. Retrieved seeds must be stored in shielded containers and disposed through approved radioactive waste protocols. Robust tracking systems and clear communication are essential to ensure safety throughout the workflow [19, 64, 67].

10.8 Implementation of RSL in the Clinic: An Example

As discussed above, there are several clinically valuable applications of integrating ^{125}I-seeds into breast cancer management. Although ^{125}I-seeds are increasingly used for tumour localization due to improved surgical planning and reduced patient

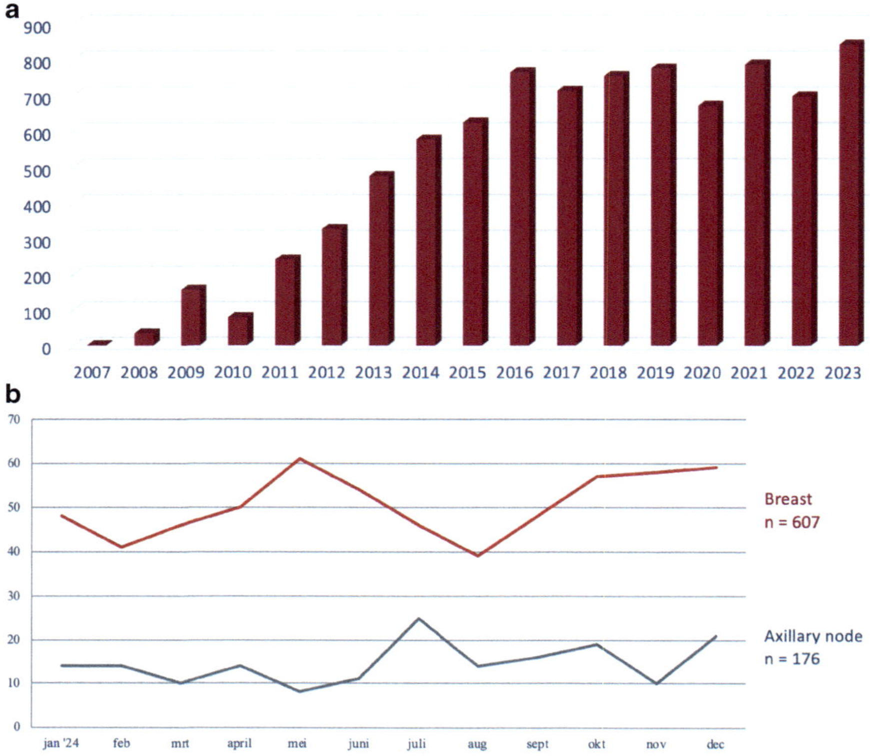

Fig. 10.6 (**a**) The total number of iodine seeds used for breast cancer care at the Netherlands Cancer Institute over the last 15 years is shown. (**b**) The total number of Iodine seeds used for breast cancer care at the Netherlands Cancer Institute in 2024 is shown. The green line represents the number of seeds placed in the breast, the blue line the number of seeds placed in an axillary node for the MARI procedure

discomfort, their use is often subject to strict regulations regarding handling and disposal of the seeds. This requires extensive protocols and administrative work, which may discourage people from starting this type of localization technique [44, 66]. However, the effort is worthwhile. These logistical challenges are most prominent during the early phase of implementation. Once workflows are established and multidisciplinary teams become familiar with the procedures, routine use becomes both feasible and efficient.

A practical illustration of this gradual implementation process is provided in Fig. 10.6a, b. At the Netherlands Cancer Institute, approximately 500–600 newly diagnosed breast cancer patients are treated annually. Since the introduction of RSL in 2008, we see that the total amount of ^{125}I seeds increases over the years (Fig. 10.6a). It also shows that full integration into routine clinical care requires approximately 5 years. Figure 10.6b further illustrates the distribution of seed use in 2024, for both breast and axilla.

A recent retrospective analysis by Miodownik et al., analysing 25.000 cases of RSL implant over 10 years, also observes a consistent upward trend of RSL implants annually in their included hospitals [19], which supports the earlier made statement that the effort of overcoming the first hassle is worthwhile.

10.9 Conclusion

Radioactive seed localization (RSL) using a ^{125}I-seed has become an increasingly popular technique to localize breast lesions and/or axillary lymph nodes.

The use of ^{125}I-seeds provide many clear advantages over other localization procedures used: (1) the point-source activity enables more precise tumour localization, improving incision planning and excision accuracy; (2) multiple seeds can be placed to bracket edges of extensive DCIS or to localize multifocal tumours; (3) it can be used in breast surgery as well as in axillary procedures like the MARI procedure; (4) its long half-life allows implantation up to months in advance, making it useful in patients receiving NST; (5) this extended half-life also provides greater flexibility in placement and surgical scheduling; (6) studies have demonstrated minimal radiation exposure to both patients, including pregnant women, and healthcare providers, provided that seed activity remains optimized and strict procedural protocols are followed; especially during pregnancy and in the postpartum period when being used in pregnancy-related BC.

In conclusion, radioactive seed localization (RSL) using an ^{125}I-seed provides a highly accurate, flexible, and safe method for the localization of breast and axillary lesions. This makes it a valuable and increasingly indispensable tool in the contemporary surgical management of breast cancer.

References

1. In 't Hout BA, Schenk KE, van der Linden AN, Roumen RM. Efficacy of localization of non-palpable, invasive breast cancer: wire localization vs. Iodine-125 seed: a historical comparison. Breast. 2016;29:8–13.
2. Hassing CMS, Tvedskov TF, Kroman N, Klausen TL, Drejøe JB, Tvedskov JF, Lambine TL, Kledal H, Lelkaitis G, Langhans L. Radioactive seed localisation of non-palpable lymph nodes – a feasibility study. Eur J Surg Oncol. 2018;44(5):725–30.
3. Dickhoff R, Peeters M-JV, Bosman PA, Alderliesten T. Therapeutic applications of radioactive sources: from image-guided brachytherapy to radio-guided surgical resection. Edizioni Minerva Medica. 2021;63(3):190–201. Gray RJ, Pockaj BA, Karstaedt PJ, et al. Radioactive seed localization of nonpalpable breast lesions is better than wire localization. Am J Surg. 2004;188:377–80
4. Al-Hilli ZGK, McLaughlin SA, Chan DM, Robinson KT, Giesbrandt JG, Slomka EL, Pizzitola VJ, Gray RJ, Jakub JW. Utilization of multiple I-125 radioactive seeds in the same breast is safe and feasible: a multi-institutional experience. Ann Surg Oncol. 2015;22(10):3350–5.

5. Luiten JD, Beek MA, Voogd AC, Gobardhan PD, Luiten EJ. Iodine seed- versus wire-guided localization in breast-conserving surgery for non-palpable ductal carcinoma in situ. Br J Surg. 2015;102(13):1665–9.
6. Janssen NNY, van la Parra RFD, Loo CE, Groen EJ, van den Berg MJ, Oldenburg HSA, Nijkamp J, Vrancken Peeters MTFD. Breast conserving surgery for extensive DCIS using multiple radioactive seeds. Eur J Surg Oncol. 2018;44(1):67–73.
7. Rebollo Aguirre AC, Fernández JF, Sánchez Sánchez R, Mendoza Arnau I, Rivas Navas DJ, Martínez Meca S. Radioguided surgery with iodine-125 seeds in breast cancer patients treated with neoadjuvant chemotherapy. Rev Esp Med Nucl Imagen Mol (Engl Ed). 2022;41(2):71–7.
8. Donker M, Straver ME, Wesseling J, Loo CE, Schot M, Drukker CA, et al. Marking axillary lymph nodes with radioactive iodine seeds for axillary staging after neoadjuvant systemic treatment in breast cancer patients: the MARI procedure. Ann Surg Oncol. 2015;261(2):378–82.
9. Caudle AS, Yang WT, Krishnamurthy S, Mittendorf EA, Black DM, Gilcrease MZ, et al. Improved axillary evaluation following neoadjuvant therapy for patients with node-positive breast cancer using selective evaluation of clipped nodes: implementation of targeted axillary dissection. J Clin Oncol. 2016;34:1072–8.
10. van Nijnatten TJA, Simons JM, Smidt ML, et al. A novel less-invasive approach for axillary staging after Neoadjuvant chemotherapy in patients with axillary node-positive breast cancer by combining Radioactive Iodine Seed Localization in the Axilla with the Sentinel Node Procedure (RISAS): a Dutch prospective multicenter validation study. Clin Breast Cancer. 2017;17:399–402.
11. van Dongen H, Voogd AC, Fentiman IS, Legrand C, Sylvester RJ, Tong D, van der Schueren E, Helle PA, van Zijl K. Long-term results of a randomized trial comparing breast-conserving therapy with mastectomy: European Organization for Research and Treatment of Cancer 10801 trial. J Natl Cancer Inst. 2001;5(2):211–2.
12. Van Riet YE, Maaskant AJG, Creemers GJ, et al. Identification of residual breast tumour localization after neo-adjuvant chemotherapy using a radioactive 125 Iodine seed. Eur J Surg Oncol. 2010;36:164.
13. Lovrics PJ, Goldsmith CH, Hodgson N, et al. A multicentered, randomized, controlled trial comparing radioguided seed localization to standard wire localization for nonpalpable, invasive and in situ breast carcinomas. Ann Surg Oncol. 2011;18:3407–14.
14. Hughes JH, Mason MC, Gray RJ, et al. A multi-site validation trial of radioactive seed localization as an alternative to wire localization. Breast J. 2008;14:153–7.
15. Gobardhan PD, de Wall LL, van der Laan L, et al. The role of radioactive iodine-125 seed localization in breast-conserving therapy following neoadjuvant chemotherapy. Ann Oncol. 2013;24:668–73.
16. Donker MDC, Valdés Olmos RA, et al. Guiding breast-conserving surgery in patients after neoadjuvant systemic therapy for breast cancer: a comparison of radioactive seed localization with the ROLL technique. Ann Surg Oncol. 2013;20:2569–75.
17. Alderliesten T, Loo CE, Pengel KE, et al. Radioactive seed localization of breast lesions : an adequate localization method without seed migration. Breast J. 2011;17:594–601.
18. Sung JS, King V, Thornton CM, et al. Safety and efficacy of radioactive seed localization with I-125 prior to lumpectomy and/or excisional biopsy. Eur J Radiol. 2013;82:1453–7.
19. Miodownik D, et al. Radioactive seed localization is a safe and effective tool for breast cancer surgery: an evaluation of over 25,000 cases. J Radiol Prot. 2024; https://doi.org/10.1088/1361-6498/ad246a.
20. Pouw B, van der Ploeg IMC, Muller SH, Valdés Olmos RA, Janssen-Pinkse LK, Oldenburg HS, Vrancken Peeters MT. Simultaneous use of an (125)I-seed to guide tumour excision and (99m)Tc-nanocolloid for sentinel node biopsy in non-palpable breast-conserving surgery. Eur J Surg Oncol. 2015;41(1):71–8.
21. Pavlicek W, Walton HA, Karstaedt PJ, Gray RJ. Radiation safety with use of I-125 seeds for localization of nonpalpable breast lesions. Acad Radiol. 2006;13:909–15.

22. Barentsz MW, van den Bosch MAAJ, Veldhuis WB, van Diest PJ, Pijnappel RM, Witkamp AJ, Verkooijen HM. Radioactive seed localization for non-palpable breast cancer. Br J Surg. 2013;100(5):582–8.
23. McGhan LJ, McKeever SC, Pockaj BA, Wasif N, Giurescu ME, Walton HA, Gray RJ. Radioactive seed localization for nonpalpable breast lesions: review of 1,000 consecutive procedures at a single institution. Ann Surg Oncol. 2011;18(11):3096–101.
24. Jakub JW, Gray RJ, Degnim AC, Boughey JC, Gardner M, Cox CE. Current status of radioactive seed for localization of non palpable breast lesions. Am J Surg. 2010;199(4):522–8.
25. Ahmed M, Douek M. Radioactive seed localisation (RSL) in the treatment of non-palpable breast cancers: systematic review and meta-analysis. Breast. 2013;22(4):383–8.
26. Dauer LT, Thornton C, Miodownik D, Boylan D, Holahan B, King V, Brogi E, Morrow M, Morris EA, Germain JS. Radioactive seed localization with 125I for nonpalpable lesions prior to breast lumpectomy and/or excisional biopsy: methodology, safety, and experience of initial year. Health Phys. 2013;105(4):356–65.
27. Gray RJ, Giuliano R, Dauway EL, et al. Radioguidance for nonpalpable primary lesions and sentinel lymph node(s). Am J Surg. 2001;2001(182):404–6.
28. Li JWL, Zhou J, Liu Y, Hu Y. Global evolution of breast cancer incidence in young women: an age–period–cohort analysis of GLOBOCAN data, 1990–2020. J Cancer Res Clin Oncol. 2025;151(2):465–74.
29. Zhang YYZ, Li J, Wang Y, Wang J, Liu J, et al. Global burden and trends of female breast cancer: a population-based study and forecast analysis from 2020 to 2035. Front Oncol. 2022;12:863282.
30. Cai YLY, Liu S, Zhang X, Zhang X, Liu Y, et al. The global burden of breast cancer among women of reproductive age from 1990 to 2019: a global burden of disease study. Sci Rep. 2025;15(1):883.
31. Bartelink H, Horiot JC, Poortmans P, Struikmans H, Van den Bogaert W, Barillot I, Fourquet A, Borger J, Jager J, Hoogenraad W, Collette L, Pierart M. Recurrence rates after treatment of breast cancer with standard radiotherapy with or without additional radiation. N Engl J Med. 2001;345(19):1378–87.
32. Clarke M, Collins R, Darby S, Davies C, Elphinstone P, Evans V, Godwin J, Gray R, Hicks C, James S, MacKinnon E, McGale P, McHugh T, Peto R, Taylor C, Wang Y. Effects of radiotherapy and of differences in the extent of surgery for early breast cancer on local recurrence and 15-year survival: an overview of the randomised trials. Lancet (London, England). 2005;366(9503):2087–106.
33. Farbera R, Marinovich ML, Pinnaa A, Houssamia N, McGeechana K, Barratta A, Bella KJL. Systematic review and meta-analysis of prognostic characteristics for breast cancers in populations with digital vs film mammography indicate the transition may have increased both early detection and overdiagnosis 2024. J Clin Epidemiol. 2024;171:111339.
34. Spronk PER, Volders JH, van den Tol P, Smorenburg CH, Vrancken Peeters M-JTFD. Breast conserving therapy after neoadjuvant chemotherapy; data from the Dutch Breast Cancer Audit. EJSO. 2018;45(2)
35. Volders JH, Negenborn VL, Spronk PE, Krekel NMA, Schoonmade LJ, Meijer S, Rubio IT, Petrousjka M, van den Tol. Breast-conserving surgery following neoadjuvant therapy-a systematic review on surgical outcomes. Breast Cancer Res Treat. 2018;168:1–12.
36. Lovrics PJ, Cornacchi SD, Vora R, Goldsmith CH, Kahnamoui K. Systematic review of radioguided surgery for non-palpable breast cancer. Eur J Surg Oncol. 2011;37(5):388–97.
37. Ahmed M, Douek M. Intra-operative ultrasound versus wire-guided localization in the surgical management of non-palpable breast cancers: systematic review and meta-analysis. Breast Cancer Res Treat. 2013;140(3)
38. Pleijhuis RG, Graafland M, de Vries J, Bart J, de Jong JS, van Dam GM. Obtaining adequate surgical margins in breast-conserving therapy for patients with early-stage breast cancer: current modalities and future directions. Ann Surg Oncol. 2009;16(10):2717–30.

39. Krekel NMA, Zonderhuis BM, Stockmann HBAC, Schreurs WH, van der Veen H, de Lange de Klerk ESM, Meijer S, van den Tol MP. A comparison of three methods for nonpalpable breast cancer excision. Eur J Surg Oncol. 2011;37(2):109–15.
40. Rahman RL, Puckett Y, Habrawi Z, Crawford S. A decade of intraoperative ultrasound guided breast conservation for margin negative resection – radioactive, and magnetic, and infrared oh my…. Am J Surg. 2020;220(6):1410–6.
41. Thind CR, Desmond S, Harris O, Nadeem R, Chagla LS, Audisio RA. Radio-guided localization of clinically occult breast lesions (ROLL): a DGH experience. Clin Radiol. 2005;60(6):681–6.
42. Moreno M, Wiltgen JE, Bodanese B, Schmitt RL, Gutfilen B, da Fonseca LMB. Radioguided breast surgery for occult lesion localization – correlation between two methods. J Exp Clin Cancer Res. 2008;27:27–9.
43. Tran VT, David J, Patocskai E, Zummo-Soucy M, Younan R, Lalonde L, Labelle M, El Khoury M, Robidoux A, Trop I. Comparative evaluation of Iodine-125 radioactive seed localization and wire localization for resection of breast lesions. Can Assoc Radiol J. 2017;68(4):447–55.
44. Sánchez Sánchez R, Jiménez ADG, Rebollo Aguirre AC, Mendoza Arnau I, Menjón Beltrán S, Vergara Alcaide ME, Osorio Ceballos JL, Llamas Elvira JM. 125I radioactive seed localization for non-palpable lesions in breast cancer. Rev Esp Med Nucl Imagen Mol (Engl Ed). 2019;38(6):343–7.
45. van der Noordaa ME, Pengel KE, Groen E, van Werkhoven E, Rutgers EJ, Loo CE, Vogel W, Vrancken Peeters MJ. The use of radioactive iodine-125 seed localization in patients with non-palpable breast cancer: a comparison with the radioguided occult lesion localization with 99m technetium. Eur J Surg Oncol. 2015;41(4):553–8.
46. Dixon J, Jasra B, Ankola A, Sharma S, Letter H. Bracketed radioactive seed localization for breast conservation surgery. Am Surg. 2020:86 90–94.
47. Kirstein LJ, Rafferty E, Specht MC, Moore RH, Taghian AG, Hughes KS, Gadd MA, Smith BL. Outcomes of multiple wire localization for larger breast cancers: when can mastectomy be avoided? J Am Coll Surg. 2008;207(3):342–6.
48. Cordiner CM, Litherland JC, Young IE. Does the insertion of more than one wire allow successful excision of large clusters of malignant calcification. Clin Radiol. 2006;61(8):686–90.
49. Straver ME, Loo CE, Alderliesten T, Rutgers EJT, Peeters MTFDV. Marking the axilla with radioactive iodine seeds (MARI procedure) may reduce the need for axillary dissection after neoadjuvant chemotherapy for breast cancer. Br J Surg. 2010;97(8):1226–31.
50. Donker M, Straver ME, Wesseling J, Loo CE, Schot M, Drukker CA, van Tinteren H, Sonke GS, Rutgers EJT, Peeters M-JTFDV. Marking axillary lymph nodes with radioactive iodine seeds for axillary staging after Neoadjuvant systemic treatment in breast cancer patients: the MARI procedure. Ann Surg Oncol. 2014;261(2):378–82.
51. Kuehn T, Bauerfeind I, Fehm T, Fleige B, Hausschild M, Helms G, Lebeau A, Liedtke C, von Minckwitz G, Nekljudova V, Schmatloch S, Schrenk P, Staebler A, Untch M. Sentinel-lymph-node biopsy in patients with breast cancer before and after neoadjuvant chemotherapy (SENTINA): a prospective, multicentre cohort study. Lancet Oncol. 2013;14(7):609–18.
52. van der Noordaa MEM, van Duijnhoven FH, Straver ME, Groen EJ, Stokkel M, Loo CE, et al. Major reduction in axillary lymph node dissections after Neoadjuvant systemic therapy for node-positive breast cancer by combining PET/CT and the MARI procedure. Ann Surg Oncol. 2018;25(6):1512–20.
53. Koolen BB, Donker M, Straver ME, van der Noordaa MEM, Rutgers EJT, Valdes Olmos RA, et al. Combined PET-CT and axillary lymph node marking with radioactive iodine seeds (MARI procedure) for tailored axillary treatment in node-positive breast cancer after neoadjuvant therapy. Br J Surg. 2017;104(9):1188–96.
54. A. Van Loevezijn, M.E.M. van der Noordaa,•F. van Duijnhoven,•E.J. Groen, M.P.M. Stokkel, C.E. Loo, P. Elkhuizen, N.S. Russell, M.J. Vrancken-Peeters. Tailored axillary treatment after neoadjuvant systemic therapy in clinically node-positive breast cancer patients is safe: 3-year follow-up of the MARI protocol. EJC Eur Breast Cancer Council 2020;138(Supplement 1), S3-S4.

55. van Hemert AKE, van Loevezijn AA, Baas M-SPD, Stokkel MPM, Groen E, Dezentje V, Loo CE, Sonke GS, Russell N, van Duijnhoven FH, Vrancken Peeters M-JTFD. Omission of axillary lymph node dissection in cN2-3 breast cancer patients with an excellent response on primary systemic treatment is safe; 4-year oncologic outcome of the MARI protocol. Breast. 2025;80:140411.
56. van Hemert AKE, van Loevezijn AA, Baas M-SPD, Stokkel MPM, Groen EJ, van der Noort V, Loo CE, Sonke GS, Russell N, van Duijnhoven FH, Vrancken Peeters M-JTFD. Response-guided axillary treatment in lymph node positive breast cancer treated with primary systemic therapy: 5-year follow-up of the MARI trial. JAMA Oncol. 11(10):1204–12.
57. Brost E, Prather A, Naik H, Jafari ME. Use of reduced activity seeds in breast radioactive seed localization. Health Phys. 2020;118(4):460–5.
58. Boere I, Lok C, Poortmans P, Koppert L, Painter R, Vd Heuvel-Eibrink MM, Amant F. Breast cancer during pregnancy: epidemiology, phenotypes, presentation during pregnancy and therapeutic modalities. Best Pract Res Clin Obstet Gynaecol. 2022;82:46–59.
59. López Allué M, et al. Image guided localization techniques for metastatic axillary lymph nodes in breast cancer; what radiologists should know. Insights Imaging. 2023;14(1):56.
60. Parazzini F, Franchi M, Tavani A, Negri E, Peccatori FA. Frequency of pregnancy related cancer: a population based linkage study in Lombardy, Italy. Int J Gynecol Cancer. 2017;27:613–9.
61. Stensheim H, Møller B, van Dijk T, Fosså SD. Cause-specific survival for women diagnosed with cancer during pregnancy or lactation: a registry-based cohort study. J Clin Oncol. 2009;27:45–51.
62. Heeling E, van de Kamer JB, Methorst M, Bruining A, van de Meent M, Vrancken Peeters MTFD, Lok CAR, van der Ploeg IMC. The safe use of 125I-seeds as a localization technique in breast cancer during pregnancy. Cancers (Basel). 2023;15(12):3229.
63. Pluim JME, van de Kamer JB, Heeling E, van der Ploeg IMC, Hulsen DJW. Assessing fetal radiation dose from iodine-125 seeds in pregnant breast cancer patients: an updated model. Phys Med Biol. 2025;70(3)
64. Goudreau SH, Joseph JP, Seiler SJ. Preoperative radioactive seed localization for nonpalpable breast lesions: technique, pitfalls, and solutions. Radiographics. 2015;35(5):1319–34.
65. Heeling E, van de Kamer JB, Bruining A, Pluim JME, Vrancken Peeters MJTFD, Lok CAR, van der Ploeg IMC. The safe use of 125I-seeds as a surgical localization technique for breast cancer patients during breastfeeding and close contact with an infant. Breast Cancer Res Treat. 2025;25(7):634–642.e4.
66. Bethesda (MD): National Institute of Child Health and Human Development: LactMed®; 2006 [updated 2021 jan 18. Available from: https://www.ncbi.nlm.nih.gov/books/NBK566932/.
67. Graham RP, Jakub JW, Brunette JJ, Reynolds C. Handling of radioactive seed localization breast specimens in the pathology laboratory. Am J Surg Pathol. 2012;36(11):1718–23.

Chapter 11
Localisation Using Radiofrequency Identification (RFID) Tags

Simon Lowes and Robert Milligan

Contents

11.1 Introduction

Radiofrequency identification (RFID) technology has been around a long time, and it was first reportedly used in aircraft during World War II. Today, it has a multitude of everyday uses, from tracking shipments and monitoring stock levels to contactless bank payments and microchipping pets.

The technology uses radiowaves to transmit information between a tag and a reader. The tag comprises two basic elements: a microchip, which contains data,

S. Lowes (✉) · R. Milligan
Northern Centre for Breast Research, Gateshead Health NHS Foundation Trust, Gateshead, Tyne and Wear, UK
e-mail: simon.lowes@nhs.net; robert.milligan@nhs.net

R. Vidya, N. Sharma (eds.), *Breast and Axilla Localisation Techniques*,
https://doi.org/10.1007/978-3-032-17995-1_11

and an antenna, which allows the microchip to be detected and read by the reader. Most RFID tags are passive, meaning that the energy source to activate and read the tag comes from the reader; the reader emits radiowaves at a given frequency, and when the tag is in range it responds by sending back its stored information. Passive RFID tags tend to be more in widespread day-to-day use, since they are small, cheap, and work over short ranges. Active RFID tags contain their own power source and are more suitable for longer range use.

Inevitably RFID technology has made its way into the healthcare setting, with a number of direct clinical applications. In surgery, it has been used to track surgical sponges [40], and in the breast setting, to track surgical instruments [36]. RFID tags are also used in certain breast implants to help assess implant position and diagnose complications such as displacements or rotation [32]. They are also now widely used to localise breast cancers and axillary nodes prior to surgery.

The current commercially available RFID system is the LOCalizer™, produced by Hologic®. The LOCalizer™ system comprises a cylindrical 10.6 × 2 mm passive RFID tag preloaded into a 12 G introducer needle, designed for percutaneous insertion into the breast (Fig. 11.1). The tags are encased in glass with a polypropylene cap, and are detected by a handheld reader, which gives a real-time distance measurement in millimetres between the detector and the tag, facilitating accurate localisation of the target lesion. Each tag carries a unique five-digit identification number, allowing discrimination between tags when multiple devices are inserted into the same breast. The handheld reader contains a built-in loop probe, which is suitable for tag detection during insertion and preoperative checks, but there is also a single-use pencil probe that attaches to the reader via a cable, which can be used for precise intraoperative localisation (Fig. 11.1). The probe is 8 mm in diameter and tapers to 7 mm at the tip. Tags can be inserted under either ultrasound or stereotactic guidance, and come in two needle lengths, 7 cm and 10 cm, for each use (Fig. 11.1).

Like other wire-free localisation devices, RFID tags can be inserted well in advance of the date of surgery, which has advantages for both the patient and the logistics of the breast service.

11.2 Evolution of the LOCalizer™ Technology

The LOCalizer system started life as an earlier technology developed by Health Beacons Inc., founded in January 2008 in California, USA [14]. The original tag reader was the TagFinder, and, like its successor, the LOCalizer reader, was battery-powered, operated at 134.2 kHz, and had two probe options, the loop reader and the pencil probe. In the earliest version of the TagFinder, the loop and pencil probes were both detachable and interchangeable, with the pencil probe attaching directly to the reader, with no extension cable [39]. A subsequent version of the TagFinder had the fixed loop reader and the detachable pencil probe with an extension cable [39], similar to the current LOCalizer reader. Both versions of the

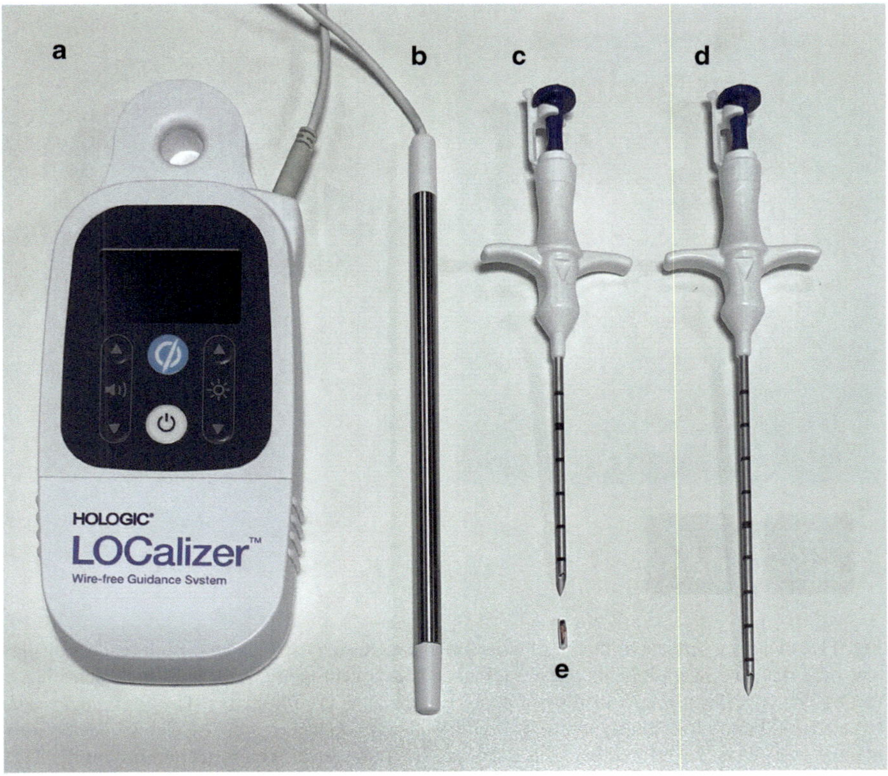

Fig. 11.1 LOCalizer system comprising tag reader with inbuilt loop probe (**a**), detachable pencil probe for intraoperative use (**b**), 7 and 10 cm introducers for ultrasound and stereotactic use, respectively (**c**, **d**), and RFID tag (**e**)

TagFinder had a Read button, which, when pressed, displayed the tag identification number ([39]; Fig. 11.2). The current LOCalizer reader displays the identification number automatically when the tag is in range. Both the TagFinder and LOCalizer reader display real-time proximity of the tag in millimetres on a liquid crystal display screen, though the TagFinder displays the distance on a scale, whereas the LOCalizer reader displays the distance numerically (Fig. 11.2). Both readers emit an audible signal that changes in pitch with proximity. The fixed loop probe detects tags at depths up to 60 mm, and the pencil probes detects tags at up to 30 mm.

A proof of concept study using the TagFinder was carried in breast phantoms, as well as in pieces of chicken breast and hotdog, to evaluate detectability at different depths, and discrimination of multiple tags placed next to one another [39]. This tested two tag sizes, differing in length only (8 and 12 mm), and both requiring a 12 G introducer. At three depths tested (10 mm, 20 mm, and 30 mm), three operators blinded to the tag positions within chicken breast were able to accurately ascertain the depth of each tag. Overall, there was no clear difference between the 8 and

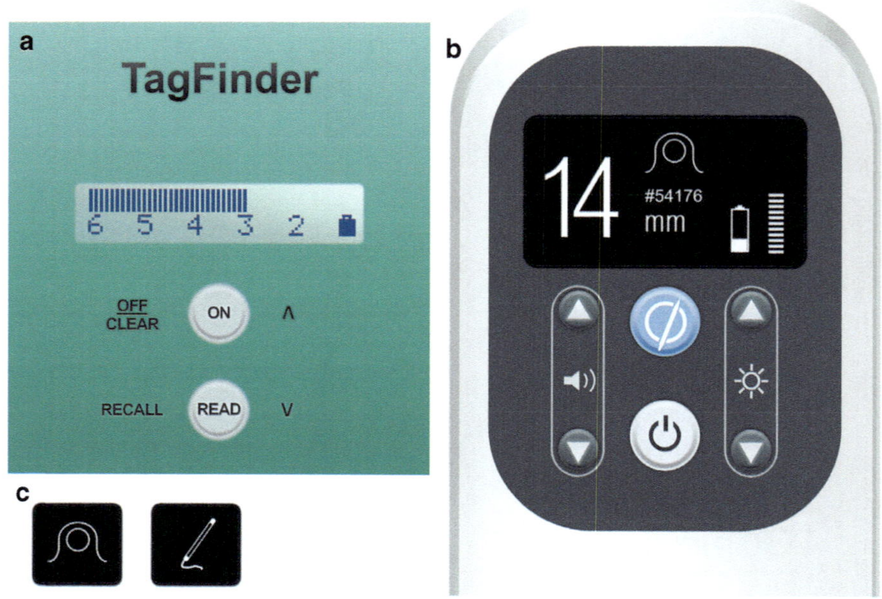

Fig. 11.2 Display screens of the Tag Finder (**a**) and LOCalizer (**b**) readers. Both readers display real-time distance in millimetres. The TagFinder uses a centimetre scale with millimetre increments. The LOCalizer reader displays a numerical distance in millimetres. The TagFinder reader has a READ button for identifying the 5-digit tag ID number, whereas the LOCalizer device automatically displays the ID number of the tag that is in closest proximity (# number on display). When the pencil probe is unattached, the LOCalizer reader defaults to the loop detector setting, which is displayed by the loop icon (**c**; left icon). When the pencil probe is attached, the reader switches to the pencil probe setting (**c**; right icon). The blue button on the handheld reader (**b**) allows toggling between the two detectors when the pencil probe is attached. (Diagram of TagFinder re-created based on a photograph of the device from Dauphine et al. [9]; diagram of LOCalizer based on current device)

12 mm tags. Because of the structure of the tags, their orientation impacts signal strength, with the strongest signal received when the reader is at the longitudinal ends of the tag, and relatively minimal signal over the tag's centre [39]. This has some influence on the ability to discriminate between multiple tags in the specimen when they lie close to one another. When two adjacent tags are oriented horizontally, the minimum distance between the two tags at which the two identification numbers are easily discernible is 20 mm, and when they are oriented vertically it is 30 mm [39]. However, the tags can be differentiated at distances as low as 5 mm apart, though this is not as easily reproducible [39]. In clinical practice, it is extremely unlikely that two tags would ever need to be placed in such close proximity.

The authors also tested the tags in a silicone breast phantom in a 1.5 T commercial MRI system and found the 12 mm tags gave a low signal intensity artefact up to 32 mm [39], and according to the current manufacturer's data sheet, the tags are MR

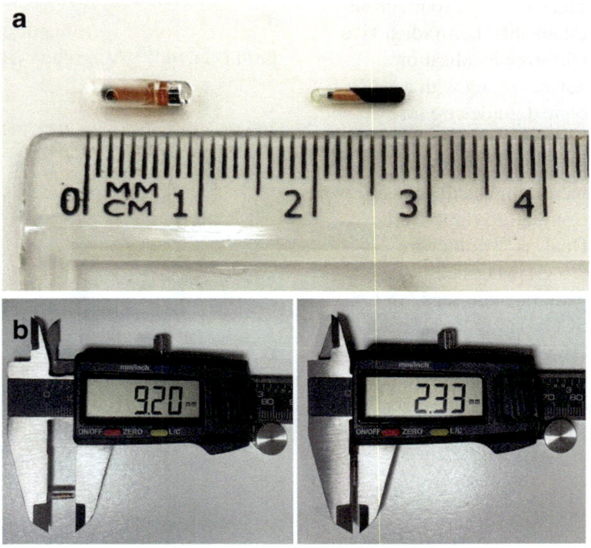

Fig. 11.3 Dimensions of the LOCalizer tag. Panel **a** shows a LOCalizer (left) next to a typical pet tag (right). Panel **b** shows the tag measured using electronic callipers; left image shows length, right image shows width

conditional for clinical use; in our own clinical experience, the tags are MRI safe and produce an artefact of approximately 35 mm in a 1.5 T MRI scanner [24]. Like other localisation devices, the RFID tags are radio-opaque, allowing visualisation on post-insertion mammography and on excised surgical specimens.

Although the manufacturer's specifications of the current LOCalizer tag are 10.6 × 2 mm, our own testing with an electronic calliper shows this consistently as 9.2 × 2.3 mm (Fig. 11.3; the tag is also shown alongside a commercially available pet RFID tag, which measures 8.2 × 1.2 mm). In terms of needle gauge, the LOCalizer tags are the largest of all commercially available wire-free devices (Fig. 11.4 and Table 11.1). This can present some challenges in device deployment, which is discussed later.

11.3 Tag Insertion

11.3.1 Localisation Planning

Where possible we aim to have a planning session for all localisations requested by the surgical team. This usually takes place at the beginning of the week and involves at least two radiologists. This involves a review of the patients' imaging, histology, and multidisciplinary team meeting outcomes, to ensure that all patients have the correct and optimal localisation procedure, and any questions or unexpected additional findings can be dealt with before the procedure. An example of our planning sheet is given in Fig. 11.5. The same sheet is completed at the time of the localisation procedure and scanned into PACS for viewing by the surgical team.

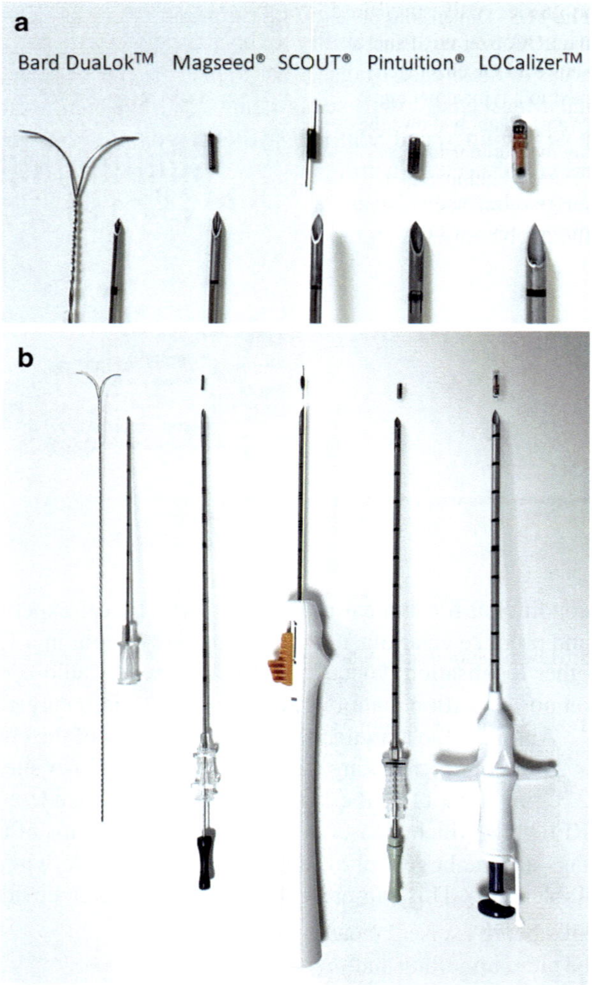

Fig. 11.4 The four current established non-radioactive wire-free localisation devices along with a typical guidewire for comparison. Introducers are arranged with increasing needle gauge from left to right: Bard DuaLok™ guidewire (20 G), Magseed® paramagnetic seed (18 G), SCOUT® radar reflector (16 G), Pintuition® permanent magnetic seed (14 G), and LOCalizer™ RFID tag (12 G)

Table 11.1 Device sizes and introducer gauges. Stated sizes refer to those freely available from the manufacturer/supplier. Measured size refers to our measurements using electronic callipers

Device	Type	Stated size (mm)	Measured size (mm)	Introducer gauge
Bard Dualok™	Guidewire	–	–	20
^{125}I seeds	Radioactive seed	4.5 × 0.8	–	18
Magseed®	Paramagnetic seed	5 × 1	5.0 × 0.9	18
SCOUT®	Radar reflector	12 × 1.6	12.2 × 1.3	16
Pintuition®	Magnetic seed	5 × 1.4	5.2 × 1.7	14
LOCalizer™	RFID tag	10.6 × 2	9.2 × 2.3	12

Localisation for Breast Surgery

Patient name.. Date of surgery......../......../20.......

Date of birth......................... Hosp. ID .... Surgeon...............................

Insertion planning: Reviewed by................................ on: ..../......../20....... No. tags.......... Ultrasound ☐ Stereo ☐

Right ☐ Left ☐ Biopsy result(s): **Site 1**......... **Site 2**........ **Site 3**......... **Axilla** .... Checklist: ICE ☐ MDM ☐ PACS ☐

Comments.. Device: GW ☐ Tag ☐ SCOUT ☐ Pin☐

....

....

....

Tag ID: Site 1 **Site 2** **Site 3** **Axilla**

....

Insertion date ..../......../20...... Inserted by.......... Check XR? ☐ Right ☐ Left ☐ Radiographer.......... (check XR)

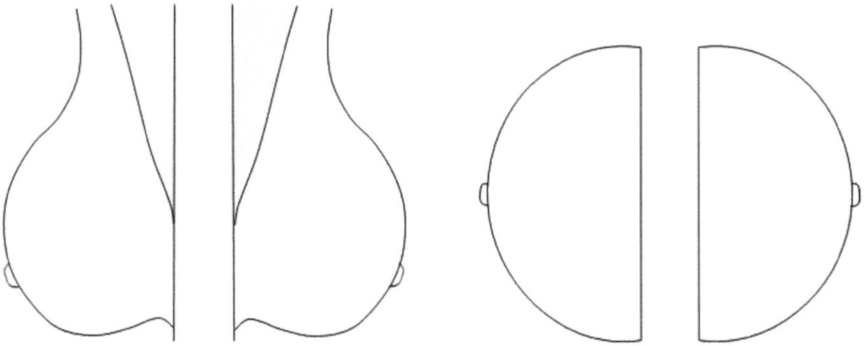

Local anaesthesia...

Localisation method: Stereo ☐ Ultrasound ☐

Depth skin to tag on US using tag reader (mm)

Site 1 .... **Site 2** .... **Site 3** ....

Comments...

....

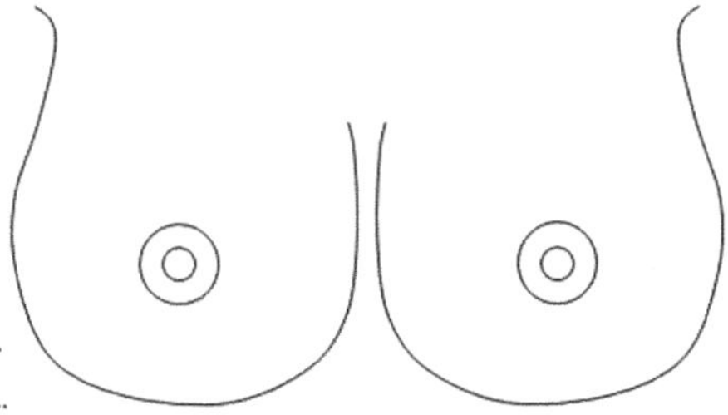

....

....

....

Fig. 11.5 Tag insertion sheet. Pre-localisation planning is documented at the top of the sheet. Details of the tag insertion are documented below at the time of the procedure. Diagrams of both breasts allow annotation of the position of the tag(s), or other localisation devices, relative to the lesion(s) and marker clip(s) based on the post-procedure mammograms. A further clinical diagram of the breasts (bottom right) is used to indicate the approximate position of the device(s) to aid preoperative device detection using the reader in the operating department

11.3.2 Insertion Technique

Insertion is the same in principle to all other localisation devices. As mentioned, RFID tags can be inserted using either ultrasound or stereotactic guidance, with the 7 cm introducer used for ultrasound-guided insertions and the 10 cm introducer used for stereotactic insertions. Once the patient is suitably positioned and the target identified, the skin is prepared using a topical antiseptic solution. A small volume of local anaesthetic (typically 1% lidocaine) is infiltrated into the skin and deeper tissues around the site of the lesion (Fig. 11.6). A small incision of a few millimetres is made in the anaesthetised skin, and the introducer needle is passed through the incision and into the target under image guidance (Fig. 11.6). Once deployed, post-procedure mammograms are done to confirm position, and to serve as a guide for

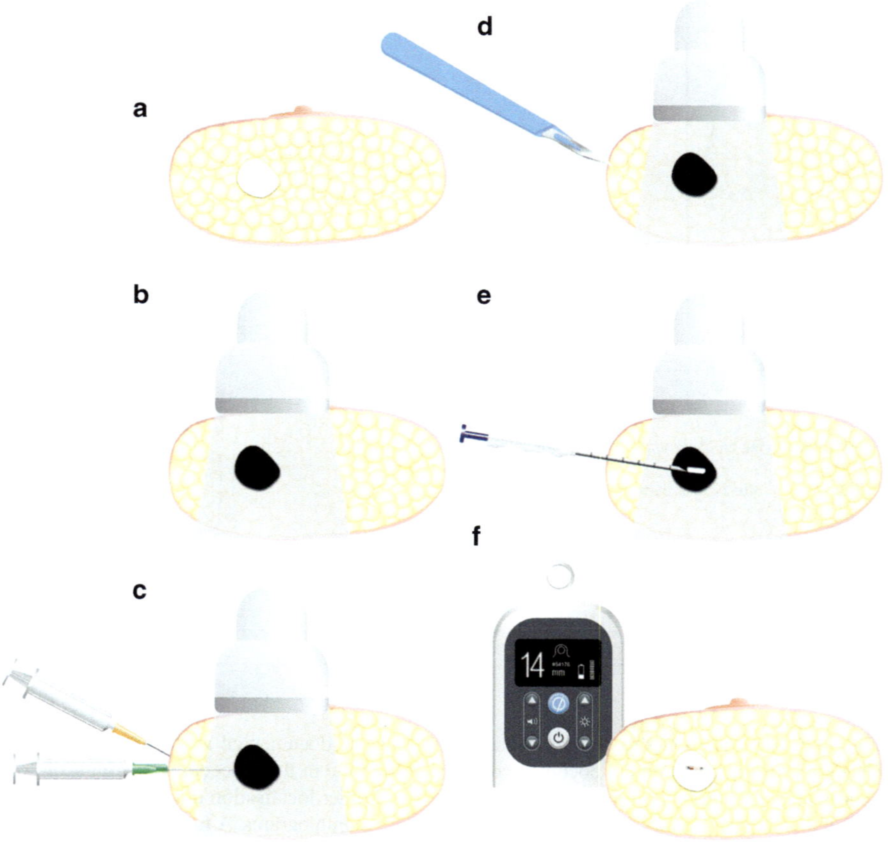

Fig. 11.6 Principles of ultrasound-guided RFID tag insertion. (**a**) Depiction of tumour in breast. (**b**) The tumour is identified using ultrasound. (**c**) After preparing the skin with antiseptic solution, local anaesthetic is infiltrated into the skin and then into the deeper tissues around the target site. (**d**) A small incision is made in the skin to facilitate passage of the introducer needle. (**e**) The introducer is passed into the tumour and the tag is deployed. (**f**) The tag is detectable using the hand-held reader

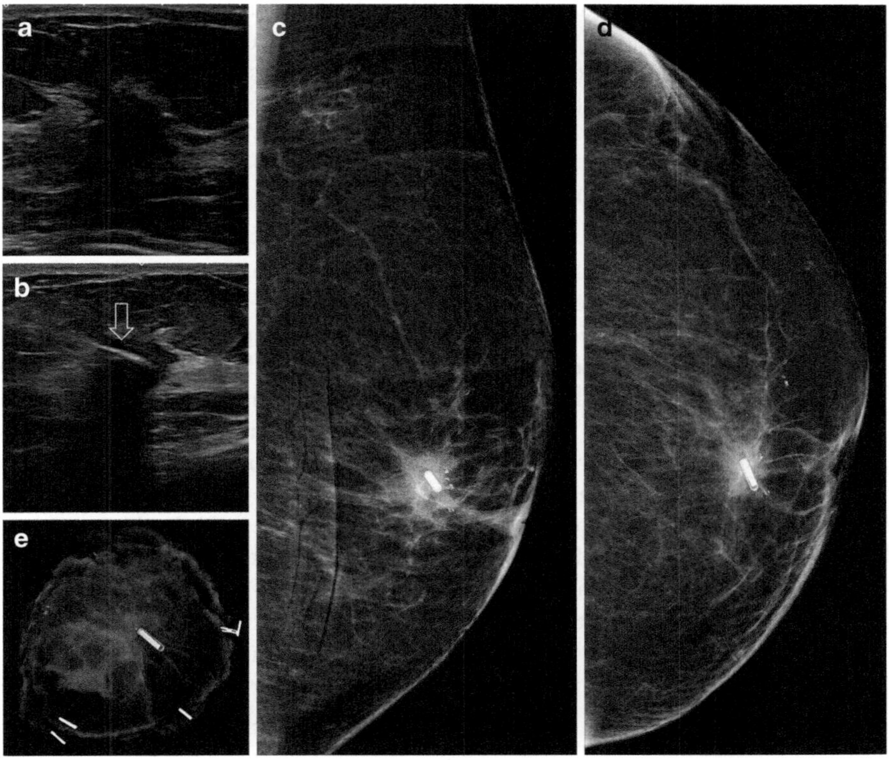

Fig. 11.7 Images from an ultrasound-guided tag insertion. Panel (**a**) shows the target lesion on ultrasound, in this case a mass, pre-tag insertion. (**b**) shows the same lesion post-tag insertion (open white arrow points to the tag). Post-procedure mediolateral oblique (**c**) and craniocaudal (**d**) mammograms show the tag within the mass. Panel (**e**) is the specimen radiograph showing the excised mass containing the tag

the surgical team (Fig. 11.7). The procedure is documented on our tag planning sheets (Fig. 11.5), including annotations of the post-procedure mammograms and any relevant comments. As well as documenting the position of the tag(s), lesions(s), and clips(s) on the mammography diagrams, the approximate position of the tag is also drawn on a clinical diagram of the breasts to assist in locating the tag (Fig. 11.5).

It is possible to insert multiple lesions into the same breast, either for targeting more than one tumour, or for bracketing larger areas, such as contiguous multifocal areas of invasive disease or fields of microcalcification [23]. In our experience, placing the tags closer than 30 mm apart is best avoided because of the potential risk of the tags being in such proximity to one another that the reader is unable to distinguish between the two tags. In any such cases, a single tag is usually sufficient to localise areas of this size [23].

Although the LOCalizer is licensed for use only in the breast, there is a good body of evidence to indicate the tags are safe and effective for use in targeting axillary nodes [24]. The principles of insertion are the same as for the breast and, as with any axillary intervention, care should be taken to avoid major vascular structures, something that is routine for experienced ultrasound operators. In any case, in practice, many nodes that are localised for targeted axillary dissection (TAD) are low-lying in the axilla and some distance from major axillary vessels [24].

11.4 Surgical Excision

Excision of breast lesions localised with the LOCalizer tags is typically a simple procedure, although there are some considerations that may differ from other localisation techniques. Prior to incision, with the patient laying supine and ipsilateral arm abducted in an non-sterile environment, the handheld reader, using the loop detector, should be used to identify the approximate location of the RFID tag within the breast. This can help to ensure the patient has optimal incision placement to remove the lesion and preserve breast cosmesis. It is incredibly rare for the surgeon to be unable to locate the tag at this stage, although this has been reported when the tag is lodged deep in the breast beneath very dense tissue [33]. In this case, it is recommended to use the reader in various positions across the breast, while manipulating the tissue to identify the position of the tag, guided by post tag insertion mammograms. Once the patient has been prepared for surgery, with sterile drapes applied, the location of the lesion should be checked again with the sterile pencil probe, after the handheld reader has been placed in a sterile cover, to confirm the exact location of the lesion, and a final decision on surgical incision is made. The superficial dissection of the parenchyma of the subcutaneous fat is performed in the mastectomy plane, taking care to be gentle with tissue handling to avoid dislodgement of the RFID tag. Once this dissection has been completed, the pencil probe is again used to identify the location of the RFID tag. This is done by stretching and flattening the superficial breast tissue, between the index and middle finger, with the probe held at 90 degrees to the surface of the breast tissue. A suture or ink mark should be placed on the breast tissue superficial to the RFID tag at the point with the lowest distance measurement between the RFID tag and probe, as indicated on the handheld reader. This allows the location of the tumour and tag to be marked in the possible event of RFID tag dislodgement. The breast excision is then performed. It is not generally necessary to use the probe to identify the RFID tag placement during further dissection of the breast tissue, nor to assess excision margins. In some cases where the surgeon is unsure of the position of the lesion within the excision sample, further checking of the position of the tag may be necessary. Where multiple RFID tags are used, the surgeon should place a suture or ink mark above each tag, and the unique identification number of the tag should be noted and correlated with the preoperative imaging and radiology tag insertion notes (Fig. 11.5). Once the specimen is removed, the surgeon should check with the probe that the tag is contained within the excised specimen. This can be further confirmed on intraoperative specimen radiograph assessment, and the resection margins checked both clinically and radiographically. In the event the tag has dislodged and is not in the excised tissue, the surgeon should use the probe to identify the position of the tag, which would typically be found in the excision cavity or on the surgical drapes. If the surgeon is unable to locate the tag in these places, then they should check the diathermy suction tube with the probe. Once the tag has been located, it may be discarded in the clinical waste. The procedure is then routinely completed with closure of the parenchymal defect following mobilisation of the tissues.

11.5 The LOCalizer System in Clinical Practice

11.5.1 A Brief Chronology of 'Firsts'

The first study in humans was conducted by the original developers of the system, evaluating the TagFinder device in 20 patients [9]. On the morning of surgery, each patient underwent insertion of a guidewire to the lesion, immediately followed by deployment of an RFID tag at the same target. Twelve underwent ultrasound localisation, and 8 stereotactic. The study excluded patients where the lesion was deeper than 60 mm from the skin when lying supine, though in practice none met this exclusion criterion. During surgery, the RFID tag was the primary method used by the operating surgeon to localise each lesion for excision, with the guidewire serving as backup in the event case of tag migration or failed localisation. Of the 20 patients, 15 had malignant lesions and 5 had non-malignant lesions containing atypical hyperplasia. All 20 lesions were successfully removed using the RFID tag as guidance, with no localisation failures. There were no cases of tag migration before incision, but in three cases, migration occurred along the insertion track as the lesion was being retracted with fingers to make the final cut along the deep surface of the specimen. In a separate case, the guidewire had been dislodged after being noted in the correct position on post-insertion mammograms. It was also found that interaction with electrocautery did not disrupt or destroy the signal of the tags. Of the 15 patients with malignancy, 4 required re-excision of a positive margin; however, additional cancer was not found in the re-excision specimens. There were no postoperative infections occurring within 30 days in any of the 20 patients [9].

Following the early experience of TagFinder system, a number of small studies in patients emerged, all subsequently using the LOCalizer system. DiNome et al. [11], based in California, USA, conducted the first study to evaluate the use of the RFID system in lieu of guidewires, inserting tags into 50 women, 33 of whom had breast cancer, and 17 with non-malignant pathology. In this cohort, all had tags alone (no simultaneous guidewire insertion), and these were inserted for an average of 1.4 days prior to surgery (range 0 to 14 days). At the time of the study (August 2017–January 2018), the LOCalizer tags were licensed for insertion up to 30 days prior to surgery [11], whereas currently there is no upper time limit provided there is intent to excise the tagged lesion. All 50 patients underwent successful placement and retrieval of the tag, with 1 of the 33 cancer cases having a positive margin on final pathology, and 2 of 33 undergoing re-excision for a close or positive margin

[11]. Patients were given a Likert-style questionnaire shortly after tag insertion, and most agreed or strongly agreed (94%) that the procedure went smoothly, and agreed or strongly agreed (78%) that the procedure was easier than expected. Radiologists and surgeons also indicated that the RFID system was as fast and reliable as guidewire-localised procedures [11].

Malter et al. [26], based in Germany, subsequently published the first reported use of the LOCalizer system in Europe, carried out in early 2019, though the cohort comprised just four patients, all with benign lesions. All tags were successfully retrieved, and all surgeons were positive about using the LOCalizer method.

McGugin et al. [30] from the USA then published a dataset of 147 LOCalizer cases from January–October 2018, which were compared against 356 guidewire cases from April–December 2016. This was the first study to compare the LOCalizer against guidewires. Of the 147 tag cases, 94 were invasive or in situ breast cancers, and 53 were atypia or other lesions (fibroepithelial lesions, papillary lesions, and imaging abnormalities). The data indicated non-inferiority of the LOCalizer compared to guidewires, with no significant difference in re-excision rates between the two techniques (19.1% versus 16.8%, respectively) [30].

The first use of the LOCalizer in the UK commenced in June 2019, published initially as a conference abstract involving 39 tags in 36 patients [20], and shortly afterwards as a larger complete dataset of 177 tags in 150 patients [23]. All cases were breast cancers, and all patients underwent breast-conserving surgery. Tags were inserted a mean 7.8 days prior to surgery (median 6, range 0–71). The vast majority of tags (173/177) were inserted under ultrasound guidance, the remaining 4 under stereotactic. The lesions comprised mostly masses (142/177), with the remaining lesions comprising microcalcification, vacuum-assisted biopsy (VAB) cavities following stereotactic biopsies, distortion of architecture, and clipped tumour beds following complete radiological response to neoadjuvant chemotherapy (NAC). In addition, in six women, biopsy-proven, clipped, metastatic axillary nodes were localised for targeted axillary dissection, and in one case a metastatic intramammary node was also targeted. Of the 150 women, 145 had tags to one breast only; 126 of these women had a single tag to a single lesion, and the others either had multiple tags to multiple lesions in the breast (± axilla), or in the case of two women, single tags to localise two adjacent lesions. Four of the 150 women had tags to both breasts (± axilla), and one woman had only a single tag insertion to localise an axillary node [23].

All tags were located and retrieved successfully, and there were no reported difficulties discriminating between different tag sites in the same breast. Thirteen patients underwent further surgery for involved radial margins where improvement was deemed feasible, equating to a re-excision rate of 8.7% per patient. Of these, ten had further margin excision and three had completion mastectomy. None of the cases of margin involvement/re-excision were attributed to the localisation technique, and there were no peri- or post-operative complications related to tag use. Although all tags were retrieved successfully, it was however reported on occasions that tags deployed to lesions superficially within the breast were often visible on intraoperative dissection, and though this did not compromise excision, it potentially places them at risk of becoming dislodged or lost; to mitigate this in the future it was recommended to deploy tags immediately deep to superficial lesions [23].

Using the LOCalizer tags to target axillary nodes in this study was thought to be the first worldwide description of this off-licence indication, but in parallel a paper from Germany showed successful use in ten patients [27]. Thus, although tags are not licensed for use in the axilla, early findings suggested this application safe and effective. This is important, because with the increasing use of targeted axillary dissection (TAD), having a single localisation device for use in both the breast and axilla is critical.

This cluster of publications over a relatively short period of time following the introduction of the LOCalizer showed not only increasing adoption of RFID tags in different parts of the world, but also increasing complexity of use. Inevitably, as adoption continued to grow, more data followed.

11.5.2 Larger Datasets and Multicentre Studies

The largest published single-centre dataset comprises a retrospective review of 1013 tags in 848 patients [19]. Unlike in most other datasets, the majority of tags (66.4%) were placed under mammographic guidance, the remainder (33.6%) using ultrasound. Most patients (84.6%) underwent localisation on the day of surgery; of those that had their localisations prior to the day of surgery, the median number of days beforehand was 3 (range 1–188). A total of 699 of the 848 patients (82.4%) had a single tag deployed, and 149 (17.6%) had more than one tag. Where multiple tags were inserted, the minimum distance apart was 20 mm. Technically, accurate placement (defined as within 10 mm of the edge of the target) was achieved for 1004 of 1013 tags (99.1%). Of the nine that were not accurately placed, seven required an additional tag or guidewire to localise the target lesion. Furthermore, in 7 of the 1004 accurately placed tags, there were some additional challenges with insertion, involving displacement or removal or the marker clip, which although did not ultimately compromise the accuracy of placement, were regarded as complications, giving overall success rate of 98.4% (997/1013). All complications happened when tags were placed under mammographic guidance. Indications for tag placement were predominantly malignancy (66.6%, both invasive and in situ), with the remainder made up of high risk (B3) lesions (28.5%), benign discordant lesions (1.5%), and benign lesions (1.3%). All but one of the 848 patients underwent surgical excision (one patient developed metastatic disease negating surgery); in all 847 cases undergoing surgery, the targets were successfully excised. Of those with a preoperative diagnosis of malignancy, 15.1% had positive or close margins requiring re-excision, which was deemed comparable to previous data from guidewires and other localisation devices available at the time [19].

In the same year, a systematic review of all published evaluations of the LOCalizer™ tags was carried out [44], analysing data from nine available studies at the time, incorporating the six dataset discussed above, and further three published datasets, in which the LOCalizer had been used in between 10 and 69 patients [7, 21, 46]. This gave a cumulative total of 1344 tags in 1151 patients, with a pooled deployment rate of 99.1%, retrieval rate of 100%, and an overall re-excision rate of 13.9% [44].

A number of other papers documenting single-centre experiences have subsequently been published, with the number of patients ranging from 123 to 445 per centre, all reporting positive clinical outcomes associated with the LOCalizer [1, 2, 8, 25, 34, 42].

The largest published multicentre dataset involving the LOCalizer was conducted by the iBRA-NET localisation group in the UK [13]. This was a retrospective study evaluating localisation of unilateral, unifocal lesions less than 50 mm in size, excluding patients having two separate lumpectomies, those with larger tumours, and those having a therapeutic mammoplasty or volume replacement with lipofilling or perforator flap. The analysis comprised 1109 patients who had undergone RFID-guided localization, recruited from 24 UK breast units. A further 1170 patients were used in a comparator cohort who had undergone guidewire localisation as part of a previously published analysis by the same group [10]. In cases of malignancy, the lesion was present in the excision specimen in 97.9% (951/971) of LOCalizer cases, compared to 99.1% (1150/1161) in the guidewire cohort, though not statistically significant [13]. There was no difference in specimen weight between the cohorts, and the positive margin rate of the main excision specimen was 11.2% for the LOCalizer and 15% for guidewires, with a re-excision rate of 15% for the LOCalizer excisions and 13.2% for guidewire excisions, again not statistically significant. There were, however, significantly more routine cavity shaves in the guidewire cohort (64.5%) than the LOCalizer group (48.3%) [13].

The largest axillary dataset is from a retrospective UK-based study involving the first 75 consecutive axillary node localisations [24]. Seventy of the 75 (93%) had a primary breast cancer, and five (7%) had no known breast cancer but had an abnormal node targeted for diagnostic excision. Of the 70 with breast cancer, 20 (29%) had undergone NAC. Tag deployment was deemed successful in all cases, and all tags and their respective nodes were excised successfully at surgery with no significant complications. There were four reported cases of tag dislodgement during excision, but, overall, this did not compromise retrieval of the tag or the node [24].

11.5.3 Margin Assessment and Re-excision Rates

Most datasets on tag use focus on accuracy of localisation and rates of surgical retrieval. As a primary outcome measure this makes sense; not only does it assess the primary function of localisation devices, it is straightforward to gauge success against an expected standard of 100% accuracy and 100% retrieval. As described above, another metric used to measure the clinical effectiveness of localisation devices is margin assessment and re-excision rates. Although on face value this is a useful surrogate for comparing the effectiveness of different localisation techniques, both are complicated by multiple factors. The heterogeneity of breast cancer means that disease extent is not always entirely predictable preoperatively, with some disease occult on imaging, even when supplemental modalities such as MRI are used. Invasive lobular carcinoma and non-calcifying ductal carcinoma in situ are just two examples, but unexpected additional disease can be found in all histological subtypes. There is also variation in clinical practice around the world, with different definitions of what constitutes close or positive margins [38], as well as controversy as to how these should be managed [4, 15, 45]. Different oncoplastic techniques will also influence other variables such as excised tissue volume.

Because of these factors, together with restricted sample size of datasets in many of the published studies to date, it is sometimes not feasible to correct fully for even the commonest variables when comparing localisation methods, necessitating pooling of data from all cases using a particular localisation technique, irrespective of disease size, histology, and oncoplastic procedure. Furthermore, there are at present very few studies that directly compare different techniques within the same centre contemporaneously, meaning that data from one localisation technique are often compared with data from another technique from a different centre or from within the same centre but from a different time frame, when other variables such as different personnel or levels of experience may contribute to heterogeneity. This can be in part mitigated by large multicentre datasets, such as those produced by the iBRA-NET localisation group, with data so far published for Magseed [10] and LOCalizer [13], both compared against a large cohort of guidewire localisations in unifocal lesions. It is anticipated that similar datasets will be published for SCOUT and Pintuition in due course; national audits for both devices have been open recently. Therefore, interpretation of positive margin rates and re-excision needs consideration of multiple potentially confounding factors.

With these caveats accepted, the range of positive margin and re-excision rates in the LOCalizer studies described above compare favourably with national re-excision rates, which based on a cohort of over 55,000 patients across the UK, average 20% [16]. In the small number of LOCalizer studies that include guidewires as a comparator, the LOCalizer shows statistical non-inferiority in all studies in terms of positive margin and re-excision rates [8, 13, 30, 42].

Using published positive margin and re-excision rates, the LOCalizer also compares favourably against other wire-free devices. In their LOCalizer study, Lamb et al. [19] reported that 15.1% of patients had close or positive margins requiring re-excision, whereas in an earlier study involving Magseed by the same authors, 21.9% had close or positive margins requiring re-excision [18]. In the iBRA-NET Magseed study, the re-excision rate was 12.3% in a cohort of 707 patients undergoing surgery for unifocal lesions [10].

Stephens et al. [42] published a cohort of 777 patients comparing the LOCalizer, ^{125}I radioactive seeds, and guidewires. Although there were no statistically significant differences in positive margins and re-excision rates between the three devices, the LOCalizer was associated with a higher specimen volume and device-to-specimen edge distance relative to ^{125}I seeds and guidewires, and showed a decreased procedure time and increased rate of ductal carcinoma in situ (DCIS) close margin compared to guidewires [42].

Lee et al. [21] published a small retrospective study comparing LOCalizer (33 patients), SCOUT (21 patients), and guidewires (50 patients), reporting no significant difference between the three methods in terms of resected volumes, positive margins, or re-excision rates. The re-excision rates were 6.1%, 9.5%, and 10.0% for LOCalizer, SCOUT, and guidewires, respectively [21]. A systematic review of 842 SCOUT cases calculated a re-excision rate of 12.8% from 624 cases where malignant lesions were targeted [17], and in a subsequent single centre study of 500 patients, Siddiqui et al. reported a re-excision rate of 7.6% [41].

Anderman et al. [2] in their dataset of 445 patients looked at potential predictors of positive margin rates. There was no significant association between tag-to-target distance or surgical specimen size; the only significant predictor of positive margins was DCIS on final pathology [2]. This finding is similar to that in studies using Magseed, where the commonest cause of re-excision is the presence of (radiologically occult) DCIS at the margin [6, 10]. This is not entirely surprising, since across large cohorts of breast-conserving surgery pre-dating the use of wire-free localisation devices, the commonest reason for re-excision is DCIS at the margin [3, 16]. It follows, therefore, that the main factor influencing margin positivity across all methods is most likely the disease characteristics rather than the localisation technique per se.

11.5.4 Technical Considerations of the LOCalizer in Clinical Practice

Overall studies report a short learning curve with device insertion, since it is similar in principle to many other image-guided breast intervention techniques, but there are certain nuances that are specific to the LOCalizer [5, 19, 23, 37]. In a number of studies, radiologists have reported difficulties with the placement of the RFID tag, partially related to the relatively large (12 G) needle applicator, and likely contributed to by the sharpness of the needle [5, 19, 23, 26, 37], something that has also been discussed in a shared learning paper published as part of the iBRA-NET Localisation Group in the United Kingdom [33]. As well as presenting difficulties in passing the needle through dense breast parenchyma and into firm tumours, sometimes upon device deployment, the tag bounces back from the mass and ends up alongside the lesion rather than within it. This does not usually pose a significant problem, since the tag remains in such proximity to the mass that it still effectively localises it, but is nevertheless suboptimal. The same phenomenon has been reported in other LOCalizer studies [19, 23]. The relatively simple work around in this situation is to advance the introducer needle a little further in the mass, about a tag's length beyond the intended deployment, then retract the needle slightly, and slowly deploy the tag into the newly created track (Fig. 11.8; [33]). A smaller device, and

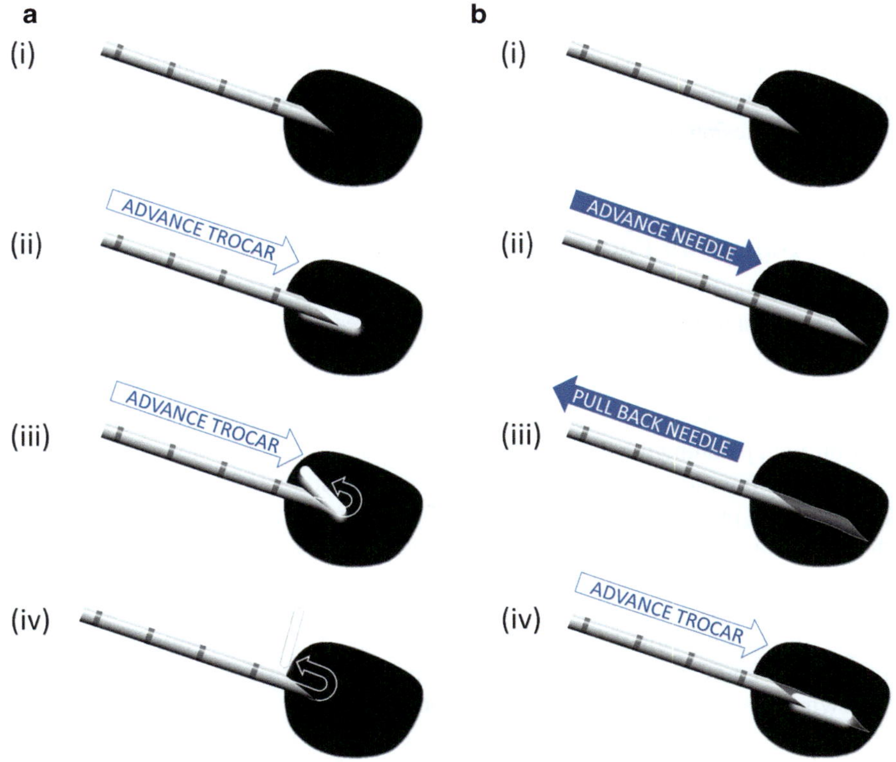

Fig. 11.8 Sometimes when the device is deployed into dense tissues and masses, the tag bounces back from the target and ends up alongside it rather than within it; Panel **a** (i–iv). This does not usually pose a significant problem, since the tag remains in such proximity to the mass that it still effectively localises it, but is nevertheless suboptimal; Panel **a** (iv). One way to try and mitigate this is to advance the introducer needle a little further into the mass, about a tag's length beyond the intended deployment (**b** i—ii), then retract the needle slightly (**b** iii), and slowly deploy the tag into the newly created track (**b** iv)

hence a needle gauge, may mitigate these issues [37]. Failed or suboptimal localisations are also felt to be more likely with stereotactic versus ultrasound-guided localisations [33].

Once at its final site of deployment, there are no reports of further migration from the target prior to surgery. Intraoperatively, however, some data suggest a higher rate of device dislodgement with tags compared to guidewires [13, 37]. This occurs mainly during manipulation of the breast tissue during lesion excision [13, 23, 33]. This seems to be most problematic when the tags are deployed in superficial breast lesions or post-biopsy haematomas [23, 33, 37]; in cases of superficial lesions, it is recommended the tag is placed more deeply within the target lesion, or even just deep to the lesion [23, 33, 37]. Another approach is to ensure early device identification, and mark the area of the tagged lesion with a stitch should the device subsequently become dislodged [33]. The higher rate of dislodgement compared to guidewires is almost certainly related to the fact that the tag has no physical anchors; the device is smooth, and its polypropylene sheath relies on adhesion to surrounding tissues through fibrosis. Despite this, in most cases, when the device does dislodge, it has already achieved its purpose of directing the surgeon towards the location of the intended lesion within the breast [33].

11.6 Impact on Patients and Breast Services

One of the main purported advantages of wire-free devices like the LOCalizer is that they can be inserted well in advance of surgery, conferring logistical advantages both for patients and clinical workflow. Having the localisation and surgery on separate days not only eases pressures on the day of surgery, it introduces much greater flexibility in planning the date of surgery and in scheduling radiology clinic lists.

By planning the localisation for an outpatient visit, patients avoid undergoing an additional procedure on the morning of surgery, an already stressful time, and no longer have a guidewire protruding from the skin, which is at potential risk of dislodgement. When localisations are done on the morning of surgery, there is also a risk of delaying start times of operating lists, particularly if unexpected difficulties arise during the localisation procedure. This is also mitigated by having the procedure at an earlier date. A UK-based survey of practice suggests that following the introduction of wire-free techniques and the resultant trend away from using guidewires, there are now fewer delays in starting operations and fewer instances of operating lists overrunning [29]. Similarly, a single-centre retrospective study in the USA involving 439 patients undergoing RFID tag localisation found that those undergoing localisation on the day of surgery (158 patients) had a significantly greater length of stay than those having their localisations on a day prior to surgery (281 patients), with cases significantly more likely to be delayed [35].

In some centres, breast radiology and breast surgery are located on different hospital sites, which can lead to logistical challenges and more stress for patients if localisations are done on the same day, something that is also avoided by having the localisation done on a separate day [33]. This was something that became a more widespread problem during the COVID-19 pandemic, when many outpatient surgical services were temporarily relocated to cold sites, necessitating different ways of working [43]. Somewhat fortuitously, the shift that was taking place around that time towards adopting wire-free localisation techniques fitted well with the enforced need to decouple localisation and surgery.

Another potential advantage of doing localisations well in advance of surgery is that, on rare occasions when localisations are carried out, additional disease is identified. In these instances, having additional time preoperatively to biopsy and re-plan the localisation might mean that the original surgical date is not delayed, whereas with guidewire localisation on the morning of surgery, the operation would have to be postponed [10].

But despite these obvious advantages, having the procedure done different days does not necessarily work in all settings. In some centres, even those who have adopted wire-free devices, it might still be better for patients to have localisation on the day of surgery. For example, in some large regional referral centres, patients have to travel long distances to the hospital, making multiple hospital visits inconvenient or impractical [19]. Furthermore, in a study using Magseed versus guidewires, patients who had a wire localisation were mostly satisfied with having it on the day of surgery, while opinion of those having the Magseed (inserted on a different day to surgery) was divided, with some expressing preference to having all procedures done on the same day [31].

There is currently very little data on patient experience of the LOCalizer. As mentioned earlier, in the first clinical cohort investing LOCalizer use by DiNome et al. [11], all 50 patients were asked to complete a Likert-style questionnaire shortly after tag insertion. The patients were asked to select whether they agreed or disagreed with one of five statements: 'The procedure was not very painful', 'The procedure was easier than the biopsy', 'I did not feel lightheaded or dizzy', 'The procedure was easier than I expected', and 'The procedure went smoothly' [11]. Most patients either strongly agreed or agreed with all five statements. Wazir et al. [46], in their dataset of ten patients, also reported highly positive feedback when patients were asked to score their experience on a visual analogue scale.

Although these data indicate the procedure is generally well-tolerated, it does not give us a relative comparison of tolerability against other localisation techniques. To date there is one study directly comparing patient satisfaction of the LOCalizer procedure against guidewires [37]. The study was set up as a single-centre, prospective, controlled, observational trial involving 80 patients: 40 undergoing guidewire localisation and 40 RFID tag localisation. Patients were asked to complete a 10-point Visual Analogue Scale, which showed a significantly greater satisfaction score for the LOCalizer cohort compared to the guidewire cohort, as well as a reduction in pain between device insertion and surgery for the LOCalizer cohort [37].

11.7 Positives and Negatives

There are trade-offs with all devices. A key advantage of RFID tags over early wire-free localisation approaches is that there is no radioactivity, and hence none of the burdensome—and sometimes prohibitive—regulatory requirements. However, the anecdotal trend is that radioactive iodine seeds are becoming obsolete in favour of the non-radioactive devices.

There are also no considerations regarding surgical equipment; with Magseed, for example, non-ferromagnetic surgical instruments are required to eliminate interference with the detection probe [12, 18].

One distinct advantage of RFID tags over the other wire-free devices is the unique tag identification numbers that allow discrimination between different tags in the same breast. This can help with specimen orientation, and differentiation of multiple sites of differing histology that may have differing surgical considerations, for example an invasive carcinoma versus a risk (B3) lesion.

A current drawback is the relatively large size of the introducer needle. At 12 G this is the largest of all current commercially available wire-free devices in the United Kingdom (Fig. 11.4 and Table 11.1), and as discussed earlier this can lead to some challenges in device deployment. A smaller version of the LOCalizer would certainly circumvent these issues. However, despite the relatively large tag size, the LOCalizer benefits from the smallest surgical probe of all current wire-free devices; at the size of a pencil, it can be used with small incisions with less risk of obscuring the lesion [11].

Another important factor to consider is cost. All wire-free devices cost significantly more than guidewires. Although clinicians may see the benefits of adopting wire-free devices for service improvement and perceived patient benefit, it may be challenging to justify this to management teams in view of the additional costs compared to guidewires. However, these devices do benefit both surgery and radiology departments, and if financial support can be shared by both divisions it may help in justification [11]. Budget analyses have been conducted for other similarly priced devices, and suggest they can be cost-efficient compared to guidewires when all factors are considered; however this will be dependent on individual institutions [22].

The LOCalizer also does not have the disadvantages that some of the other devices have. The SCOUT, for example can be de-activated by electrocautery, which is not the case with RFID tags [9]. SCOUT detection can also be impeded by post-biopsy haematoma, which can absorb the infrared wavelength utilised by the console probe [41]. However, this can be avoided by placing the SCOUT adjacent to, rather than within, any large haematomas [28, 41].

Unlike guidewires, wire-free devices cannot be repositioned once deployed, and therefore may require additional device deployment to ensure successful localisation, either an additional wire-free device or guidewire [18, 19, 23].

Despite being MRI safe, it is advisable not to insert the LOCalizer into the breast or axilla before doing MRI because of the large bloom artefact. A similar artefact has been reported for Magseed [6], and a similar artefact would be expected for the Pintuition device, since it is also magnetic. With an artefact of around 20–40 mm, this will obscure any abnormality within the field of the artefact, limiting its diagnostic use in MRI staging, as well as in assessing response to neoadjuvant chemotherapy if any of these devices were deployed prior to completion of treatment. The SCOUT on the other hand has a much smaller artefact on MRI, potentially making it more amenable to deployment either at the time of biopsying suspicious unifocal lesions in lieu of a standard tissue biopsy clip, or prior to neoadjuvant chemotherapy, both potentially saving patients a future hospital visits for preoperative localisation [41].

Since all wire-free devices are clearly visible on mammography without artefact, the emerging use of contrast enhanced mammography (CEM) to assess response to neoadjuvant chemotherapy, could potentially mean that any of the wireless localisation devices could be inserted prior to neoadjuvant chemotherapy without compromising response assessment, however further studies are needed to evaluate this.

11.8 Concluding Remarks

The RFID system represents an effective wire-free localisation device for localising breast cancers prior to surgery. Although not currently licensed for axillary use, there is a strong body of evidence to demonstrate its safety and effectiveness at targeting lymph nodes.

It has significant advantages over guidewires in terms of logistics and the patient pathway, and has advantages over the other currently available wire-free localisation devices in that is radiation-free, the tags' 5-digit identification numbers allow discrimination between multiple tags in the same breast, the handheld reader makes the system more portable, and the surgical pencil probe is much smaller than that of its competitors. Its main potentially modifiable drawback is the size of the tag, which necessitates a 12 G introducer, and can present challenges in device deployment. A narrower tag, and hence a smaller gauge introducer, would likely make significant improvements in its practicality.

Declarations of Interest SL has received speaker honoraria and standard class travel expenses from Hologic (LOCalizer™ and Magseed®), Merit (SCOUT®), and Sirius (Pintuition®).

RM has received speaker honoraria and standard class travel expenses from Hologic (LOCalizer™).

References

1. Almalki H, Rankin AC, Juette A, Youssef MG. Radio-frequency identification (RFID) tag localisation of non-palpable breast lesions a single centre experience. Breast Edinb Scotl. 2023;69:417–21.
2. Anderman KJ, Daly AE, Newman AM, Dang PA, Smith BL, Gadd MA, Lamb LR, Specht MC. Placement of radiofrequency identification tags: is there an optimal tag-to-target distance? Eur Radiol., [published online ahead of print; awaiting final citation details]. 2025; https://doi.org/10.1007/s00330-025-11817-5.
3. Boundouki G, Wong Sik Hee JR, Croghan N, Stocking K, Pieri A, Critchley A, Kirwan CC, Harvey JR. Comparing long-term local recurrence rates of surgical and non-surgical management of close anterior margins in breast conserving surgery. Breast Cancer Res Treat. 2019;176(2):311–9. https://doi.org/10.1007/s10549-019-05242-8.
4. Bundred JR, Michael S, Stuart B, Cutress RI, Beckmann K, Holleczek B, Dahlstrom JE, Gath J, Dodwell D, Bundred NJ. Margin status and survival outcomes after breast cancer conservation surgery: prospectively registered systematic review and meta-analysis. BMJ. 2022;378:e070346. https://doi.org/10.1136/bmj-2022-070346.
5. Christenhusz A, den Dekker BM, van Dalen T, Jongen L, van der Schaaf MC, Alic L, Ten Haken B, Pijnappel RM, Dassen AE. Radiofrequency localization of nonpalpable breast can-

cer in a multicentre prospective cohort study: feasibility, clinical acceptability, and safety. Breast Cancer Res Treat. 2023;201(1):67–75. https://doi.org/10.1007/s10549-023-07006-x.

6. Constantinidis F, Sakellariou S, Chang SL, Linder S, MacPherson B, Seth S, Gill N, Seth A. Wireless localisation of breast lesions with MagSeed. A radiological perspective of 300 cases. Br J Radiol. 2022;95(1133):20211241. https://doi.org/10.1259/bjr.20211241.
7. Cullinane CM, Byrne J, Akmenkalne L, O'Leary DP, Connors AM, Corrigan MA, Redmond HP, Kelly L, O'Sullivan MJ. The LOCalizer radiofrequency identification system: an effective new technology for localizing non-palpable breast lesions for surgery. Surg Innov. 2021;28(4):473–8. https://doi.org/10.1177/1553350620967853.
8. Daly GR, Hamza E, Singh S, Patterson R, Hassett C, Hembrecht S, Crilly E, O'Brien A, Downey E, Hegarty A, Mhuircheartaigh NN, Power C, Healy NA, Duke D, Hill ADK. Wire-guided localisation vs HOLOGIC® LOCalizer™ radiofrequency identification (RFID) tag localisation of non-palpable breast lesions; a comparative analysis of ease of use and accuracy of localisation. Surgeon. 2025;23(4):248–53. https://doi.org/10.1016/j.surge.2025.04.052.
9. Dauphine C, Reicher JJ, Reicher MA, Gondusky C, Khalkhali I, Kim M. A prospective clinical study to evaluate the safety and performance of wireless localization of nonpalpable breast lesions using radiofrequency identification technology. AJR Am J Roentgenol. 2015;204(6):W720–3. https://doi.org/10.2214/AJR.14.13201.
10. Dave RV, Barrett E, Morgan J, Chandarana M, Elgammal S, Barnes N, Sami A, Masudi T, Down S, Holcombe C, Potter S, Somasundaram SK, Gardiner M, Mylvaganam S, Maxwell A, Harvey J, iBRA-NET Localisation Study collaborative. Wire- and magnetic-seed-guided localization of impalpable breast lesions: iBRA-NET localisation study. Br J Surg. 2022;109(3):274–82. https://doi.org/10.1093/bjs/znab443.
11. DiNome ML, Kusske AM, Attai DJ, Fischer CP, Hoyt AC. Microchipping the breast: an effective new technology for localizing non-palpable breast lesions for surgery. Breast Cancer Res Treat. 2019;175(1):165–70. https://doi.org/10.1007/s10549-019-05143-w.
12. Gera R, Tayeh S, Al-Reefy S, Mokbel K. Evolving role of Magseed in wireless localization of breast lesions: systematic review and pooled analysis of 1,559 procedures. Anticancer Res. 2020;40(4):1809–15. https://doi.org/10.21873/anticanres.14135.
13. Harvey J, Morgan J, Lowes S, Milligan R, Barrett E, Carmichael A, Elgammal S, Masudi T, Holcombe C, Masannat Y, Potter S, Dave RV, iBRA-Net Localization Study Collaborative. Wire- and radiofrequency identification tag-guided localization of impalpable breast lesions: iBRA-NET localization study. Br J Surg. 2024;111(2):znae007. https://doi.org/10.1093/bjs/znae007.
14. Health Beacons Inc. https://gust.com/companies/Health_Beacons_Inc. Accessed 13th July 2025.
15. Houssami N, Macaskill P, Marinovich ML, Morrow M. The association of surgical margins and local recurrence in women with early-stage invasive breast cancer treated with breast-conserving therapy: a meta-analysis. Ann Surg Oncol. 2014;21(3):717–30. https://doi.org/10.1245/s10434-014-3480-5.
16. Jeevan R, Cromwell DA, Trivella M, Lawrence G, Kearins O, Pereira J, Sheppard C, Caddy CM, van der Meulen JH. Reoperation rates after breast conserving surgery for breast cancer among women in England: retrospective study of hospital episode statistics. BMJ. 2012;345:e4505. https://doi.org/10.1136/bmj.e4505.
17. Kasem I, Mokbel K. Savi Scout® radar localisation of non-palpable breast lesions: systematic review and pooled analysis of 842 cases. Anticancer Res. 2020;40(7):3633–43.
18. Lamb LR, Bahl M, Specht MC, D'Alessandro HA, Lehman CD. Evaluation of a nonradioactive magnetic marker wireless localization program. AJR Am J Roentgenol. 2018;211(4):940–5. https://doi.org/10.2214/AJR.18.19637.
19. Lamb LR, Gilman L, Specht M, D'Alessandro HA, Miles RC, Lehman CD. Retrospective review of preoperative radiofrequency tag localization of breast lesions in 848 patients. AJR Am J Roentgenol. 2021;217(3):605–12. https://doi.org/10.2214/AJR.20.24374.

20. Leaver A, Amonkar S, Milligan R, Potterton J, Hamilton P, Lowes S. A new breast localisation technique: use of the Hologic LOCalizer radiofrequency ID tag system in a UK breast unit. Breast Cancer Res. 2019;20(Suppl 1):0086.
21. Lee MK, Sanaiha Y, Kusske AM, Thompson CK, Attai DJ, Baker JL, Fischer CP, DiNome ML. A comparison of two non-radioactive alternatives to wire for the localization of non-palpable breast cancers. Breast Cancer Res Treat. 2020;182(2):299–303. https://doi.org/10.1007/s10549-020-05707-1.
22. Lindenberg M, van Beek A, Retèl V, van Duijnhoven F, van Harten W (2020). Early budget impact analysis on magnetic seed localization for non-palpable breast cancer surgery. PLoS One, 13;15(5):e0232690. doi:https://doi.org/10.1371/journal.pone.0232690.
23. Lowes S, Bell A, Milligan R, Amonkar S, Leaver A. Use of Hologic LOCalizer radiofrequency identification (RFID) tags to localise impalpable breast lesions and axillary nodes: experience of the first 150 cases in a UK breast unit. Clin Radiol. 2020;75(12):942–9. https://doi.org/10.1016/j.crad.2020.08.014.
24. Lowes S, El Tahir S, Koo S, Amonkar S, Leaver A, Milligan R. Pre-operative localisation of axillary lymph nodes using radiofrequency identification (RFID) tags: a feasibility assessment in 75 cases. Clin Radiol. 2023;78(9):e668–75. https://doi.org/10.1016/j.crad.2023.05.017.
25. Malik M, Brookes P, Kasana MI, Tromans L, Audrey Chew WY, Green MJ. Radiofrequency as a method of localizing impalpable breast lesions. Surgeon. 2024;22(5):296–300. https://doi.org/10.1016/j.surge.2024.08.001.
26. Malter W, Holtschmidt J, Thangarajah F, Mallmann P, Krug B, Warm M, Eichler C. First reported use of the Faxitron LOCalizer™ radiofrequency identification (RFID) system in Europe – a feasibility trial, surgical guide and review for non-palpable breast lesions. In Vivo. 2019;33(5):1559–64. https://doi.org/10.21873/invivo.11637.
27. Malter W, Eichler C, Hanstein B, Mallmann P, Holtschmidt J. First reported use of radiofrequency identification (RFID) technique for targeted excision of suspicious axillary lymph nodes in early stage breast cancer – evaluation of feasibility and review of current recommendations. In Vivo. 2020;34(3):1207–13. https://doi.org/10.21873/invivo.11894.
28. Mango VL, Wynn RT, Feldman S, Friedlander L, Desperito E, Patel SN, Gomberawalla A, Ha R. Beyond wires and seeds: reflector-guided breast lesion localization and excision. Radiology. 2017;284(2):365–71. https://doi.org/10.1148/radiol.2017161661.
29. Mavor F, Somasundaram SK, Carmichael AR, Elgammal S, Foster R, Lowes S, Masannat Y, Milligan R, Morgan JL, St John ER, Vidya R, Dave RV, Harvey J. Adoption of nonwire localisation devices in UK breast units: an iBRA-NET survey to assess changes in practice. Ann R Coll Surg Engl., [published online ahead of print; awaiting final citation details]. 2025; https://doi.org/10.1308/rcsann.2024.0106.
30. McGugin C, Spivey T, Coopey S, Smith B, Kelly B, Gadd M, Hughes K, Dontchos B, Specht M. Radiofrequency identification tag localization is comparable to wire localization for non-palpable breast lesions. Breast Cancer Res Treat. 2019;177(3):735–9. https://doi.org/10.1007/s10549-019-05355-0.
31. Micha AE, Sinnett V, Downey K, Allen S, Bishop B, Hector LR, Patrick EP, Edmonds R, Barry PA, Krupa KDC, Rusby JE. Patient and clinician satisfaction and clinical outcomes of Magseed compared with wire-guided localisation for impalpable breast lesions. Breast Cancer. 2021;28(1):196–205. https://doi.org/10.1007/s12282-020-01149-1.
32. Munhoz AM, Chala L, de Melo GG, Marques Filho AA, Tucunduva T, Gemperli R. Usefulness of radio frequency identification device in diagnosing rotation of Motiva SmoothSilk implants after augmentation mammoplasty. Plast Reconstr Surg Glob Open. 2019;7(11):e2497. https://doi.org/10.1097/GOX.0000000000002497.
33. Morgan JL, Harvey J, Lowes S, Milligan R, Krizak S, Masannat Y, Carmichael A, Elgammal S, Youssef M, Petralia G, Dave RV, iBRA-NET Localisation Study Group. Results of shared learning of a new radiofrequency identification localization device-a UK iBRA-NET breast cancer localisation study. Clin Radiol. 2024;79(11):e1288–95. https://doi.org/10.1016/j.crad.2024.06.014.

34. Munday C, Malhotra A, Taif S, Omotade A, Menon A, Mokbel K. Evaluation of Hologic LOCalizer™ RFID tags for preoperative localization of breast lesions: a single-center experience. Diagnostics (Basel). 2025;15(6):746. https://doi.org/10.3390/diagnostics15060746.
35. Newman AM, Daly AE, Anderman KJ, Dang PA, Nguyen AT, Smith BL, Gadd MA, Specht MC. Timing of radiofrequency identification tag placement: can early placement save time and patient experience? Breast Cancer Res Treat. 2025;211(3):669–74. https://doi.org/10.1007/s10549-025-07681-y.
36. Olivere LA, Hill IT, Thomas SM, Codd PJ, Rosenberger LH. Radiofrequency identification track for tray optimization: an instrument utilization pilot study in surgical oncology. J Surg Res. 2021;264:490–8. https://doi.org/10.1016/j.jss.2021.02.049.
37. Pete R, Pinard C, Sirodot F, Molnar I, Dressaire M, Ginzac A, Abrial C, Durando X, Tekath M. Patient satisfaction with radio-frequency identification (RFID) tag localization compared with wire localization for nonpalpable breast lesions: the RFID trial. BMC Cancer. 2025;25(1):123. https://doi.org/10.1186/s12885-025-13453-0.
38. Rakha EA, Quinn C, Masannat YA, Lee AHS, Tan PH, Karakatsanis A, Matrai ZT, Al Shaibani SHM, Gehani SA, Shaaban A, Khout H, Chagla L, Cserni G, Varga Z, Yong WF, Meattini I, Kulka J, Yang W, Tse GM, Pinder SE, Fox S, Dixon JM. Revisiting surgical margins for invasive breast cancer patients treated with breast conservation therapy – evidence for adopting a 1 mm negative width. Eur J Surg Oncol. 2024;50(10):108573. https://doi.org/10.1016/j.ejso.2024.108573.
39. Reicher JJ, Reicher MA, Thomas M, Petcavich R. Radiofrequency identification tags for preoperative tumor localization: proof of concept. AJR Am J Roentgenol. 2008;191(5):1359–65. https://doi.org/10.2214/AJR.08.1023.
40. Rupp CC, Kagarise MJ, Nelson SM, Deal AM, Phillips S, Chadwick J, Petty T, Meyer AA, Kim HJ. Effectiveness of a radiofrequency detection system as an adjunct to manual counting protocols for tracking surgical sponges: a prospective trial of 2,285 patients. J Am Coll Surg. 2012;215(4):524–33. https://doi.org/10.1016/j.jamcollsurg.2012.06.014.
41. Siddiqui S, Povey M, Rowland M, Sharma S. SCOUT® radar reflectors for impalpable lesion localisation in the breast and axilla: our experience in the first 500 patients. Clin Radiol. 2025;81:106777. https://doi.org/10.1016/j.crad.2024.106777.
42. Stephens KR, Patel L, Malik DA, Wilson M, Gaskins JT, McMasters KM, Ajkay N. Comparison of radiofrequency identification, radioactive seed, and wire localization techniques for nonpalpable breast cancer. J Am Coll Surg., [published online ahead of print; awaiting final citation details]. 2025; https://doi.org/10.1097/XCS.0000000000001368.
43. Strickland J, Elsberger B, Lip G, Fuller M, Masannat Y. Impalpable breast cancer and service delivery during the COVID-19 pandemic e the role of radiofrequency tag localization. Arch Breast Cancer. 2021;8:247e50.
44. Tayeh S, Wazir U, Mokbel K. The evolving role of radiofrequency guided localisation in breast surgery: a systematic review. Cancers (Basel). 2021;13(19):4996. https://doi.org/10.3390/cancers13194996.
45. Vos EL, Siesling S, Baaijens MHA, Verhoef C, Jager A, Voogd AC, Koppert LB. Omitting re-excision for focally positive margins after breast-conserving surgery does not impair disease-free and overall survival. Breast Cancer Res Treat. 2017;164(1):157–67. https://doi.org/10.1007/s10549-017-4232-6.
46. Wazir U, Tayeh S, Perry N, Michell M, Malhotra A, Mokbel K. Wireless breast localization using radio-frequency identification tags: the first reported European experience in breast cancer. In Vivo. 2020;34(1):233–8. https://doi.org/10.21873/invivo.11765.

Chapter 12
Localisation Using Pintuition

Azra Khatun, Walid Abou-Samra, Avi Agrawal, and Edward St John

Contents

12.1 Background

Breast cancer is the most common cancer in women worldwide [1]. In the UK, aided by the national screening programme, 33% of all breast cancer cases are non-palpable at the time of diagnosis [2]. For early-stage breast cancer, breast conserving surgery (BCS) with radiotherapy is most commonly performed. The aim of the

A. Khatun · A. Agrawal
Breast Department, Portsmouth Hospitals University NHS Trust, Portsmouth, UK
e-mail: azra.khatun2@nhs.net; avi.agrawal@nhs.net

W. Abou-Samra
Breast Department, Glan Clwyd Hospital, Bodelwyddan, North Wales, UK
e-mail: walid.a.samra@wales.nhs.uk

E. S. John (✉)
Breast Department, Portsmouth Hospitals University NHS Trust, Portsmouth, UK

Breast Department, University of Portsmouth, Portsmouth, UK
e-mail: edward.stjohn3@nhs.net

R. Vidya, N. Sharma (eds.), *Breast and Axilla Localisation Techniques*,
https://doi.org/10.1007/978-3-032-17995-1_12

surgery includes complete excision of the tumour, staging of the axilla, and satisfactory cosmetic results. The treatment of impalpable tumours has long posed challenges in accurately identifying tumour margins during surgery. Radiologists play an important role in facilitating image-guided localisation of non-palpable lesions in everyday clinical practice.

Localisation technologies have evolved over time to optimise breast conserving surgery. Traditional localisation methods include wire-guided localisation (WGL) where radiologists implant an anchor wire into the breast lesion to guide surgeons. Despite its safe, effective, and inexpensive use, WGL has several limitations both to clinicians and patients. This has subsequently led to the development of alternative localisation techniques as described in previous chapters.

12.2 Sirius Pintuition

Developed by Sirius Medical (High Tech Campus 41, 5656 AE, Eindhoven, North Brabant, Netherlands), a Dutch medical company, the Pintuition device is a wire-free, magnetic seed-based technology designed to improve tumour localisation during surgery.

12.2.1 Radiological Insertion

The goal of the radiological insertion is to place the Pintuition marker into or near a target lesion within the breast so that it can later be located during surgery using the magnetic detection probe. The device currently utilises a 5 mm magnetic seed, which is percutaneously implanted into the breast via a sterile, preloaded 14G needle (Figs. 12.1 and 12.2). Pre-procedure preparation involves a review of imaging to determine the best approach, ultrasound or stereotactic (mammographic), depending on lesion visibility, then patient consent is obtained and a sterile technique is used during the placement. Local anaesthetic is administered to numb the skin and tissue. A Pintuition introducer needle is used to insert the localiser into the lesion site. The magnetic marker is inserted under imaging control (ultrasound or stereotactic). Once deployed, the needle is rotated and removed, leaving the marker in situ. Placement is confirmed with post-insertion imaging (usually with a craniocaudal and mediolateral mammogram). The patient is monitored briefly for any immediate complications. The location of the marker is documented for the surgical team. Surgery can be scheduled flexibly as the marker is not radioactive and has no time constraints (though it is advisable to insert the marker a week before surgery to allow the tract to close and minimise migration at the time of surgery).

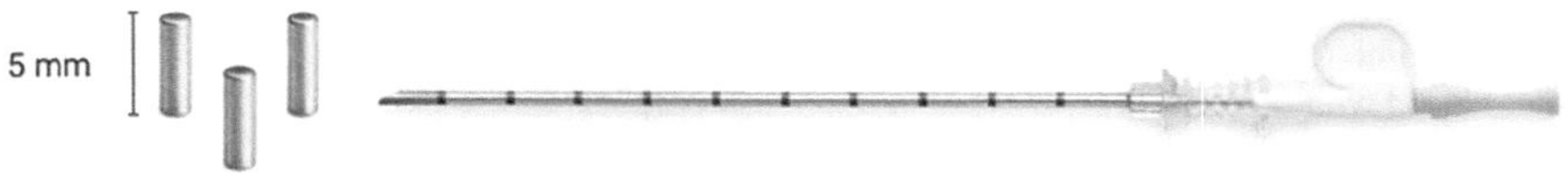

Fig. 12.1 The Pintuition Marker (5mm) is deployed with a 14G pre-loaded needle (7cm, 12cm variants) with an ultrasound-enhanced tip. (Image reproduced with permission from Sirius Medical, 2025)

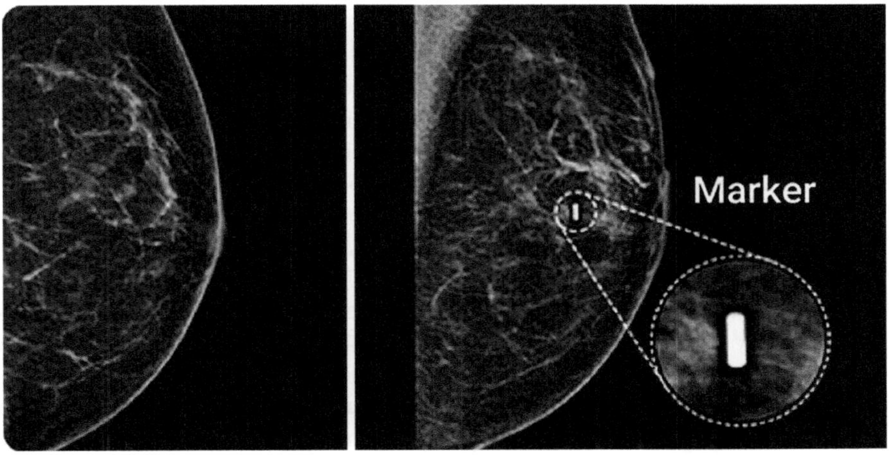

Fig. 12.2 Pintuition marker within breast tissue. (Image reproduced with permission from Sirius Medical, 2025)

12.2.2 Surgical Technique

Preoperative planning includes confirming the number and location of Pintuition markers using preoperative mammography and/or ultrasound. The details provided by radiology regarding the position of the marker should be checked before surgery. Prior to use, the Pintuition device is calibrated once in the operating room before use and a sterile cover applied over the probe. During surgery, the precise position of the seed is detected by the handheld Pintuition probe connected to a table-top base unit (Fig. 12.3). The system provides a metric detection (maximum 50 mm distance) with visual and audible feedback enabling surgeons to pinpoint the tumour location with high accuracy and without the need for wires or radioactive materials [24]. Dissection is performed through subcutaneous and breast tissue towards the signal; as the marker is approached, the proximity (in mm) decreases. The lesion and magnetic marker are excised in a single en bloc specimen, with appropriate margins based on oncological intent. Haemostasis is achieved and the specimen is sent for imaging. Intraoperative specimen assessment with specimen X-ray is recommended and can confirm the presence of the magnetic marker and lesion (if calcifications or clip present). The Pintuition system can differentiate markers at different locations

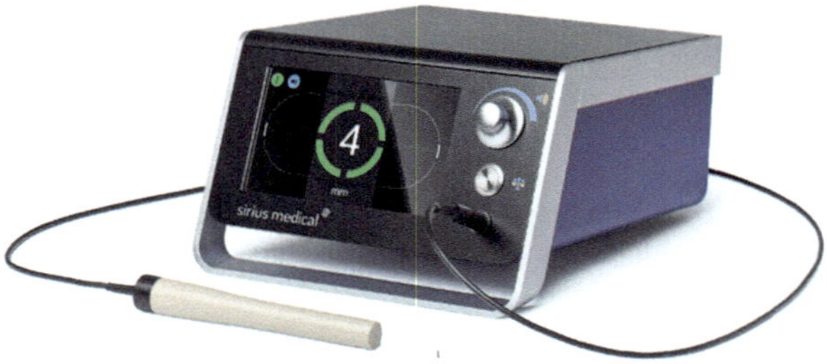

Fig. 12.3 Pintuition probe and base unit. (Image reproduced with permission from Sirius Medical, 2025)

(approved for lesions >5 cm apart) based on signal strength and probe orientation. If excising multiple lesions/markers, the surgeon should carefully isolate each signal and plan the excisions accordingly. For single lesions, one marker in the specimen confirms success, for multiple lesions, each should contain one marker and specimen imaging should confirm all. Margins should be marked according to local practice. Post-operative reports should include the number of markers retrieved.

As no radioactivity is involved, localisation and seed placement can be performed up to 180 days before surgery in the EU and without a time limit in the USA. The decoupling of radiology and surgery schedules enables greater scheduling flexibility and overall workflow efficiency [4]. The aim of Pintuition was to develop a device that would simplify the localisation process, improve surgical outcomes, and enhance the patient experience. To achieve this, the Sirus Link program was launched—a surgical care pathway centred on activities, outcomes, and quality of care, rather than merely cost reduction, aligning with the principles of the Value-Based Healthcare model.

12.3 Evolution of the Technology

The early research related to the Pintuition technology was conducted at the Netherlands Cancer Institute, leveraging an existing clinical magnetic detection technology which had evidential benefits over wire localisation. The aim of developing the Pintuition device was to overcome the limitations experienced in the existing magnetic localisation technologies such as a lack of range, lack of directionality and challenges with repeated re-calibration during use, and interference with metallic instruments.

The initial work went into developing a unique magnetic marker known as the Magnetic Marker Localisation device (MaMaLoc) 2014–2018. Differences in marker shape, volume, material, and assembly were explored to determine the optimal characteristics required. The prototypes were then subjected to ex vivo testing in comparison to another commercially available para-magnetic seed (EndoMagnetics Ltd., Cambridge, UK) [22]. Early first-in-woman trials coupled the detection of the MaMaLoc with a third-party detection probe (SentiMag,

EndoMagnetics Ltd., Cambridge, UK). Results were obtained from 15 patients with non-palpable breast cancer in a single breast that had both a radioactive iodine seed and a magnetic marker inserted. A magnetic probe and gamma probe were used to localise the markers with identification rate of 100% for both devices [23]. Between February 2017 and May 2018, the MaMaLoc seed was also tested together with the Sentimag detection probe (EndoMagnetics Ltd., Cambridge, UK), by placing the marker within the index metastatic lymph node of 12 patients with resectable stage III melanoma. Markers remained in situ for a median of 23 days (i.q.r. 21–27). All of the markers were detected transcutaneously, and all were successfully removed with the correct (index) lymph node. A system usability scale score of 98/100 was achieved, as rated by surgeons and the process was deemed to be intuitive (4.8/5) [21]. Between October 2017 and December 2018, the MaMaLoc marker was coupled with the Sentimag detection probe (EndoMagnetics Ltd., Cambridge, UK) and compared to wire-guided localisation in women with early-stage breast cancer ($n = 32$ in the MaMaloc group and $n = 35$ in the WGL group). One hundred per cent of both the wires and the Mamaloc were correctly identified and retrieved. The usability of the device as reported by the surgeon was higher for MaMaLoc: 70.2 ± 8.9 vs.58.1 ± 9.1, $p < 0.001$. Patient overall satisfaction was higher with MaMaLoc (median score 5/5) versus WGL (score 4/5), $p < 0.001$ [25].

Sirius Medical was founded as a company in 2017, and work started on developing a unique detector specifically designed to detect the magnetic marker. The aim was to ensure the probe and the software algorithm was sensitive enough to detect the seed's magnetic field with sufficient precision to allow mm distance detection and directional information to be read out.

The marker previously known as MaMaLoc, was renamed 'Pintuition'. In 2020, the Pintuition device received CE marking, a regulatory certification for medical devices to be sold in the European Union. The technology was quickly adopted in hospitals and clinics across Europe due to its advantages over traditional localisation methods. The first presented clinical report of the Pintuition detector being used in patients was from the European Society of Surgical Oncology (ESSO) 2020, with the abstract published in 2021 [6]. This study included 2 surgeons and 25 female patients diagnosed with an ultrasound-visible unifocal pathologically confirmed breast cancer. In 2021, in the Netherlands, the Pintuition detector was also used successfully to localise an ectopic parathyroid adenoma [8]. From then on, further studies used both the Pintuition marker and the Pintuition detector as described in the literature review below. The Sirius Pintuition marker and device was first used surgically in the UK in February 2021 to aid localisation of breast cancer Reference: https://www.royalmarsden.nhs.uk/Sirius-Pintuition.

Following its success in Europe, the Pintuition device received clearance from the US Food and Drug Administration (FDA) in 2021, enabling its sale and use in the US market. This approval opened doors for the technology to be adopted by leading cancer centres and hospitals in the USA, further validating its clinical effectiveness and patient-centred design.

12.4 Advancements and Improvements

Sirius Medical continued to enhance the Pintuition device based on feedback from surgeons, radiologists, and clinical data. Newer versions of the technology have evolved with features such as GPSDetect, where the multi-sensor probe allows for real-time directional feedback using audio and visual guidance. The onscreen displays a white bar that narrows as you approach the marker, becoming a green circle when very close ('on-target') and a hashed green circle when directly over the marker ('TargetLOC'). Throughout this process, the distance from the marker in millimetres is also displayed on the screen (Figs. 12.4 and 12.5). The easy-to-use, reusable detection system only requires a single calibration per procedure. The TargetLOC feature enables easier navigation and perfect alignment to enable greater accuracy and localisation of tumours.

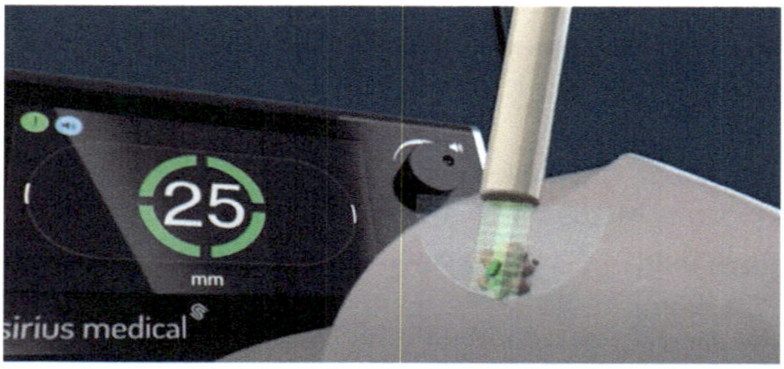

Fig. 12.4 On screen TargetLOC display once the probe is pointing directly at the Pintuition marker. (Image reproduced with permission from Sirius Medical, 2025)

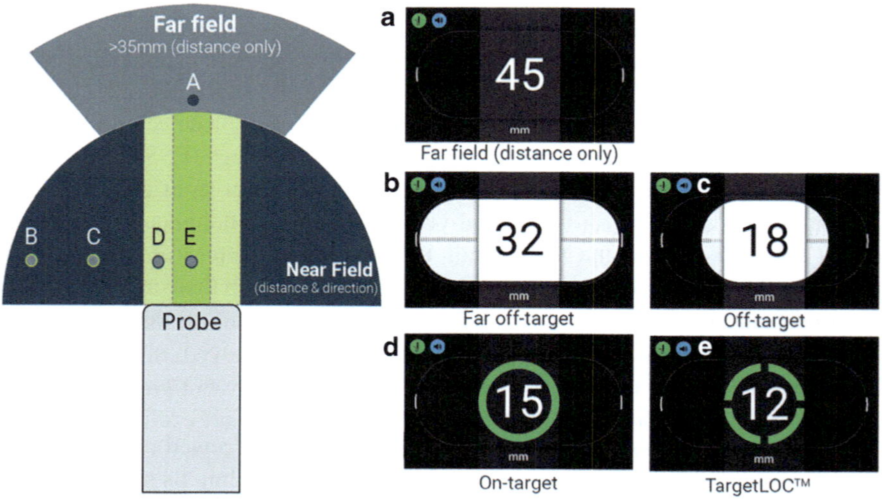

Fig. 12.5 Schematic diagram of TargetLOC function. (Image reproduced with permission from Sirius Medical, 2025)

The 'Slim' probe (Figs. 12.6 and 12.7) was first introduced to Europe in October [20] at the 43rd European Society of Surgical Oncology (ESSO) Congress, Antwerp, Belgium. The probe is 55% slimmer (12 mm diameter) than the standard probe (18 mm diameter) but with the same performance and precision (Table 12.1). It features a working length of 10 cm and is easier to use when access is limited, such as through small incisions or within the axilla (Fig. 12.8).

Furthermore, Sirius Pintuition can be used in conjunction with other imaging modalities such as ultrasound and mammography to guide the surgeon. This integration aims to offer a comprehensive tumour localisation solution, particularly for complex cases where multimodal imaging can enhance surgical precision.

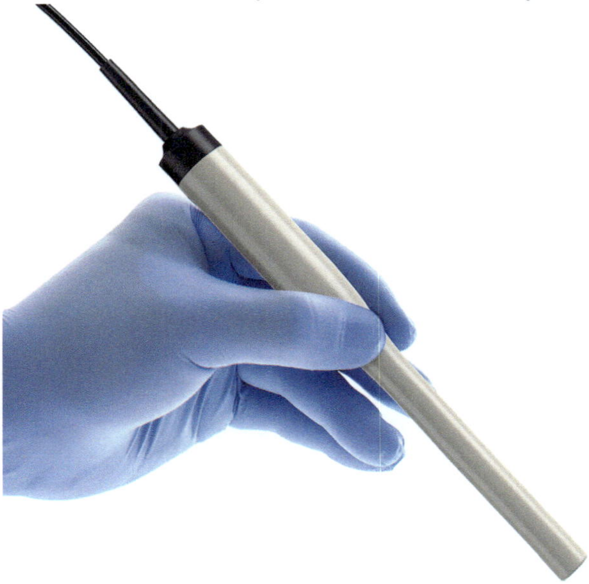

Fig. 12.6 The Pintuition Slim Probe. (Image reproduced with permission from Sirius Medical, 2025)

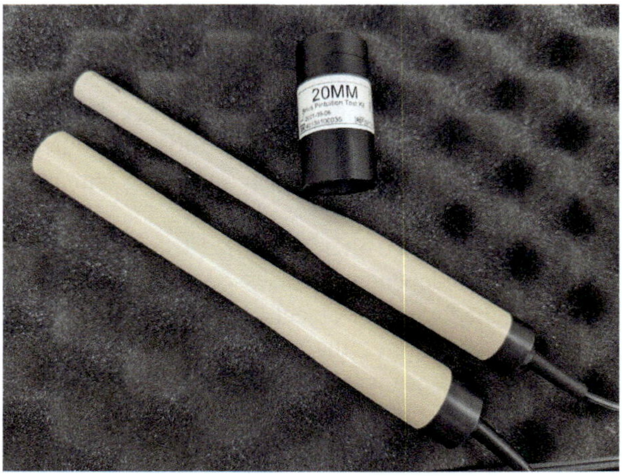

Fig. 12.7 The normal probe (bottom) and the slim probe (top), with the black 20mm calibration cap above the slim probe. (Photo by E. St John—Portsmouth Hospitals University NHS Trust)

Table 12.1 Specification of Pintuition and Pintuition slim probe

Features	Pintuition Slim Probe	Pintuition probe
Diameter (tip of probe)	12 mm	18 mm
Length of probe	19 cm	18 cm
Multi-sensor detection	Yes	Yes
GPS*Detect*™	Yes	Yes
TargetLOC™	Yes	Yes
Re-sterilization (only in FDA-regulated regions)	Yes	Yes

Table reproduced with permission from Sirius Medical, 2025

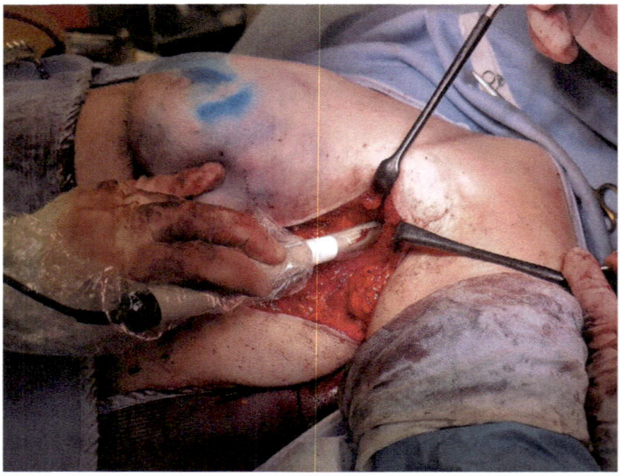

Fig. 12.8 Pintuition slim probe being used in the left axilla for Targeted Axillary Dissection. (Photo by E. St John—Portsmouth Hospitals University NHS Trust)

12.5 Literature Review

A literature review was conducted using Pubmed and GoogleScholar as primary sources, for studies published between January 2010 and December [20]. MeSH terms in the inclusion criteria included: Magnetic seed localisation, Sirius Pintuition, localisation of non-palpable breast lesions and outcomes. Further inclusion criteria were studies available in English, involving human subjects and including participants aged 18 and above.

Following this, we filtered by title, abstract, and full text availability. The included articles were independently assessed, and studies not satisfying the inclusion criteria, misaligned with our objectives, or providing insufficient data were excluded.

In early literature, the originally developed Magnetic Marker Localisation Device (MaMaLoc) was compared to WGL in a small randomised controlled trial (RCT) ($n = 70$) [25]. Retrieval rates were 100% for both groups, with a significantly lower positive margin rate in the MaMaLoc arm (8% vs. 18% in the WGL group), while reoperation rates were similar (4% vs. 6%). Surgical usability was rated higher for MaMaLoc, and patients reported greater satisfaction (median score 5/5 vs. 4.5/5 in WGL). However, this RCT did not include data on the Pintuition localisation device.

A German study conducted a comparative analysis of wire-guided localisation (WGL) and non-radioactive seed (NRS) localisation techniques available in Germany, including Pintuition, SAVI SCOUT, LOCalizer, and Magseed [18]. While the primary focus of the study was on logistical factors and carbon footprint, the findings demonstrated that magnetic seed localisation presents a viable and safe alternative to WGL. The study concluded that NRS techniques offer logistical advantages, particularly in facilitating surgical scheduling and enhancing patient comfort. Additionally, the results suggested that the adoption of NRS may contribute to a reduced environmental impact.

Sirius Pintuition has been evaluated in several single-centre studies with small cohorts. In an Italian study of 20 patients, Pintuition was deemed safe, easy to use, and precise [14]. Similarly, a US cohort of 29 patients reported 100% marker retrieval, with only one re-excision for positive margins and no seed migration [12].

A series from southern England included 42 patients, where 41 had successful lesion identification, and one had a complete pathological response post-neoadjuvant chemotherapy. The reoperation rate for margin re-excision was 21%, with seed migration observed in three patients [15]. A continuation of this series with 170 patients reported a 98.2% tumour identification rate, an 18% re-excision rate, and 4% postoperative complications [17]. Complications included seroma or wound infection. This larger cohort study involved nine surgeons; however, results were from abstracts, highlighting the need for multicentre trials.

A Dutch study compared Pintuition ($n = 85$) to WGL ($n = 52$), finding no significant differences in re-excision rates (3.5% vs. 3.8%) or complication rates (5.8%). Importantly, there were no cases of seed migration [24]. A Spanish series evaluated Pintuition in 77 breast lesions and 7 axillary lymph nodes, reporting 100% retrieval and a 15.6% re-excision rate in breast cases. This study was the first to assess lymph node localisation, though larger samples are needed for generalisability.

The largest cohort study to date, from a French cancer centre, evaluated 200 procedures. Tumour and marker retrieval rates were 100%, with a 9% re-excision rate, lower than the 10–20% observed internationally [16]. Notably, patients with ductal carcinoma in situ (DCIS) with microcalcifications were excluded, potentially affecting re-excision rates. This could be attributed to higher rates potentially linked to the presence of DCIS associated with an invasive carcinoma or DCIS alone. In this study, patients with DCIS with microcalcifications on mammography were excluded, only ten patients had DCIS alone and one re-excision for clear margins.

The Pintuition device's application is expanding to non-breast tumours. A Dutch study assessed ten patients with non-palpable soft tissue lesions including melanoma, soft tissue carcinoma, and recurrent rectal cancer demonstrating safety and feasibility despite small numbers [11]. Another Dutch study evaluated 58 patients; non palpable melanoma ($n = 45$), Merkel cell carcinoma ($n = 2$), and soft tissue sarcoma ($n = 11$), reporting 100% localisation and comparable resection margins with no seed migration. However, its retrospective design and low subgroup sizes limit the findings [7].

Recent literature increasingly supports the de-escalation of axillary surgery in breast cancer patients who convert from node-positive to node-negative status following neoadjuvant chemotherapy (NACT). Conventional axillary lymph node dissection (ALND), once standard in such cases, is now being supplemented or replaced by less invasive techniques such as sentinel lymph node biopsy (SLNB) and targeted axillary dissection (TAD). These approaches aim to reduce surgical morbidity without compromising oncologic safety. One critical aspect of TAD involves the accurate localisation and retrieval of previously biopsied metastatic lymph nodes, which has led to the development of various marking technologies, including magnetic seed localisation devices such as Sirius Pintuition [27].

In a US-based retrospective study involving 24 breast cancer patients undergoing NACT, the Sirius Pintuition device achieved a 100% retrieval rate of marked axillary lymph nodes, highlighting its precision and reliability in intraoperative localisation in both NACT and non-NACT patients [13]. A similar single-centre Austrian study evaluated 20 patients with biopsy-proven nodal disease who had magnetic markers placed prior to systemic treatment. All marked nodes were successfully retrieved, and no complications related to marker placement were reported [10]. While these early findings suggest that the Pintuition system offers a feasible, wire-free, and minimally invasive alternative to conventional localisation methods, both studies are limited by small sample sizes and potential selection bias. Larger prospective trials are needed to validate these results and assess long-term outcomes, including recurrence rates.

In conclusion, studies show promising early results with Pintuition compared to competing technologies. However, most data are from single centres with small cohorts, and cost-effectiveness remains unclear. Multicentre trials are needed to confirm oncological safety and patient outcomes. The ongoing MELODY (MEthods for LOcalization of Different types of breast lesions) study, initiated by EUBREAST and iBRA-NET, aims to address these knowledge gaps [9]. Additionally, the iBRA-NET localisation study with Sirius Pintuition is nearing completion, with results expected in 2025.

12.6 Summary of Clinical Evidence (Table 12.2)

Table 12.2 Summary of clinical evidence and publications on Pintuition

Title (reference)	Publication year	No. of patients	Design	Objective	Target/ device
Magnetic surgical marker navigation for excision of non-palpable ultrasound visible breast lesions: first 200 cases in a French cancer center [28]	2025	200	Monocentre, prospective	Outcomes	Breast cancer Pintuition
Magnetic seed localization is feasible for non-palpable melanoma, Merkel cell carcinoma, and soft tissue sarcoma lesions [7]	2024	61	Monocentre, retrospective	Feasibility	Melanoma, Merkel cell carcinoma, soft tissue sarcoma Pintuition
Targeted axillary dissection using surgical marker navigation after Neoadjuvant systemic treatment in breast cancer patients: A single-center experience [10]	2024	20	Monocentre, retrospective	Safety and performance	Lymph nodes Pintuition
Combining contrast-enhanced mammography and radioactive-free magnetic seed localization of non-palpable breast tumors: A feasibility study [26]	2024	20	Prospective, observational	Safety and feasibility	Breast cancer Pintuition

(continued)

Table 12.2 (continued)

Title (reference)	Publication year	No. of patients	Design	Objective	Target/ device
Surgical marker navigation system in breast conserving surgery and excision of non-palpable lesions: First Spanish single-center experience [20]	2024	84	Retrospective, observational	Safety and feasibility	Breast cancer, lymph nodes Pintuition
A novel surgical marker navigation system to localise and remove non-palpable breast lesions. A Dutch Centre experience. [24]	2023	Pintuition [$n = 85$], WGL [$n = 52$]	Monocentre, retrospective case series vs. WGL	Safety and performance (margin status, satisfaction, etc.)	Breast cancer Pintuition and WGL
Safety and performance of Sirius Pintuition - a novel wire-free and non-radioactive localization system for breast cancer surgery. [6]	2021	33 (25 treated with device)	Monocentre prospective, single-arm	Safety and performance (user satisfaction, RR, operative time)	Breast cancer Pintuition
Intraoperative localisation of ectopic parathyroid adenoma with a magnetic marker. [8]	2021	1	Case report	Safety and performance	Soft tissue Pintuition
Randomised controlled trial comparing magnetic marker localisation with wire guided localisation in the treatment of early-stage breast cancer [25]	2020	70 (35 × 2)	Monocentre randomised controlled prospective. Comparison to WGL	Safety and performance (margin status, satisfaction)	Breast cancer MaMaLoc

Adapted from Sirius Medical Clinical Evidence with permission 2025

12.7 Tips, Tricks, Pitfalls

Surgical innovation has transformed the way clinical care is delivered. New techniques, devices, and instruments often require the development of new skills. To get the most out of the Pintuition localisation device, here are a few key tips and tricks to optimise its performance and ensure accuracy:

Neoadjuvant Chemotherapy (NACT) is increasingly being employed as the initial treatment for locally advanced breast cancer and for women with axillary lymphadenopathy. Tumour size reduction to facilitate breast conservation is often an indication for neoadjuvant therapy, making an accurate method for detecting residual cancer essential for surgical planning.

Artefact on MRI For patients who undergo NACT, MRI is regarded as the imaging reference standard for response monitoring during NACT. Though there is no contraindication to Pintuition during NACT, one of the main disadvantages of all metallic markers is the creation of an MRI signal void artefact surrounding the marker thus hampering accurate MR imaging. The size of the artefact depends on the specific properties of the marker, but is quoted at 2.5–6 cm for Pintuition and depends on local imaging systems and settings. If tumour response is to be assessed by the MRI, then magnetic markers should not be placed in the vicinity of the tumour area before NACT. Instead, a radiologically inserted clip can be placed to mark the area of concern, and the Pintuition marker can be inserted prior to surgery. The potential issue with this is that some have reported [5] that it is more difficult to insert a marker into a treated node that has responded to NACT, because it becomes smaller and more fibrotic. Therefore, some centres use Ultrasound or Contrast-Enhanced Mammography (CEM) to assess treatment response to NACT instead of MRI. It is acceptable to insert Pintuition upfront prior to NACT, providing the tumour in the breast is away from the upper outer quadrant, and would not be affected by a 6 cm diameter artefact originating from the low axilla.

Contrast-Enhanced Mammography (CEM) While MRI is currently the most sensitive and specific imaging modality for determining response to neoadjuvant therapy in breast cancer patients, multiple studies have demonstrated that CEM is comparable to MRI in assessing complete pathological response and identifying the extent of residual disease (5–6). This evidence suggests that CEM offers advantages over breast MRI, which may have limited clinical utility due to its high cost, prolonged scan times, limited availability, and restrictions in patients contraindicated for MRI. CEM provides an effective imaging modality for response monitoring while magnetic markers are in situ. CEM is a breast imaging technique that utilises an iodine-based intravenous contrast agent in combination with standard mammography to enhance the visibility of certain breast lesions. Since CEM does not rely on magnetic fields, no image distortion occurs when CEM is combined with magnetic seed localisation (Fig. 12.9). A recent study conducted in the Netherlands showed promising results in evaluating whether Pintuition seeds caused imaging artefacts in

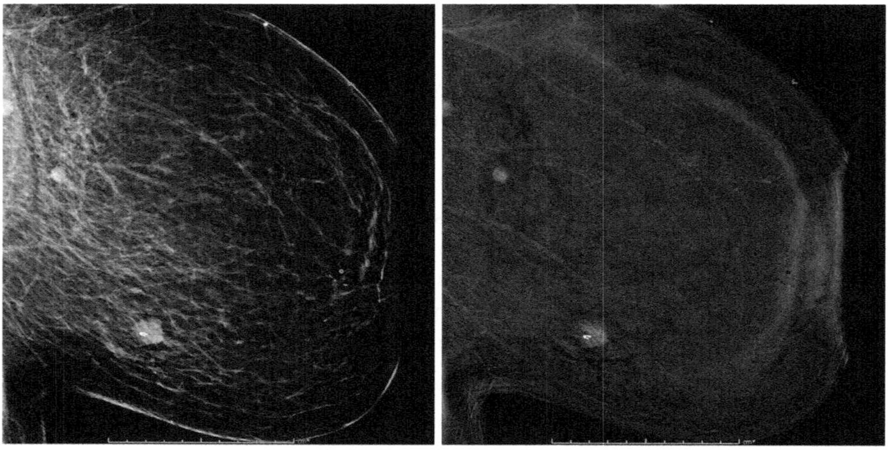

Fig. 12.9 Contrast-enhanced mammogram demonstrating a tumour with a clip in situ. (Photo by W. Abou-Samra—Betsi Cadwaladr University LHB, Glan Clwyd Hospital)

CEM examinations. The results indicated that no imaging artefacts were observed on CEM, in contrast to MRI [26].

Seed Migration In early iterations of the Pintuition delivery needle, it was possible for the seed to drop out under gravity and prior to being deployed in the correct position. The addition of a hashed element to the needle tip solved this problem. However, as is the case with all marker and clips, migration along the needle tract is a problem that is not infrequently encountered. Some markers have aimed to reduce this by the addition of anchors, spikes, or ridges. The Pintuition seed is smooth, hence is susceptible to this phenomenon. One technique described to reduce seed migration during stereotactic deployment is to wait a few minutes after deployment before slowly releasing the compression. Another tip is to rotate the needle as the seed is deployed and during retraction.

Magnetisation Unlike paramagnetic seed detection systems (Magseed) that will interact with all ferrous containing instruments, the Pintuition probe only detects magnetised material and therefore in theory is compatible with standard metal instruments. However, some surgical instruments do become magnetised during their lifetime, often when they have been placed on a magnetic mat as used in some theatres for instrument organisation. Once an instrument is magnetised, it can cause interference with the probe. Thus, it may be prudent to have one set of non-magnetic instruments available, such as polymer, carbon fibre, or titanium.

Furthermore, as the seed is magnetic, upon interaction with the tissue and manoeuvring close to the seed (within ~5 mm), it may dislodge from the target lesion and adhere to a metallic instrument. To overcome this, during initial dissection, it is recommended to place a stitch over the site of the seed. This allows the surgeon to safely localise the tumour site if the seed was to get dislodged.

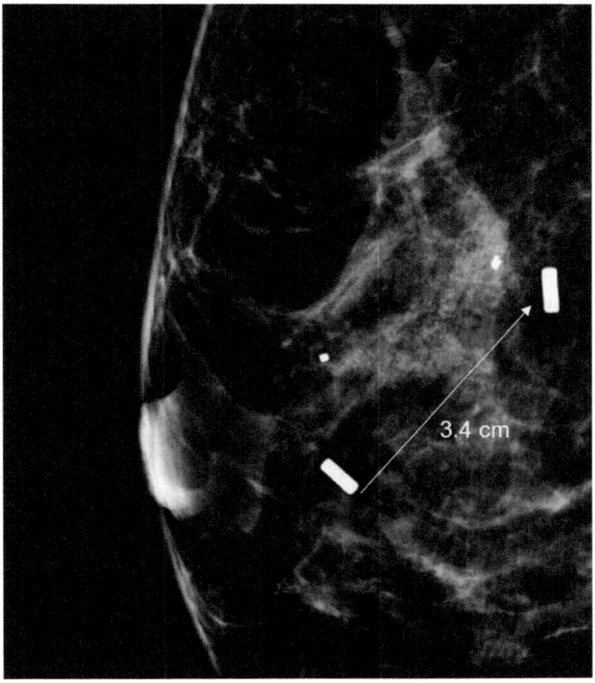

Fig. 12.10 Bracketing of lesion using two Pintuition marker seeds. (Photo by permission of Dr Erica Giblin)

Bracketing In larger lesions two or more seeds can be placed within >5 cm of each other to define the extent of the lesion that require excision [19] (Fig. 12.10). The 5 cm distance is recommended by the manufacturer but others have reported successful bracketing using Pintuition seeds at smaller distances. However, the closer the seeds are together, the increased likelihood the signals from the seeds will clash, hence confusing the probe device and leading to inaccurate readings. Furthermore, if multiple markers are required, there are increasing cost benefits for utilising wires in these settings.

Learning Curves As with all novel technologies, there is a learning curve for both the radiologist placing the marker and the surgeons finding it. An advantage of the Pintuition is it is intuitively designed. The deployment needle works much like other needles the radiologists are familiar with; however, the size (14 g) is larger than most clips that are routinely deployed. For the surgeon, there is a simple on/off button and it only needs calibration once at the beginning of the operation. It is not susceptible to the 'drift' that hampers other devices. The onscreen display is clear and the audible tone appropriate. As with all probe-based detection systems, there is an additional skill to learn to watch and check the detection system whilst operating, though this is not dissimilar to the technique used when using a gamma probe to locate the sentinel lymph node, and therefore is a familiar technique to most surgeons.

12.8 Future Scoping

It is reasonable to expect this product category will evolve in a similar manner to gamma-probe technology, which has gradually advanced over time. This includes developments such as the introduction of thinner probes, wireless functionality, a broader range of probe options (including angled and laparoscopic probes), and enhanced versatility for a wider array of clinical indications.

For the GPSDetect platform specifically, there are numerous potential improvements that can be integrated. Sirius Medical are working towards the launch of GPSDetect360, a feature that will allow users to seamlessly assess the depth of a seed relative to the probe's surface by providing a clear view of the area 'behind the probe tip'. In the future, the incorporation of more advanced 3D data regarding the precise location of the seed in relation to the probe is both feasible and likely to further improve the usability of the system. Novel methods integrating 3D localisation with augmented reality offer a new level of precision for surgeons. Such an approach has the potential to provide a better understanding of the operating scene, especially for lumpectomies where magnetic seeds are already being utilised [3].

12.9 Conclusion

The Sirius Pintuition device is an intuitive, easy-to-use localisation technology designed for the surgical removal of breast tumours and other soft tissue cancers. Available across Europe and the USA, it provides precise, intuitive guidance with on-screen directional support. Surgeons and radiologists have reported greater satisfaction with this system compared to traditional wire-guided localisation, and cohort studies have shown promising results. This device enhances surgical outcomes and improves patient satisfaction, making it a valuable addition to breast cancer management.

References

1. Sung H, Ferlay J, Siegel RL, et al. Global cancer statistics 2020: GLOBOCAN estimates of incidence and mortality worldwide for 36 cancers in 185 countries. CA Cancer J Clin. 2021;71:209–49. https://doi.org/10.3322/caac.21660.
2. Ahmed M, Rubio IT, Klaase JM, Douek M. Surgical treatment of nonpalpable primary invasive and in situ breast cancer. Nat Rev Clin Oncol. 2015;12:645–63. https://doi.org/10.1038/nrclinonc.2015.161.
3. Ambrosini P, AzizianAmiri S, Zeestraten E, et al. 3D magnetic seed localization for augmented reality in surgery. Int J Comput Assist Radiol Surg. 2024;19:723–33. https://doi.org/10.1007/s11548-024-03066-6.
4. Banys-Paluchowski M, Kühn T, Masannat Y, et al. Localization techniques for non-palpable breast lesions: current status, knowledge gaps, and rationale for the MELODY study

(EUBREAST-4/iBRA-NET, NCT 05559411). Cancer. 2023;15:1173. https://doi.org/10.3390/cancers15041173.
5. Barry PA, Harborough K, Sinnett V, et al. Clinical utility of axillary nodal markers in breast cancer. Eur J Surg Oncol. 2023;49:709–15. https://doi.org/10.1016/j.ejso.2022.12.019.
6. Bessems M, Van Breest Smallenburg V, Van Bebber I, et al. Safety and performance of Sirius Pintuition – a novel wire-free and non-radioactive localization system for breast cancer surgery. Eur J Surg Oncol. 2021;47:e1. https://doi.org/10.1016/j.ejso.2020.11.148.
7. van der Burg SJC, Kuijpers A, Baetens T, et al. Magnetic seed localization is feasible for non-palpable melanoma, Merkel cell carcinoma, and soft tissue sarcoma lesions. Eur J Surg Oncol. 2024;50. https://doi.org/10.1016/j.ejso.2024.108485.
8. Clement C, DM Hoed, Jansen P. Intraoperative localisation of ectopic parathyroid adenoma with a magnetic marker. J Surg Endocrinol. 2021;3. https://doi.org/10.36959/608/452.
9. Dave RV, Barrett E, Morgan J, et al. Wire- and magnetic-seed-guided localization of impalpable breast lesions: iBRA-NET localisation study. Br J Surg. 2022;109:274–82. https://doi.org/10.1093/bjs/znab443.
10. Egle D, Brunner C, Ritter M, et al. Targeted axillary dissection using surgical marker navigation after neoadjuvant systemic treatment in breast cancer patients: a single-center experience. Breast Care. 2025;20:57–65. https://doi.org/10.1159/000541704.
11. Galema H, Mulder EEAP, Grunhagen DJ, et al. Successful use of a magnetic localisation system for non-palpable malignant lesions: a single centre experience. Eur J Surg Oncol. 2022;48:e141. https://doi.org/10.1016/j.ejso.2021.12.270.
12. Giblin E, Aaron J. First experience with Sirius Pintuition® in the United States- an innovative navigation system for targeted surgical excision of non-palpable breast cancer. Eur J Surg Oncol. 2023;49:e76. https://doi.org/10.1016/j.ejso.2022.11.242.
13. Giblin E, Govert K. Targeted axillary node dissection using Sirius Pintuition GPSDetect™ marker navigation: a retrospective multicenter case series. Breast. 2024;74:103651. https://doi.org/10.1016/j.breast.2023.103651.
14. Giovanazzi R, Pellitteri C, Gisabella M, et al. First Italian experience with Sirius Pintuition system for localization of small non-palpable breast lesions (<9 mm): preliminary data. Eur J Surg Oncol. 2022;48:e66–7. https://doi.org/10.1016/j.ejso.2021.12.058.
15. Hassan I, Abdelaziz Y, Sheehan L, et al. Early UK experience of Pintuition localiser device within a representative large UK breast unit. Eur J Surg Oncol. 2023;49:e239. https://doi.org/10.1016/j.ejso.2023.03.092.
16. Jamaris S, Akpolat-Basci L, Stephanou M, et al. Re-excision rates in breast-conserving surgery for invasive breast cancer after neoadjuvant chemotherapy with and without the use of a radiopaque tissue transfer and X-ray system. Breast Care. 2019;14:302–7. https://doi.org/10.1159/000493017.
17. Khatun A, Khokher A, Ghosh A, et al. First year data regarding use of Pintuition localisation device for non-palpable breast lesions in a large UK breast unit. Eur J Surg Oncol. 2024;50. https://doi.org/10.1016/j.ejso.2024.108114.
18. Lukac S, Leinert E, Kühn T, et al. Eco-logistical comparison of non-radioactive seeds and the wire-guided localization for intraoperative detection of breast lesions. Eur J Surg Oncol. 2025;51. https://doi.org/10.1016/j.ejso.2024.108779.
19. Parks R, Mckay M, Abbasi A, et al. Sirius Pintuition™ localisation device for impalpable breast lesions – the UHDB experience. Eur J Surg Oncol. 2024;50. https://doi.org/10.1016/j.ejso.2024.108215.
20. Santana Valenciano Á, Rivas Fidalgo S, Corral Moreno S, et al. Surgical marker navigation system in breast conserving surgery and excision of non-palpable lesions: first Spanish single-center experience. Breast Cancer Res Treat. 2024;207:533–40. https://doi.org/10.1007/s10549-024-07382-y.
21. Schermers B, Franke V, Rozeman EA, et al. Surgical removal of the index node marked using magnetic seed localization to assess response to neoadjuvant immunotherapy in patients with stage III melanoma. Br J Surg. 2019;106:519–22. https://doi.org/10.1002/bjs.11168.

22. Schermers B, ten Haken B, Muller SH, et al. Optimization of an implantable magnetic marker for surgical localization of breast cancer. Biomed Phys Eng Express. 2018;4:067001. https://doi.org/10.1088/2057-1976/aadb53.
23. Schermers B, van der Hage JA, Loo CE, et al. Feasibility of magnetic marker localisation for non-palpable breast cancer. Breast Edinb Scotl. 2017;33:50–6. https://doi.org/10.1016/j.breast.2017.03.003.
24. Stengs L, van Veen S, Moormann G. A novel surgical marker navigation system to localise and remove non-palpable breast lesions: a Dutch Centre experience. Breast Glob J. 2023;1:49. https://doi.org/10.4103/bgj.bgj_2_23.
25. Struik GM, Schermers B, Mares I, et al. Randomized controlled trial comparing magnetic marker localization (MaMaLoc) with wire-guided localization in the treatment of early-stage breast cancer. Breast J. 2021;27:638–50. https://doi.org/10.1111/tbj.14262.
26. Theunissen JEM, van Haaren ERM, Frotscher CNA, et al. Combining contrast-enhanced mammography and radioactive-free magnetic seed localization of non-palpable breast tumors: a feasibility study. J Cancer. 2024;15:6177–84. https://doi.org/10.7150/jca.98597.
27. Banys-Paluchowski M, de Boniface J. Axillary staging in node-positive breast cancer converting to node negativity through neoadjuvant chemotherapy: Current evidence and perspectives. Scand J Surg. 2023;112(2):117–25. https://doi.org/10.1177/14574969221145892. Epub 2023 Jan 15. PMID: 36642957.
28. Ceccato V, Wallaert L, Michel S, Gaillard T, Girard N, Darrigues L, Pauly L, Gauroy E, Raimond E, Menouer I, Graesslin O, Rosa J, Laas E, Reyal F, Grandal B, Hotton J. Magnetic surgical marker navigation for excision of non-palpable ultrasound visible breast lesions: first 200 cases in a French cancer center. Sci Rep. 2025;15(1):5002. https://doi.org/10.1038/s41598-025-88430-5. PMID: 39930014; PMCID: PMC11811009.

Chapter 13
Pathology Perspective of Analysing Histology Following Localisation of Impalpable Breast Cancer

Abeer M. Shaaban and Elyse Rigby

Contents

13.1 Introduction

The diagnosis of an impalpable breast lesion involves the combined use of advanced skills in diagnostic radiology, surgical precision, and pathological expertise. Without this collaboration of specialties, many of these asymptomatic cases might otherwise remain undiagnosed and untreated. Advances in breast imaging modalities, such as

A. M. Shaaban (✉)
University Hospitals Birmingham NHS Foundation Trust, Birmingham, UK
e-mail: Abeer.shaaban@uhb.nhs.uk; a.shaaban@bham.ac.uk

E. Rigby
University Hospitals Birmingham NHS Foundation Trust, Birmingham, UK

Department of Pathology, University Hospital Birmingham, Birmingham, UK

R. Vidya, N. Sharma (eds.), *Breast and Axilla Localisation Techniques*,
https://doi.org/10.1007/978-3-032-17995-1_13

mammography, ultrasound, and magnetic resonance imaging (MRI), have significantly increased the detection of impalpable lesions through breast screening programmes and incidental radiological discovery, less commonly lesions can be identified incidentally during pathological examination. Impalpable lesions frequently account for early-stage breast cancers and high-risk abnormalities, which pose distinct challenges in localisation, surgical excision, and pathological assessment.

From a pathology perspective, accurate handling and macroscopic evaluation of the specimens are central to ensuring that the lesion is excised, margins are clear, and diagnostic markers are accurately assessed. Once identified, preoperative localisation techniques such as localisation wire, dye, radioactive and magnetic markers are essential for ensuring precise surgical removal and consequent pathological examination. Intraoperative specimen radiography should be completed to confirm excision of the suspicious lesion and images should be made available to the pathologist for radiological–pathological correlation to verify the presence and nature of the lesion, and anatomical relationships within the excised specimen.

Here, we provide an update on the pathology-specific considerations involved in managing impalpable breast lesions; discussing the types of breast specimens, localisation techniques, macroscopic handling, microscopic examination, and the overall integration of radiological and surgical findings in the pathological assessment. Through discussing challenges and current best practices in diagnostic histology of impalpable breast lesions, this chapter highlights the essential role of pathology in the multidisciplinary care of impalpable breast cancer.

13.2 Localisation Techniques and Radiological-Pathological Correlation

13.2.1 Impact of Wire-Guided Versus Wire-Free Techniques

As the starting point for treatment and diagnosis, lesion localisation can impact the approach from a pathological perspective including both macroscopic and microscopic examination. For macroscopic examination, localisation techniques are best divided into wire-guided and wire-free methods as the external appearance of the guide wires provides two potential identifiers for the pathologist to find the excised lesion(s), with the guide wire providing a direct tract to the lesion as well as the internal marker clips. The wire-guided localisation technique also requires coupling of radiology and surgery on the day of the operation, which may lead to extra preoperative images compared to wire-free techniques.

In contrast to these advantages, wire-guided methods also have the potential of causing extra challenges to radiological–pathological correlation as there is a risk of wire displacement and tissue injury, particularly on extracting the wire from the tissue during macroscopic dissection. Pre- or intraoperative wire displacement is more concerning as it may lead to incomplete excision. Intraoperative specimen X-raying is considered the best practice to confirm marker clip placement and reduce such risks. Post-operative displacement is more likely to occur during specimen transit or handling and poses less of a challenge due to the use of laboratory X-ray imaging, which can readily locate the target lesion and clip markers.

The most popular methods of wire-free localisation can be further sub-categorised into radioactive and non-radioactive techniques, which from a pathology perspective can bring the addition of laboratory compliances with handling and disposing of radiolabelled specimens. However, due to the low radiation exposure from these specimens, there is no impact or required adaptations to the examination and dissection. In contrast to wire-guided methods, there is a low risk of seed misplacement or displacement once inserted, as the marker remains deep within the breast tissue and cannot be pulled or knocked by external objects. However, occasionally, the seeds can migrate away from the biopsy site between the time of implantation and the time of excision.

13.2.2 Alternative Localisation Techniques

In addition to the most common wire-guided and wire-free localisation techniques, there are several alternative and less commonly used techniques, which are worth noting. Several of these techniques involve injecting a marker substance, which can cause microscopic changes to the breast tissue (Table 13.1).

Table 13.1 Summary of less common localisation methods and their histological appearances

Technique	Description	Histological findings
Cryolocalisation	Uses a frozen cryo-marker to identify lesions during surgery	Minimal freezing-related tissue changes, including ice-crystal damage, may cause focal cellular disruption
Electromagnetic localisation	Employs radiofrequency tags detected with a handheld reader for precise lesion localisation	No tissue reactions or histological artefacts
Ultrasound-guided localisation	Provides real-time intraoperative guidance for lesions visible on ultrasound without requiring markers	No tissue reaction or artefacts due to absence of marker placement
Hydrogel markers	Biodegradable injectable markers for long-term lesion tracking	Gelatinous material that may elicit a mild foreign body reaction involving macrophages, histiocytes, and multinucleated giant cells
Carbon localisation	Utilizes a sterile carbon suspension to create a visible mark near the lesion for surgical guidance	Black pigment deposits visible microscopically; excessive carbon may obscure underlying cellular details
Collagen markers	Biocompatible markers injected during biopsy that integrate into tissue and remain detectable for future localisation	Amorphous or fibrous material; may cause a mild foreign body reaction with macrophages, histiocytes, and multinucleated giant cells

13.3 Histopathology Specimen Request Forms

Adequate clinical information is paramount on dealing with surgical specimens. Knowledge of the core biopsy diagnosis is essential as it determines how pathologist deal with the surgical specimen including requirements for specimen X-raying and extent of sampling. For example, a diagnostic excision following a B3 uncertain diagnosis is generally processed in its entirety. Lesions associated with mammographic calcification, mammographically occult lesions, multifocal lesions, and residual tumours that have been modified by prior therapy require extensive and thorough sampling.

An important and useful way of providing relevant and concise clinical information is by filling histopathology surgical request forms. Illustration by diagrams is extremely helpful particularly for non-straightforward specimens. Tick boxes of relevant parameters serve as aid memoire and ensure that important parameters are not missed. An example of a good histopathology request form is provided (Fig. 13.1a). Other relevant information such as pregnancy/lactation, previous/concurrent cancer, enrolment in a clinical trial is also useful to include on the request form.

13.4 Specimen Transport and Cold Ischaemic Time

Care should be taken to transfer surgical specimens to the pathology laboratory as soon as possible. A delay in transport leads to a long cold ischaemic time with subsequent deterioration of specimen quality [1]. Small specimens can be placed in sufficient amount of formalin to fix. Larger specimens should be inked and sliced. For large specimens, if rapid transport cannot be done for logistical reasons (such as weekend surgeries), they can be left in pots in theatre fridges, without immersion in formalin, until transport to pathology is arranged. This preserves the quality of specimen DNA and proteins and avoids the detrimental effect of delayed fixation on tissue.

13.5 Specimen Orientation, Inking, and Fixation

Orientation is particularly important if malignancy is suspected. Specimens that are sent without orientation, such as lumpectomies and breast reductions, are generally inked in one colour and representative sections taken. Inking ensures that surgical resection margins can reliably be identified microscopically and the distance between malignancy accurately measured.

A standard method for orientation, agreed between the surgical and pathology teams is preferable. Where full orientation sutures/clips are present, such as in wide

a

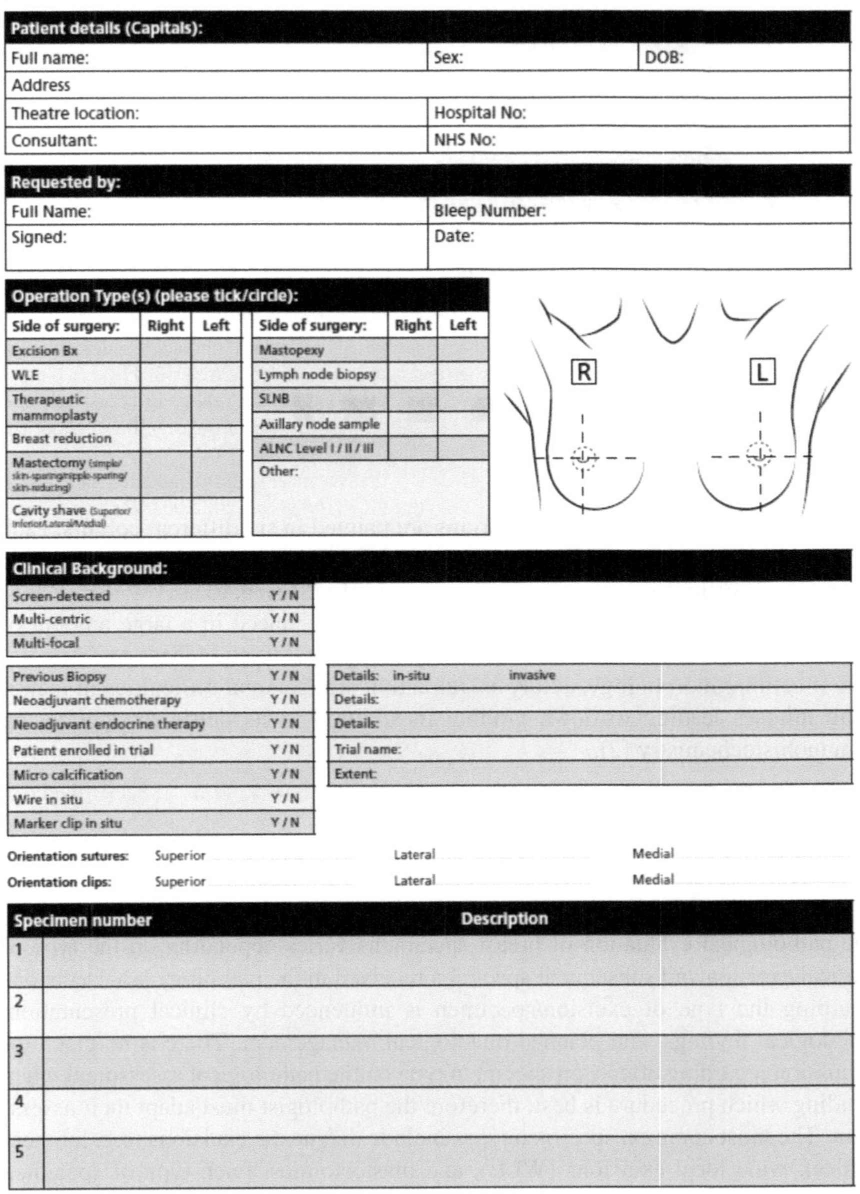

Patient details (Capitals):		
Full name:	Sex:	DOB:
Address		
Theatre location:	Hospital No:	
Consultant:	NHS No:	

Requested by:	
Full Name:	Bleep Number:
Signed:	Date:

Operation Type(s) (please tick/circle):

Side of surgery:	Right	Left	Side of surgery:	Right	Left
Excision Bx			Mastopexy		
WLE			Lymph node biopsy		
Therapeutic mammoplasty			SLNB		
Breast reduction			Axillary node sample		
Mastectomy (simple/ skin-sparing/nipple-sparing/ skin-reducing)			ALNC Level I / II / III		
Cavity shave (Superior/ Inferior/Lateral/Medial)			Other:		

Clinical Background:		
Screen-detected	Y / N	
Multi-centric	Y / N	
Multi-focal	Y / N	
Previous Biopsy	Y / N	Details: in-situ invasive
Neoadjuvant chemotherapy	Y / N	Details:
Neoadjuvant endocrine therapy	Y / N	Details:
Patient enrolled in trial	Y / N	Trial name:
Micro calcification	Y / N	Extent:
Wire in situ	Y / N	
Marker clip in situ	Y / N	

Orientation sutures: Superior .... Lateral .... Medial ....

Orientation clips: Superior .... Lateral .... Medial ....

Specimen number	Description
1	
2	
3	
4	
5	

Fig. 13.1 Clinicopathological correlation for breast specimens. (**a**) An example of surgical specimen histopathology request form containing relevant clinical details. A breast diagram is available to indicate laterality, site, and any other features of the lesion(s) of interest. (**b**) Wide local excision specimen showing standard orientation sutures and clips. (**c**) Schematic representation of standard inking and slicing of an orientated wide local excision specimen. (**d**) Lumpectomy specimen inked in one colour (black) and sliced for embedding and processing. It contains a greyish white lesion in the middle slice

b

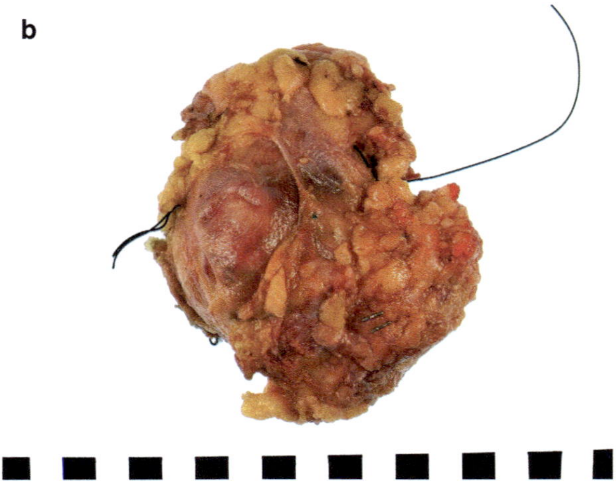

Fig. 13.1 (continued)

local excision (WLE) specimens, margins are painted in six different colours; each representing one surface for accurate microscopic margin identification and measurements of distance to margins where required (Fig. 13.1b, c).

Following inking, specimens are sliced to fix and placed in a large amount of formalin. Adequate fixation time is 7–72 h. Sub-optimal fixation leads to deterioration of cellular morphology, autolysis, retraction artefact, and difficulties in identifying mitoses leading to down grading in addition to its detrimental effect on immunohistochemistry [2].

13.6 Specimen Types and Gross Assessment

The pathological evaluation of breast specimens varies depending on the type of surgical excision and subsequent specimen received in the pathology lab. Decisions regarding the type of excision/specimen is influenced by clinical presentation, radiological findings, and planned oncological management. There is no place for discussion regarding effects on specimen type on the pathological assessment when deciding which procedure is best; therefore the pathologist must adapt their assessment. The most common specimen types include diagnostic excisions (e.g. lumpectomies), wide local excisions (WLE), and mastectomies. Each type of specimen requires a different approach to orientation and handling as part of the pathological assessment. Guidelines or specimens macroscopic handling and dissection are provided by the UK Royal College of Pathologists (RCPath) [3].

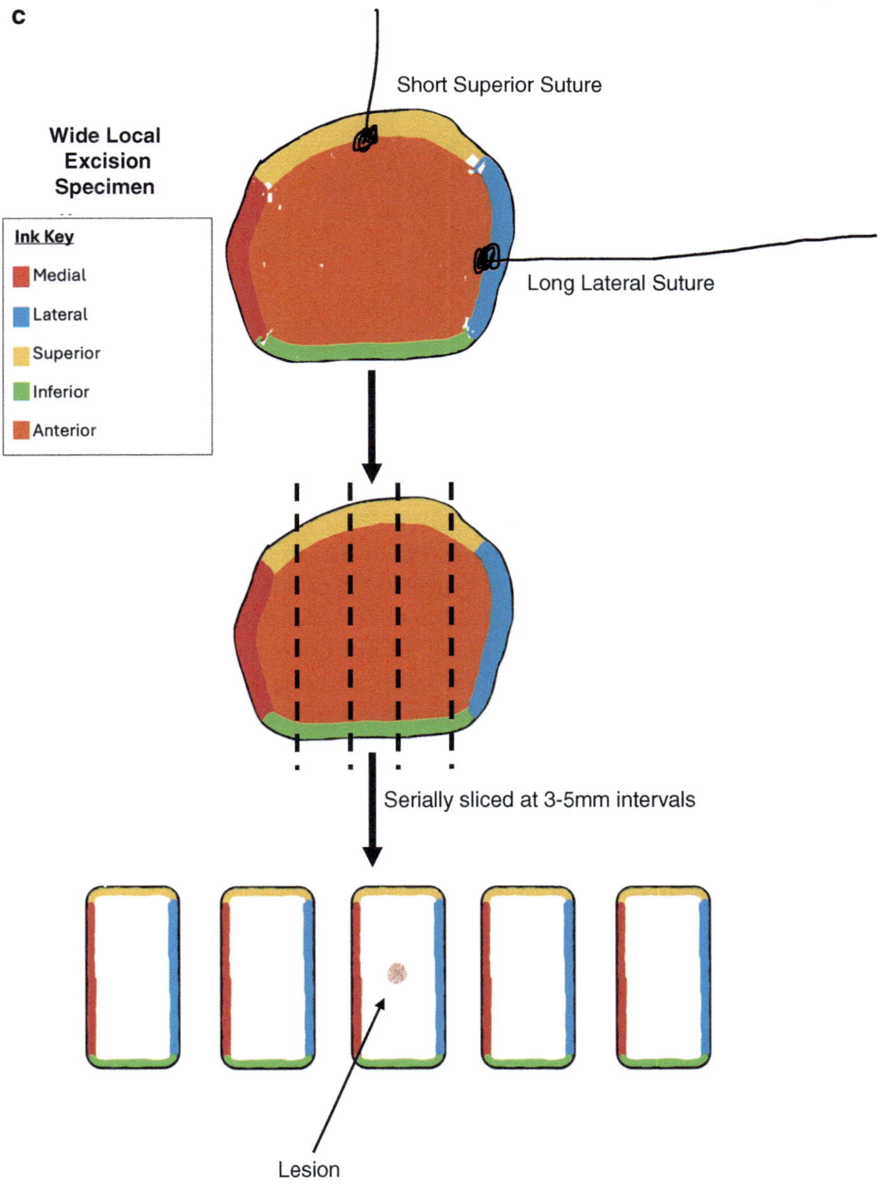

Fig. 13.1 (continued)

(a) *Lumpectomy/Diagnostic Excision*

Diagnostic excision specimens are typically completed to remove radiologically suspicious small, localised lesions or indeterminate preoperative diagnoses (e.g. C3/B3 or C4/B4 lesions) [4, 5]. These specimens may include a range of findings,

d

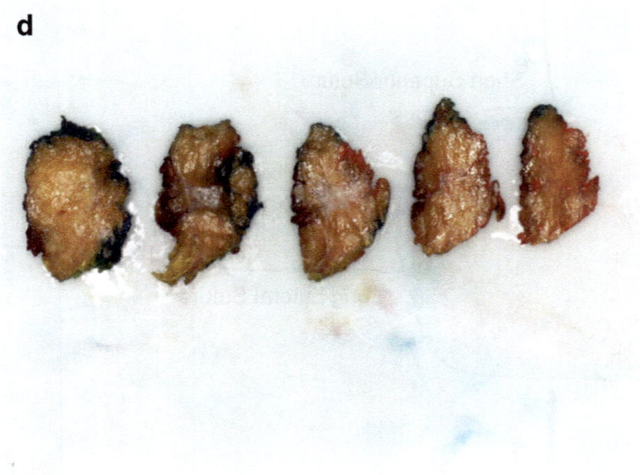

Fig. 13.1 (continued)

such as benign lesions, atypical hyperplasia, or early-stage malignancies such as ductal carcinoma in situ (DCIS). A systematic approach is essential; specimens should be inked, weighed, and measured in three dimensions before being serially sliced at intervals of 3–5 mm (Fig. 13.1d). Proper orientation and thorough documentation of any surgical markers in these cases are crucial to ensure accurate pathological assessment and to therefore guide subsequent treatment decisions.

For small specimens (less than 30 mm), it is generally recommended to embed and examine all tissues. In larger specimens, blocks should be taken to measure the histological size of the lesion and sampling must adequately include the extremes of mammographic abnormalities, plus adjacent tissue to avoid underestimating the lesion size, particularly in cases of DCIS.

(b) *Wide Local Excision (WLE)*

Wide local excisions are performed to remove malignant lesions along with an adequate margin of surrounding normal tissue. Orientation of these specimens is critical and is typically achieved using techniques like sutures or clips, which also help to identify the spatial relationship of the lesion to surgical margins (Fig. 13.1b, c). On initial examination, markers such as sutures are identified, with local protocol dictating orientation methods, agreed locally between the surgeon and pathologist, e.g. long suture for lateral, short suture for superior, and looped suture for nipple are commonly used. Accurate assessment of the margins is essential for determining whether additional surgical procedures are necessary to achieve clear margins; therefore, identifying the location of the lesion within the WLE and assessing the relationship to margins is essential.

From a pathology perspective, the approach to examining impalpable breast lesions in WLEs, particularly those associated with ductal carcinoma in situ (DCIS), requires meticulous coordination between radiological and pathological evaluation. DCIS frequently presents as mammographic abnormalities, such as microcalcifications, which may not be visible macroscopically. Therefore, a combined radiological–pathological approach is essential to ensure accurate lesion identification and sampling.

Specimens should be thoroughly documented, including weight, three-dimensional measurements, and detailed inking of excision margins. Different coloured inks are used to distinguish specific margins, though radio-opaque inks should be avoided if specimen radiographs are likely to be required. Serial slicing at 3–5 mm intervals facilitates radiographic mapping, where each slice is X-rayed to map the entire specimen, therefore enabling accurate localisation of the lesion(s) and minimizing the risk of underestimation of its size or overestimation of distances to margins. This process is particularly important for microcalcifications to produce mapped documentation of the lesions within a specimen. Alternatively, the whole specimen can be embedded for histological examination.

(c) *Mastectomy Specimens*

1. *Therapeutic Mastectomy*

Mastectomy specimens, which consist of the entire breast, are significantly larger than WLEs in the vast majority of cases but, on principle, are orientated similarly, often using the same local orientation methods involving sutures or clips. The posterior surface is typically inked using India ink; however, some centres or individual pathologists may use differential colour inking for anterior, posterior, and radial margins to help preserve orientation during and after block taking, particularly for skin sparing cases (Fig. 13.2a). Sampling must include a nipple block to assess for DCIS, and the remainder of the specimen is typically sliced in the sagittal plane, although in some instances coronal slicing is completed. The specimen may be X-rayed prior to slicing and/or once dissected into slices, to identify lesions and radiological markers and to provide detailed mapping. Several systems such as Faxitron® Path Specimen Radiology system and XPERT® Specimen Radiography Systems are available to purchase and use by pathology laboratories. The use of such laboratory image systems allows instant accessibility for the pathologist to X-ray images before and during macroscopic assessment, to identify impalpable lesions and ensure appropriate sampling of relevant tissues (Fig. 13.2b, c). Specimen X-ray findings form part of the patient records and help correlate with the preoperative diagnostic imaging such as during multidisciplinary team (MDT) discussions.

The extent of tissue sampling for pathological evaluation of DCIS is guided by the radiological size of the lesion, with careful attention to capturing the extremes of radiographic calcifications and adjacent tissues to avoid underestimating the lesion's size. A minimum of 1–2 conventional tissue blocks per 10 mm of calcification is recommended, with radiological correlation required to map the total lesion size.

Thorough sampling of any mass is essential to exclude an invasive component. Large tissue blocks may be beneficial for evaluating extensive DCIS and determining lesion size accurately. The entire mastectomy specimen, including areas of apparent normal tissue, should be sliced at 10 mm intervals and examined both

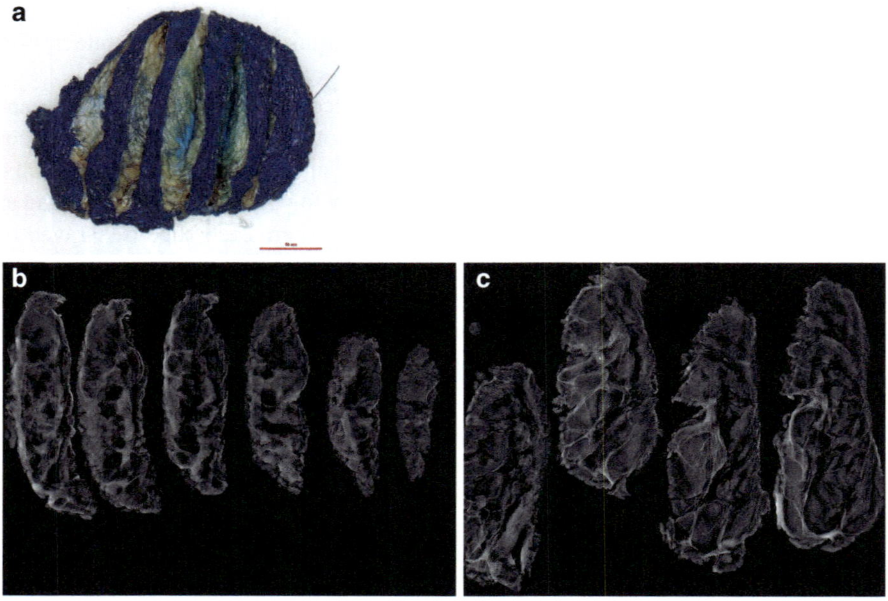

Fig. 13.2 Macroscopic handling of breast specimens. (a) Mastectomy specimen inked and sliced from the deep aspect. (b) X-rays of slices of a mastectomy in the pathology laboratory showing calcifications in two slices (first two slices from left). (c) Sliced, X-rayed mastectomy specimen. A marker clip is confirmed in second slice from left

visually and by palpation to identify and sample all abnormalities. Representative sampling of the nipple-areolar complex is required to assess for DCIS and look for mammary Paget's disease. The lateral end of the specimen should be examined for intramammary or low axillary lymph nodes. Additional quadrant sampling should be performed to ensure evaluation of all areas of the breast.

2. *Post-Neoadjuvant Mastectomy*

Pathological evaluation of breast specimens for tumour response from patients treated with neoadjuvant therapy poses unique challenges due to the reduction in size of the original tumour, frequently downstaging disease, including reduced numbers of nodal involvement. Although neoadjuvant therapy is commonly employed for high-grade, large, locally advanced, or inflammatory breast cancers, the tumour response therefore means that residual disease in the post-neoadjuvant mastectomy tends to present to the pathologist similarly to an impalpable lesion. These changes can complicate both macroscopic and microscopic handling of excision specimens, particularly in cases when treatment has been highly effective and there may not be any visual or palpable evidence of the original lesion [6].

Effective pathological evaluation depends heavily on detailed clinical imaging and pathological history including the tumour's original location, tumour type, and grade. This information can be crucial for identifying the tumour bed, which as forementioned, may be difficult to locate macroscopically. Specimen handling should follow standard protocols as for wide local excision or mastectomy, with prompt fixation and precise orientation. Localisation of the tumour bed can be aided by markers placed in the tumour before treatment or by pre-treatment lesion images. Skin markings such as a pre-chemotherapy tattoo, which externally maps the tumour size before therapy can also be valuable in guiding pathological evaluation in cases of non-skin spring mastectomy specimens. When the tumour shows an incomplete response to therapy, a residual mass may be apparent on palpation or slicing, allowing the specimen to be examined as with any primary resection. Significant tumour regression often presents as pale, ill-defined fibrotic areas, which may be identified on examination however; as discussed, there may be an absence of any visual or palpable area in the specimen, in which case detailed examination guided largely by radiological markers or residual microcalcifications must still be used.

The tumour bed is thoroughly sampled to detect any residual disease, with additional blocks taken from areas corresponding to the pretreatment extent of the lesion. In cases of focal regression, the tumour may appear as scattered foci within the bed, requiring extensive sampling to capture all the residual disease. Large tissue blocks, when available, are particularly valuable for preserving architecture and evaluating multiple foci, helping to assess the residual tumour volume and response to therapy. For larger tumours, assessment of the tumour bed may involve estimating slice thickness, counting consecutive blocks, and correlating histological dimensions.

Margins in therapeutic post-neoadjuvant wide local excision specimens must be sampled meticulously to ensure tumour clearance. Lymph nodes, which may be affected by neoadjuvant therapy, often present additional challenges in macroscopic identification as the original or the residual disease may only be represented by micrometastases or isolated tumour cells. Residual disease can be subtle and requires detailed microscopic examination with optional use of broad-spectrum cytokeratin immunohistochemical stains. Pathological evaluation of sentinel lymph nodes or axillary clearances should follow standard guidelines; however, it should be noted that node yield may be reduced in patients receiving neoadjuvant chemotherapy.

(d) *Oncoplastic Specimens*

Oncoplastic surgery combines cancer excision with cosmetic techniques during one or multiple operations to maintain breast aesthetics, allowing the surgeon to excise larger portions of tissue and often resulting in wider tumour-free margins. Oncoplastic excision specimens are typically completed for larger tumours; however, due to the large volume of tissue taken, they may result in incidental findings of impalpable lesions. From a pathology perspective, the principles of examination align with conventional specimens, and tumour sampling is performed similarly; however, margins typically require less thorough evaluation due to the increased amount of tissue, especially if the lesion is more than 30 mm from the margin. This is because it is rare for disease to be present in these areas without multifocal or extensive disease being detected preoperatively or during dissection using radial blocks or serial slicing.

Pathological evaluation of contralateral breast reduction specimens in cancer patients and prophylactic mastectomies in high-risk individuals requires more comprehensive sampling as there is an increased likelihood of identifying a high risk or precursor lesion, such as in situ carcinoma or atypical hyperplasia. Any abnormal areas should be sampled with a minimum of two tissue blocks including fibrous areas or parenchymal-rich tissue; however, additional blocks may be taken for patients aged over 40 or those with dense fibrous breast tissue to complete a more thorough assessment.

(e) *Handling of the Axilla*

The axillary lymph nodes are crucial in breast cancer staging, prognosis, and treatment planning. Sentinel lymph node biopsy (SLNB) is used to diagnose metastatic involvement whilst minimising the need for more extensive procedures such as full axillary dissection, which is associated with greater morbidity. Sentinel lymph nodes are typically identified using radioactive tracers or dyes like methylene blue or isosulphan blue and are then selectively excised during surgery for histological examination. If the patient undergoes neoadjuvant therapy, localisation techniques, such as the placement of clips or tattoos may be used to help identify previously involved nodes once the treatment is complete. Sentinel nodes undergo meticulous microscopic analysis through serial sectioning at 2 mm intervals and optional staining with immunohistochemical (pan-cytokeratin) markers, increasing the detection rate of micrometastases and isolated tumour cells.

In cases requiring complete axillary dissection, levels I and II lymph nodes are generally removed, and pathological evaluation includes detailed nodal count, measurement of metastatic deposits, and detection of extranodal extension, which are critical factors for accurate staging and therapeutic decision-making. If the apical node was marked, this is identified and reported separately. The axillary clearance is manually dissected by careful inspection and palpation. Following NACT, lymph nodes undergo atrophy resulting in lower lymph node yields.

13.7 Microscopic Findings and Reporting of Impalpable Breast Lesions

Microscopic assessment of impalpable breast lesions is fundamental to establishing a definitive diagnosis and determining prognostic factors. Where localisation methods such as clips or seeds are inserted, pathologists must document and confirm the presence of these macroscopically and, more importantly, microscopically to further verify target lesion excision. There are cases where it may be difficult to estimate the location with radiological–pathological correlation, and where macroscopic identification is not always possible; therefore, histological findings must be reported as an additional verifying factor. Tissue changes related to previous biopsy and a clip reaction are usually identified microscopically in the form of fat necrosis, multinucleated giant cell reaction, and chronic inflammation (Fig. 13.3a–c). These

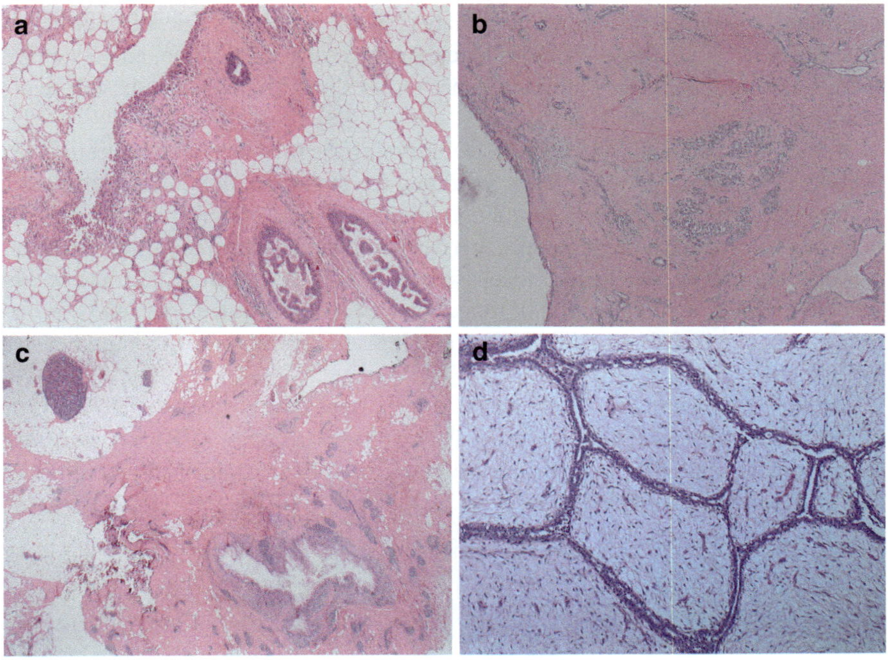

Fig. 13.3 Microscopic H&E features of some impalpable breast lesions. (**a**) A marker clip (upper left) associated with reactive stromal changes and fat necrosis with adjacent micropapillary DCIS. (**b**) Clip cavity with an adjacent mammary lobule containing atypical lobular hyperplasia (ALH). (**c**) Section from a tumour bed (post-neoadjuvant chemotherapy) showing two different marker clips (upper left, lower right) representing two previously biopsied areas. (**d**) Section of an intracanalicular fibroadenoma presenting as impalpable lesion

findings indicate evidence of the initial biopsy site, thus providing reassurance that the targeted lesion has been excised.

Benign and atypical lesions include flat epithelial atypia, lobular in situ neoplasia, fibroadenomas, papillomas, and radial scars. The impalpable malignant lesions include ductal carcinoma in situ (DCIS) [7], invasive ductal carcinoma (IDC), and invasive lobular carcinoma (ILC). Classification begins by identifying the lesion type, with DCIS characterized by malignant cells confined to the ductal system and invasive carcinomas characterised by malignant cells showing stromal invasion. Tumour grading is performed using the Nottingham criteria, which includes nuclear pleomorphism, mitotic activity, and tubule formation, which reflects tumour differentiation and aggressiveness [3]. Microscopic classification and grading provide crucial information for diagnosis, risk stratification, and therapeutic planning.

Microscopic assessment of margins ensures tumour clearance, with ≥2 mm clear margins being typically recommended for DCIS to reduce the recurrence risk. Accurate measurement of tumour size is critical for tumour staging (pT stage), particularly for small, impalpable lesions, as size influences decisions regarding adjuvant therapy. It is important to assess lymphovascular invasion in impalpable malignant tumours, due to its association with a higher risk of metastasis. Calcifications are assessed for radiological–pathological correlation, and if not initially found on histology, multiple deeper levels should be cut to assess a greater quantity of tissue.

If multiple specimens are received, determining the total extent of the lesion may become challenging. In these cases, summing the maximum dimensions from each tissue piece provides an estimate, though orientation markers may be more helpful in these cases to take more reliable size measurements. The written pathology report should describe all the factors discussed including the macroscopic and radiographic findings, documentation of the lesion size in three dimensions, and correlation of histological findings with the imaging features, giving a comprehensive assessment.

Immunohistochemistry (IHC) plays an important prognostic role and must be completed at the time of microscopy for oestrogen receptor (ER), progesterone receptor (PR), and HER2 expression. Pathologists follow established guidelines of cancer data set and biomarker reporting [3, 8–10].

13.8 Conclusion

The pathological analysis of histology following localisation of impalpable breast cancer highlights the complex interactions between surgical, radiological, and pathological specialties. Accurate evaluation of impalpable breast lesions, which often represent early-stage cancers or high-risk abnormalities, requires a meticulous and collaborative approach. Advances in imaging and localisation techniques have improved lesion identification, yet challenges remain in achieving precise excision, radiological–pathological correlation, and comprehensive histological assessment.

Pathologists play a crucial role in diagnosis, starting with the macroscopic handling of localised tissue to the microscopic evaluation of margins, tumour grading, and hormone receptor profiling with immunohistochemistry. Each step contributes to a thorough assessment, with one of the most significant differences in approach being through radiological specimen mapping. The detection of subtle or residual disease in neoadjuvant cases, although most likely not related to an impalpable primary lesion, presents similar challenges.

Through the discussed methods, pathologists work to ensure that impalpable lesions are identified and comprehensively assessed. This multidisciplinary approach highlights the important role of pathology in early detection, accurate diagnosis, and ultimately guiding treatment strategies in impalpable breast lesions.

References

1. Yildiz-Aktas IZ, Dabbs DJ, Bhargava R. The effect of cold ischemic time on the immunohistochemical evaluation of estrogen receptor, progesterone receptor, and HER2 expression in invasive breast carcinoma. Mod Pathol. 2012;25(8):1098–105.
2. Lee AH, Key HP, Bell JA, Kumah P, Hodi Z, Ellis IO. The effect of delay in fixation on HER2 expression in invasive carcinoma of the breast assessed with immunohistochemistry and in situ hybridisation. J Clin Pathol. 2014;67(7):573–5.
3. Guidelines Working Group of the UK National Coordinating Committee for Breast Pathology. G.148. Dataset for histopathological reporting of breast disease in surgical excision specimens of breast cancer. https://www.rcpath.org/static/d255f34c-176a-490d-9b5a7d58ac85f3a6/G148-Dataset-for-histopathological-reporting-of-breast-disease-in-surgical-excision-specimens-of-breast-cancer.pdf. The Royal College of Pathologists; 2024.
4. Rubio IT, Wyld L, Marotti L, Athanasiou A, Regitnig P, Catanuto G, et al. European guidelines for the diagnosis, treatment and follow-up of breast lesions with uncertain malignant potential (B3 lesions) developed jointly by EUSOMA, EUSOBI, ESP (BWG) and ESSO. Eur J Surg Oncol. 2024;50(1):107292.
5. Pinder SE, Shaaban A, Deb R, Desai A, Gandhi A, Lee AHS, et al. NHS breast screening multidisciplinary working group guidelines for the diagnosis and management of breast lesions of uncertain malignant potential on core biopsy (B3 lesions). Clin Radiol. 2018;73(8):682–92.
6. Pinder SE, Rakha EA, Purdie CA, Bartlett JM, Francis A, Stein RC, et al. Macroscopic handling and reporting of breast cancer specimens pre- and post-neoadjuvant chemotherapy treatment: review of pathological issues and suggested approaches. Histopathology. 2015;67(3):279–93.
7. Maxwell AJ, Clements K, Dodwell DJ, Evans AJ, Francis A, Hussain M, et al. The radiological features, diagnosis and management of screen-detected lobular neoplasia of the breast: findings from the Sloane project. Breast. 2016;27:109–15.
8. Fox SB, Webster F, Chen CJ, Chua B, Collins L, Foschini MP, et al. Dataset for pathology reporting of ductal carcinoma in situ, variants of lobular carcinoma in situ and low-grade lesions: recommendations from the International Collaboration on Cancer Reporting (ICCR). Histopathology. 2022;81:467.
9. Rakha EA, Tan PH, Quinn C, Provenzano E, Shaaban AM, Deb R, et al. UK recommendations for HER2 assessment in breast cancer: an update. J Clin Pathol. 2022;76:217.
10. Wolff AC, Somerfield MR, Dowsett M, Hammond MEH, Hayes DF, McShane LM, et al. Human epidermal growth factor receptor 2 testing in breast cancer: ASCO-College of American pathologists guideline update. J Clin Oncol. 2023;41(22):3867–72.

Chapter 14
Cost-Effectiveness of Non-Wire Localisation Techniques: Comparing Different Techniques Commonly Used

Stefan Lukac and Thorsten Kühn

Contents

14.1 Introduction

Comparing the cost-effectiveness of different localization techniques for breast and axillary lesions is complicated because of the usual healthcare triangle: the one providing is not paid by the one receiving, the one paying is neither receiving nor providing, and the one receiving is not paying directly. The cost-effectiveness for the healthcare provider is highly dependent on the reimbursement system, which varies widely between countries and may include payment for services or bundle payment. Moreover, different systems for outpatient or inpatient care, or the

S. Lukac
Department of Obstetrics and Gynecology, University Hospital Ulm, Ulm, Germany

T. Kühn (✉)
Department of Obstetrics and Gynecology, University Hospital Ulm, Ulm, Germany

Breast Cancer Center, Die Filderklinik, Filderstadt, Germany

R. Vidya, N. Sharma (eds.), *Breast and Axilla Localisation Techniques*,
https://doi.org/10.1007/978-3-032-17995-1_14

insurance status (private vs. public), can impact the cost-effectiveness of the same approach.

Factors affecting reimbursement generally:

- Type of reimbursement system: Payment for services or bundle payment
- Separate reimbursement for out- and inpatient for the same case or individual payments
- Type of insurance
- Existence of alternatives
- Evidence for clinical use

Different reimbursement systems largely affect economic considerations and the use of different surgical techniques. For example, the tertiary hospital with bundle-payment could have a low interest in the application of modern techniques, which are more expensive compared to the standard procedure due to high acquisition costs and lower profitability. On the other hand, the private clinic with direct payment and advertising modern technologies would be interested in new approaches to strengthen its market position. In addition, the prices for localization materials (seeds, wire, equipment, ultrasound/mammography) and personnel costs (physicians, nurses) vary among countries. Cost-effectiveness for different marking and localization procedures must therefore be distinguished from clinical efficiency, which is characterized by the effectiveness of the clinical workflow [1–3].

Given the complex impact of reimbursement systems on economic aspects, we focus in this chapter on the clinical efficiency of different marking and localization techniques and the cost-effectiveness from the perspective of a healthcare provider.

14.2 Logistical Considerations

14.2.1 Breast

Wire-based localization (WBL) represents the current standard of care in the surgical treatment of non-palpable breast lesions in many countries [4, 5]. This relates to small solid tumours scheduled for primary surgery, areas of microcalcifications, or lesions that are marked with a clip before neoadjuvant chemotherapy (NACT) to identify the original tumour bed thereafter. Due to its simple technology, no specific equipment is needed for the localization and removal of the lesion. Mammography and ultrasound for image-guided localization are widely available, rendering WBL an easily accessible and utilizable tool [5].

One limitation of the WBL is the necessity to place the wire shortly before surgery to avoid dislocation and minimize patients' discomfort [6]. The wire should ideally be placed on the day of surgery. This can lead to logistical challenges in the collaboration between the departments for radiology and surgery, and requires additional personnel expenses due to another contact of the patient with a healthcare provider [7]. Moreover, scheduling the surgical intervention may be complicated due to the coordination of the localization procedure with the surgery.

If non-palpable breast lesions or clips are localized with a wire, specimen imaging is mandatory to ensure adequate resection of the target volume. While small, solid tumours can be visualized by the surgeon through the use of intraoperative ultrasound, microcalcifications or clips require specimen radiography, which is again associated with the need to coordinate clinical procedures of two departments (radiology, surgery) and consumes additional resources with regard to personnel and material [5]. In addition, intraoperative specimen imaging is often associated with waiting times in the operating room.

Probe-guided localization techniques (PGL) have been introduced as an alternative to WBL to improve the surgical procedure by allowing more precise and targeted surgery and reducing the surgical trauma [8–10]. In addition, these procedures significantly improve the workflow for the healthcare provider since the coordination of diagnostic and therapeutic procedures is reduced or eliminated.

The most frequently used devices for PGL are radioactive seeds. This technique allows placement of the device independently from surgery, but still requires the availability of a department of nuclear medicine to prepare, store, and dispose of radioactive materials. Radioactive seeds cannot be used in many countries due to radiation protection regulations [5].

Non-radioactive seeds (NRS) using magnetic or radar signals have recently been developed as an alternative. The identification rates for the seeds and the target lesions have shown similar results compared to radioactive seeds. The NRS can be placed up to 180 days before the surgery, does not cause a radioactive burden, and can be detected with specific localizing probes. NRS uses ferromagnetic (Magseed) or paramagnetic (Sirius Pintuition) signals or radar-based technologies (SaviScout, LOCalizer) [5, 7]. Due to their highly developed technologies, NRS are associated with higher costs for the marking devices.

14.2.2 Axilla

Sentinel Lymph Node Biopsy

Complete axillary dissection has been replaced by sentinel-node biopsy (SNB) as the standard of care to assess the lymph node status in clinically node-negative breast cancer patients. For the localization of an ipsilateral sentinel node, different techniques are available [11].

The most popular detection method uses radioactive colloids ($Tc^{99)}$) [12, 13]. These are injected into the breast tissue or the overlying skin. The tracer accumulates in the first draining node(s), which are identified with the use of a gamma probe. The technique is logistically challenging as it requires a specialized team of nuclear physicians and a department for nuclear medicine to store, prepare, and display radioactive material. Due to the half-time of 6 h associated with radioactive tracers, the injection time has to be closely coordinated with the surgical schedule in order to achieve an adequate activity for the detection of an SLN. An additional appointment in a department for nuclear medicine is required, which is often located outside of the surgical clinic, resulting in high expenditure for manpower and time, and leads to logistic challenges. The procedure requires a specific gamma probe and a console.

An alternative approach for the detection of an SLN is the intraoperative use of coloured fluids such as blue dye or indocyanine green (ICG) [14]. These techniques allow the tracer injection directly in the operating theatre during the surgery. From the patients' perspective, this approach is associated with less discomfort because additional appointments are avoided and the injection is performed during anaesthesia directly in the operating room. For the use of blue dye, no specific equipment is required, which is advantageous compared to the ICG-technique, where a special camera and monitor is required to display the SN. Moreover, the cameras for SN detection have to be sterilized after each surgery.

Another option is the use of superparamagnetic iron oxide (SPIO) [15]. A volume of 1–2 ml of the tracer can be injected by the surgeon up to several weeks before the intervention, which makes the surgical schedule independent from other departments and allows short-term postponement of surgery. The SLN is detected intraoperatively with the use of a magnetic probe and can also be identified by its brownish colour. This technique requires a specific magnetic probe and a console to indicate the magnetic activity.

Finally, according to the recently published results of the INSEMA and the SOUND study, it can be expected that omission of SNB will become more popular in early breast cancer.

Targeted Axillary Dissection

NACT is increasingly being used in the treatment of breast cancer. While SNB is accepted as a standard of care to assess the lymph node status after NACT in patients with clinically negative lymph nodes at presentation, the procedure is associated with an unacceptable false negative rate (FNR) in patients who have biopsy-proven lymph nodes before the start of treatment. In these patients, marking the most prominent node and removing it along with the SLN after NACT (Targeted Axillary Dissection, TAD) has become a popular procedure that reduces the FNR to <5%. Different techniques for marking a tumour-involved lymph node (target lymph node, TLN) and its localization after NACT are available [13]. These include the use of charcoal solution for the intraoperative visual detection of a TLN, metallic clips for a preoperative image-guided needle localization, or different seeds for the intraoperative probe-guided identification of a TLN.

The use of a charcoal solution is associated with the lowest costs with regard to material and personnel. A simple ultrasound-guided injection of a charcoal solution by the treating radiologist or surgeon before the start of NACT is required. Since the technique is often associated with large areas of colouration and a higher surgical trauma, many surgeons prefer the use of clips or seeds for the localization of TLNs.

Clips can be placed into a biopsy-proven node before NACT. The clip is inserted either by a needle or a seed before surgery. The detection of metallic clips after NACT can be challenging once the lymph node metastasis has shrunk and lost its hypoechogenic structure. Therefore, detection rates for the post-NACT identification of clips vary widely between 70% and 99% and are largely dependent on experience.

The use of radioactive, (para-)magnetic, or radar-based seeds for marking and localizing a TLN has shown reliable detection rates of >95% and has become increasingly popular. The seeds available for marking a breast lesion can be placed in the TLN as well. In contrast to the WGL, the removal of a TLN can be confirmed directly by the surgeon using a detection device instead of intraoperative radiography.

14.3 Economical Aspects

According to the economic activity-based costing method [16], the expenses associated with localization techniques can be divided into two categories: activity-related costs and activity-neutral costs. The latter includes two subgroups: personnel costs and equipment costs (including ultrasound and facility-related expenses). From an economic perspective, we adhere to direct costing instead of full cost accounting to focus on comparing different techniques while omitting overhead cost inclusion. Therefore, we distinguish only between personnel costs and material costs. A general comparison of direct costing and full cost accounting for localization techniques is presented in Table 14.1.

Conventional wire-guided procedures and modern probe-guided technologies have different advantages and disadvantages in terms of cost-effectiveness. Here, we attempt to create a simplified model to compare the costs of different methods. Since there are various combinations for the localization of breast and axillary lesions, they will be discussed separately.

Table 14.1 Comparison of different costing in the localization of breast lesions

Cost category	Direct costing (only variable costs)	Full cost accounting (all costs included)
Material (incl. consumables)	Wires, radioactive seeds, markers, sterile packaging	Procurement, storage, disposal
Personnel	Direct staff costs (physician, assistant)	Training, administrative costs
Equipment	Usage of ultrasound/mammography	Depreciation, maintenance costs
Room costs	n.a.	Facility maintenance, energy costs

14.3.1 Breast

Initial Consultation

After biopsy and histological confirmation of a malignant disease or a lesion at risk, two treatment options are available. The patient can either undergo primary surgery or NACT, depending on histology and the subtype of invasive disease. In patients with non-palpable lesions undergoing primary surgery, the tumour has to be located before surgery. In patients scheduled for NACT, the tumour should be marked in the early stage of systemic treatment to identify the tumour bed in case of a good clinical response to chemotherapy.

If WGL is planned for patients undergoing primary surgery, no additional intervention at the initial consultation is required since the wire placement is performed on the day of surgery. Patients undergoing NACT or those scheduled for PGL in primary surgery need an additional appointment for the placement of a clip or a seed, which is independent from the day of surgery.

Expenditure includes costs for the seed/clip, disinfection, local anaesthesia, and material (surgical compresses, needle, and the cannula for the anaesthesia). Personnel costs include the physicians' and nurses' working time of approximately 10 min for the ultrasound-guided detection of the lesion and placement of the seed/clip.

Surgery

On the day of surgery, medical staff in the radiology or surgery department are required to place the wire in the case of WGL. The costs are similar to those described above for seed or clip placement.

During surgery, the target lesion is removed using standard instruments, without the need for additional materials or instruments. If a clip is placed, the specimen must be transported to the radiology department for specimen radiography, which incurs costs for transportation, radiology staff (nurses and doctors), and specimen radiography (device-related costs).

For PGL, the adequate removal of the target lesion is confirmed directly intraoperatively by the surgeon. In contrast to WGL, additional equipment, such as the detecting/navigating probe and the console for seed localization, is required. However, no additional personnel costs are incurred. These one-time costs for the seed-localizing device are offset by an increasing number of performed surgeries. An exception applies to microcalcifications, which must be confirmed by specimen radiography as well.

The costs for different seeds, clips, and localization devices vary between countries, making a general comparison difficult, particularly in light of the two different reimbursement systems mentioned above. We provide an overview of cost-triggers related to breast surgery in Table 14.2.

Table 14.2 Comparison of cost-triggers in localization of breast lesion for breast-conserving surgery

		Preoperative consultation		Preoperative period		Surgery		After removal	
		WGL	PGL	WGL	NRS	WGL	NRS	WGL	NRS
Material costs	Activity-related	None	Seed and placement device, disinfection, local anaesthesia, surgical compresses, needle and the cannula for the anaesthesia	Wire and placement cannula Disinfection, local anaesthesia, surgical compresses, needle and the cannula for the anaesthesia	None	None	None with exception of LOCaliser (single-use detecting device), energy of detecting device	Ev. Mammography, if clip was placed	None
	Activity independent	None	Ultrasound, facility-related-costs	Ultrasound, facility-related-costs	None	None	Detecting device	None	Detecting device
Personnel costs	Physician	None	Placement time (approx. 10 min)	Placement time (approx. 10 min)	None	Unaffected surgery time	Unaffected surgery time	Ev. Time for specimen radiography if clip was placed[a]	None
	Nursing	None	Placement time (approx. 10 min)	Placement time (approx. 10 min)	None	Unaffected surgery time	Unaffected surgery time	Ev. Time for specimen radiography if clip was placed[a]	None

WGL Wire-guided localization, *PGL* probe-guided localization

[a]The working time is doubled as the surgeon with the scrubbing nurse needs to wait for confirmation from the radiology (waiting time) and the radiological nurses perform the specimen radiography that need to be confirmed by the radiologist

14.3.2 Axillary Interventions: Sentinel Node Biopsy

Consultation

For SNB localization with the use of radioactive colloids, blue dye, or ICG, no additional intervention from the surgeon is required before surgery.

For SPIO, the application is often performed several days before surgery to improve SLN identification compared to the application on the day of surgery. Expenditure includes the cost of 1–2 ml of SPIO, local anaesthesia (needle, syringe, disinfection, compresses), and personnel costs for the physician and assisting personnel, which is similar to the preoperative breast lesion localization. Synergistic effects on the overall costs can be expected if the breast lesion is marked with a paramagnetic seed at the time point of consultation, together with the injection of SPIO for SLN detection.

Preoperative Period

If radioactive colloids are used for SLN localization, the patient needs an appointment in the department for nuclear medicine to inject the tracer and for lymphoscintigraphy, if needed. This includes additional costs for the patient's transportation and personnel costs for the nuclear medicine staff (physicians and nurses), as well as material costs for the injection. Significant costs arise from the storage of technetium, which can be categorized as activity-neutral costs. Finally, the costs for lymphoscintigraphy could be included, depending on clinical standards and national radiation protection regulations.

Intraoperative Period

The most cost-effective SNB detection technique is the use of blue dye, which incurs only material costs for the liquid, needle, and syringe, as its application is performed intraoperatively.

For the use of ICG, the costs of the camera and monitor are obligatory, activity-neutral costs. The necessity of re-sterilizing the camera after each surgery leads, however, to additional activity-triggered costs. Multiple cameras may be necessary to enable more than one SNB procedure per day.

For radioactive-guided SN detection, a gamma probe is used to detect the technetium-labelled SLN. Radioactive seeds used for breast lesion or lymph node localization can be detected with the same probe. The probe incurs only acquisition costs and expenditure for sterile covers as activity-triggered costs.

Similarly, for paramagnetic seeds and SLN labelled by SPIO, both SLNs and seed-marked lesions can be detected using the same magnetic probe, covered with a sterile sheath.

14.3.3 Axillary Interventions-Targeted Axillary Dissection (TAD)

In TAD, SNB is combined with the removal of an additional, biopsy-proven marked lymph node metastasis. Charcoal, clip/wires, and seeds can be used for lymph node marking. TAD integrates lesion localization techniques with SNB procedures in the axillary space. From a cost perspective, the use of a single technique for TAD, rather than combining multiple methods, would be the most effective procedure.

The overview of cost-triggers in axillary surgery can be found in the Table 14.3.

Table 14.3 Comparison of cost-triggers in localization of axillary sentinel node during breast surgery

		Preoperative consultation				Pre-surgery				During surgery			
		Technetium	SPIO	ICG	Blue dye	Technetium	SPIO	ICG	Blue dye	Technetium	SPIO	ICG	Blue dye
Material costs	Activity-related	None	SPIO and disinfection, surgical compresses, needle and the cannula for application	None	None	Technetium, application equipment	None	None	None	Sterile cover	Sterile cover, energy of the detecting device	ICG, needle and syringe, sterilization of the ICG-camera, sterile cover, energy of the camera	Blue dye, needle and syringe
	Activity independent	None	Ultrasound, facility-related-costs	None	None	Gama-camera, storage cost of technetium	None	None	None	Geiger-probe	Plastic surgical instruments, detector probe	ICG-camera for 1 SNB, ICG-tower with monitor	None

Personal costs	Physician	None	10 min	None	None	Physician in the nuclear medicine	None	None	None	Unaffected surgery time	Unaffected surgery time	Possibly slightly increased time of surgery due to intraoperative application of ICG	Possibly slightly increased time of surgery due to intraoperative application of blue dye
	Nursing	None	10 min	None	None	Nurse in nuclear medicine	None	None	None	Unaffected surgery time	Unaffected surgery time	Possibly slightly increased time of surgery due to intraoperative application of ICG	Possibly slightly increased time of surgery due to intraoperative application of blue dye

14.4 Ecological Aspects

Financial aspects play an important role in the decision process for the implementation of new technologies. Nowadays, in the times of climate change, new aspects are arising, especially from the ecological perspective. Every human activity leads to an emission of greenhouse gases and to a particular carbon footprint (CF). This includes waste analysis or, in the broader spectrum, enviro-logistical analysis, which covers the travel and process-triggered CF as well. According to recent studies, novel technologies such as PGL are associated with lower CF compared to WGL [7]. Therefore, not only economic aspects, but also ecological issues should be considered.

14.5 Conclusions

Our findings highlight a marked variability in the costs of seeds and localization devices in different countries, adding to the complexity introduced by differing reimbursement systems. This economic heterogeneity, which also will be part of the evaluation of the EUBREASTs/MELODY study suggests that cost-effectiveness analyses must be interpreted within specific healthcare contexts and cannot be calculated generally.

Although modern probe-guided marking technologies are associated with higher acquisition costs, the overall cost-effectiveness may be more favourable compared to the classical gold standard of wire localizations. Savings of personal and material costs can outweigh the initial cost by optimizing the workflow flow leading to indirect cost-saving.

References

1. Law W, Look Hong N, Ravi A, Wright FC, Curpen B. ASO author reflections: which preoperative breast localization method is more economical: radioactive seed or wire-guided localization? Ann Surg Oncol. 2021;28:1379–80. https://doi.org/10.1245/S10434-020-09163-5/METRICS.
2. Wright CM, Moorin RE, Saunders C, Marinovich ML, Taylor DB, Bourke AG, et al. Cost-effectiveness of radioguided occult lesion localization using 125I seeds versus hookwire localization before breast-conserving surgery for non-palpable breast cancer. Br J Surg. 2021;108:843–50. https://doi.org/10.1093/BJS/ZNAA160.
3. Nguyen CL, Cui R, Zhou M, Ali F, Easwaralingam N, Chan B, et al. Cost-effectiveness of radar localisation versus wire localisation for wide local excision of non-palpable breast cancer. Ann Surg Oncol. 2024;31:3916. https://doi.org/10.1245/S10434-024-15142-X.
4. Lovrics PJ, Goldsmith CH, Hodgson N, McCready D, Gohla G, Boylan C, et al. A multi-centered, randomized, controlled trial comparing radioguided seed localization to standard wire localization for nonpalpable, invasive and in situ breast carcinomas. Ann Surg Oncol. 2011;18:3407–14. https://doi.org/10.1245/S10434-011-1699-Y.

5. Banys-Paluchowski M, Kühn T, Masannat Y, Rubio I, de Boniface J, Ditsch N, et al. Localization techniques for non-palpable breast lesions: current status, knowledge gaps, and rationale for the MELODY study (EUBREAST-4/iBRA-NET, NCT 05559411). Cancers. 2023;15:1173. https://doi.org/10.3390/CANCERS15041173.
6. Heindl F, Schulz-Wendtland R, Jud S, Erber R, Hack CC, Preuss C, et al. Evaluation of a wireless localization system for nonpalpable breast lesions — feasibility and cost-effectiveness in everyday clinical routine. In Vivo. 2022;36:2342. https://doi.org/10.21873/INVIVO.12965.
7. Lukac S, Leinert E, Kühn T, Dayan D, Ebner F, Pfister K, et al. Eco-logistical comparison of non-radioactive seeds and the wire-guided localization for intraoperative detection of breast lesions. Eur J Surg Oncol. 2024:108779. https://doi.org/10.1016/J.EJSO.2024.108779.
8. Gera R, Tayeh S, Al-Reefy S, Mokbel K. Evolving role of magseed in wireless localization of breast lesions: systematic review and pooled analysis of 1,559 procedures. Anticancer Res. 2020;40:1809–15. https://doi.org/10.21873/ANTICANRES.14135.
9. Bessems M, van Breest Smallenburg V, van Bebber I, van Dijk E-J, van der Giessen A, Schermers B, et al. Safety and performance of Sirius Pintuition – a novel wire-free and non-radioactive localization system for breast cancer surgery. Eur J Surg Oncol. 2021;47:e1. https://doi.org/10.1016/J.EJSO.2020.11.148.
10. Srour MK, Kim S, Amersi F, Giuliano AE, Chung A. Comparison of wire localization, radioactive seed, and Savi scout® radar for management of surgical breast disease. Breast J. 2020;26:406–13. https://doi.org/10.1111/TBJ.13499.
11. Ahmed M, Purushotham AD, Douek M. Novel techniques for sentinel lymph node biopsy in breast cancer: a systematic review. Lancet Oncol. 2014;15:e351–62. https://doi.org/10.1016/S1470-2045(13)70590-4.
12. Chang W-D, Liu R-S, Tseng L-M, Chang C-P, Wang S-J, Yeh S-H. Detection of sentinel lymph nodes in patients of breast cancer by Technetium-99m-phytate lymphoscintigraphy and comparison of peri-tumor and subareolar injection. J Nucl Med. 2010;51:1593.
13. Kontos M, Kanavidis P, Kühn T, Masannat Y, Gulluoglu B, Gonzalez E, et al. Targeted axillary dissection: worldwide variations in clinical practice. Breast Cancer Res Treat. 2024;204:389–96. https://doi.org/10.1007/S10549-023-07204-7.
14. Papathemelis T, Jablonski E, Scharl A, Hauzenberger T, Gerken M, Klinkhammer-Schalke M, et al. Sentinel lymph node biopsy in breast cancer patients by means of Indocyanine green using the Karl Storz VITOM® fluorescence camera. Biomed Res Int. 2018;2018:6251468. https://doi.org/10.1155/2018/6251468.
15. Shams S, Lippold K, Blohmer JU, Röhle R, Kühn F, Karsten MM. A pilot study evaluating the effects of Magtrace® for sentinel node biopsy in breast cancer patients regarding care process optimization, reimbursement, surgical time, and patient comfort compared with standard Technetium99. Ann Surg Oncol. 2021;28:3232. https://doi.org/10.1245/S10434-020-09280-1.
16. Lievens Y, Van Den Bogaert W, Kesteloot K. Activity-based costing: a practical model for cost calculation in radiotherapy. Int J Radiat Oncol Biol Phys. 2003;57:522–35. https://doi.org/10.1016/S0360-3016(03)00579-0.

Chapter 15
Advances in Breast Lesion Localisation: Evidence-Based Technologies and Future Directions

Daniel Ahari and James Harvey

Contents

D. Ahari (✉)
Manchester University Foundation Trust, Manchester, UK
e-mail: Daniel.ahari@mft.nhs.uk

J. Harvey
Nightingale Breast Unit, Manchester University Foundation Trust, Manchester, UK
e-mail: James.Harvey@mft.nhs.uk

R. Vidya, N. Sharma (eds.), *Breast and Axilla Localisation Techniques*,
https://doi.org/10.1007/978-3-032-17995-1_15

15.1 Introduction

Wire-guided localisation (WGL) of impalpable breast lesions under mammographic guidance was first carried out in 1965, with the addition of a hooked tip introduced in 1976 [1]. Spurred by successful reductions in mortality reported in the 1980s, screening programmes proliferated, and with that grew the importance of WGL in removing non-palpable cancers [2]. WGL has therefore come to be regarded as the gold standard in breast cancer localisation, serving as the comparator and point of reference for modern RCTs, systematic reviews, and Cochrane reviews [3]. It is inexpensive, familiar to most surgeons, and supported by a large body of evidence. This translates to its benefit and risk profile being well understood, so that patients can be fully briefed to be able to give informed consent.

However, as the problems and drawbacks of the technique have become well documented, and given the importance of improving the technology that enables breast conserving surgery (BCS), new localisation techniques have been developed and are available for use by surgeons across the globe. This chapter will cover emerging localisation techniques, how the evidence base for modern localisation devices has been gathered, and the direction of future technologies.

15.2 Wire Guided Localisation: Gold Standard or Flawed Technique?

WGL is limited by the logistical need to place the wire on the day of surgery. This has led to the development of technologies that have uncoupled the placement of a localisation device from the date of surgery. One of the first studies to report a change in National practice was the Netherlands Breast Cancer Audit [4]. This study retrospectively reviewed patients from 2012 to 2018 who had BCS for non-palpable breast cancer, with any documented localisation technique. There were over 28,000 patients. Strikingly, in just 5 years, from 2013 and 2018, they found that WGL usage dropped from 75% to 32%. A more modern technique on the other hand—radioactive seed localisation (RSL)—rose from 16% to 61%.

The authors speculated that it may be the logistic advantages driving this change: that RSL can be associated with shorter operations and smaller excision samples.

A national practice questionnaire of 98 units ran soon after in the United Kingdom (UK) from October 2018 to April 2019, which aimed to identify attitudes towards WGL and the need for future technologies. They found that the dominant localisation technique in 83% of units ($n = 82$) was WGL, with Magseed®—a magnetic marker—being the second most used technique, represented by 9 units (9.2%) [5].

The UK questionnaire explored the perceived limitations of current techniques. The most reported issue (74 units, 75.5%) was a logistical one: the effect the technique has on theatre scheduling such as delays and cancellations. The second most common concern was the technique not being patient friendly (46 units, 52.0%).

The third and fourth limitations were directly related to WGL: 46 units (46.9%) reported wire migration as a limitation, and 42 units (42.9%) also reported difficulties locating the tip of the wire. Immediately it can be seen that the most reported perceived limitations are multifaceted, affecting the preoperative phase (as regards efficiency and patient satisfaction), as well as concerns over efficacy intraoperatively.

The next most reported perceived limitations were intraoperative: excising too much tissue (39 units, 39.8%); interference and/or delays when combined with sentinel lymph node localisation (33 units, 33.7%); depth sensing in large or dense breasts (29 units, 29.6%), and concerns about failure to excise the index lesion (20 units, 20.4%). Overall, 55 units (56.1%) of the 98 expressed a desire to change their main technique, and of the 82 WGL units specifically, 60% (49 units) wished to change to a different technique.

The same questionnaire was repeated in the UK just 3 years later in 2022 and found that localisation device use had significantly changed. WGL usage as the primary technique was 84% in 2019, but just 18% in 2022. The 2022 results also showed that paramagnetic seeds were now used by 49% of units, radiofrequency devices by 20%, and radar, RSL, and magnetic seeds being used by a further 13% in total, demonstrating the appetite for new localisation devices [6].

15.3 Modern Localisation Techniques

Research into new techniques has culminated in a marked change in the landscape of breast cancer localisation techniques within a very short time period, with all of these technologies having their own inherent pros and cons. While below is not an exhaustive list of available technologies, it does illustrate the breadth of new techniques. Several emerging technologies are discussed later in this chapter.

15.3.1 Radioactive Techniques

These techniques rely upon a radioactive marker placed into the breast, followed by detection with a gamma probe intraoperatively. These markers are most commonly radioactive seeds or radiocolloids (for ‘radioactive occult lesion localisation’—ROLL). Seeds can be placed into any lesions with radiological guidance, and the half-life of the seed’s isotope allows this to be performed well in advance of any operation. The radiocolloid for ROLL on the other hand is injected on the day before, or of, surgery, and can also be used for simultaneous sentinel lymph node localisation [7].

15.3.2 Magnetic Techniques

The Magnetic Marker Localisation (MaMaLoc) is a magnetic marker with a commercially available detection system called Pintuition® (Sirius Medical, Eindhoven, The Netherlands). Another magnetic marker is the Magnetic Occult Lesion Localisation Instrument (MOLLI™—Stryker Medical, Michigan, United States of America). Both markers can be placed ahead of the surgery, then intraoperatively the handheld probe of the respective system can provide information on the direction and distance to the magnetic marker [7].

15.3.3 Paramagnetic Techniques

Magnetic markers are permanent markers, whereas paramagnetic markers become magnetic only when a magnetic field is applied to them. Magseed® (Endomag, Cambridge, UK) can be inserted days to weeks before surgery and then becomes magnetised when the Sentimag® probe is used intraoperatively. The probe's low-level magnetic field makes the Magseed® magnetised, and therefore detectable—with numerical and audible feedback on direction and proximity [7].

15.3.4 Radar Techniques

SCOUT® (Merit Medical, Utah, United States of America) reflectors can be placed inside the tissue and generate an electromagnetic signal after being activated by infrared light. The infrared pulses are generated by a probe, and the resultant electromagnetic wave is captured by a console that gives real-time information on distance between the probe and SCOUT® reflector [7].

15.3.5 Radiofrequency Tag Techniques

Radiofrequency identification (RFID) tags can be used to mark lesions. LOCalizer™ tags (Hologic Inc., California, United States of America) can be detected intraoperatively by a probe that detects the RFID tags and gives information on the distance to a tag. The RFID tags have unique identifiers, so that multiple tags can be used without interference when more than one isinserted [7].

15.4 The Ideal Localisation Device

By looking at the various technologies that are currently available, we can extrapolate certain themes. Generally, they do not have a protruding element like WGL, aid decoupling with radiology services, and can provide information on depth and direction.

When deciding to use a new technology, there is a need to work out the reason for the said change and what users—and patients—would like from a new device. On reading the first iBRA-NET questionnaire, there are clear reasons that have pushed clinicians away from WGL and towards other techniques [5]. The participants were asked what improvements they would like to see when changing to a new localisation technique, summarised below:

- '*Improved patient experience*'—this was the most common response (70.4%, 69 units)
- '*Better organisation of lists/theatre scheduling*'—second most common (68.4%, 67 units)
- '*Better use of radiology time*'—third most common (66.3%, 65 units)

These three answers speak to two clear priorities: the patient's satisfaction and the need to decouple radiology services with theatre listings.

The common theme among the next most common answers is efficacy—removing the target lesion in totality to avoid re-excisions, while leaving as much healthy tissue as possible behind.

- '*Accuracy in localisation*' (55 units, 56.1%)
- '*Decrease in re-excision rate*' (42 units, 42.9%)
- '*Smaller specimen weights*' (41 units, 41.8%)

The final component of the questionnaire was on the perceived barriers when changing techniques. Here, the most common factors were:

- '*Cost*' ($n = 63$, 64.3%),
- '*Organisational issues*' ($n = 60$, 61.2%)
- '*Training*' ($n = 39$, 39.8%)
- '*The learning curve that comes with trying to change to a new technique*' ($n = 38$, 38.8%)

The follow-up questionnaire in 2022 (which demonstrated significant change in the landscape of device usage in the UK) directly asked participating surgeons and radiologists to assign a satisfaction score to different devices for different attributes [6]. The attributes in question were informed by focus groups in the network's prior research into Magseed® [8]. All clinicians were asked on the ease of logistics with the device. Surgeons alone were asked about the risk of the device dislodging, ease of detection in surgery (both generally and for deep breasts), the signal's focus intra-operatively, the ability to judge distance from the probe during surgery, and the ease for bracketing a lesion. Radiologists were asked about the reliability of the device and then the ease of insertion and deployment both with ultrasound and with stereotactic means.

The results of the surveys allow us to paint a picture of what the next-generation device—or even, the 'ideal' device—should look like. As per the priorities of the clinicians, such a device would be comfortable for the patient, and would enable the decoupling of theatre schedules from radiology activity. The radiological experience could be further improved by easy insertion and deployment under different modalities. The device would of course be easy to find intraoperatively with low dislodgement rates and reliable feedback to the surgeon about distance to the device regardless of the depth of the lesion. When a lesion requires bracketing, any ideal device would be able to facilitate this. In totality, this would enable low re-excision rates, and the removal of as little tissue as necessary. When adopting this new device, it should be affordable to do so (beyond the savings made by reduced re-excision rates). Moreover, the learning curve and training required should be minimal in terms of time and money invested.

As mentioned at the start of this section, patients are important stakeholders and should be central to the process of designing new devices. However, though some papers comparing new devices to WGL have looked into patient attitudes towards the device that was used during and after their breast cancer journey, there are no large papers looking at patient perspectives on multiple non-WGL devices compared to each other. This is also more difficult to study than clinician attitudes: a surgeon may use multiple devices over the course of their career, whereas a patient—unless experiencing recurrence or another breast cancer—is unlikely to experience more than one device. Studies are underway both in the UK and EU (MELODY [7]) to gain some insights into patient experience.

15.5 Device Surveillance

So just how do we get to the ideal device? As shown in the Netherlands Breast Cancer Audit and the iBRA-NET surveys, the pace of change can be significant over just a few years. However, widespread adoption requires careful consideration—the need for additional training, regulatory hurdles (particularly for radiation-based systems), and the current relative lack of large-scale evidence present real barriers. But care must also be taken to ensure a device is truly safe and, when available on the market, adverse outcomes and concerns must be proactively communicated, collected, and shared. Although such devices are deployed only temporarily within the breast, one must be mindful that this could still have long-term effects, Hence, successful integration of new localisation methods ultimately requires not only technical performance, but also robust evidence to support patient consent and long-term clinical confidence. One surgical device that unfortunately acts as a learning point, especially as regards surveillance for adverse outcomes, is surgical mesh used for pelvic organ prolapse.

Surgical mesh was banned by the USA's Food and Drug Administration in 2019, and the UK enacted a pause pending a review. This came following frequent reports and concerns over side effects including pain, infection, and erosion of internal organs, with patients eventually requiring partial or total removal of the mesh [9]. The UK review (The Cumberlege Report) was published in 2020 and highlighted significant weaknesses in both the marketing and oversight of the mesh roll-out that contributed to patient harm. Moreover, there was a systemic reluctance to collect evidence on potential harm, and a lack of coordination to allow both clinicians and government agencies to be aware of, and act upon, such evidence information. The review suggested that patient databases should be created to enable the research and auditing of outcomes, specifically in terms of device safety and patient reported outcomes [10].

One might therefore argue that to ensure there is a safe roll-out of any device, we should ensure there are large international randomised control trials (RCTs) with a database to record short- and long-term outcomes, but this approach has pitfalls that may not be immediately obvious.

15.6 Barriers to Research and The IDEAL Framework

One framework to study new innovations and overcome issues with traditional research is IDEAL, developed by the Balliol Collaboration. Noticing that new medicines were only introduced after a large body of evidence, the group questioned why the same standards are not applied to surgical devices or techniques—why are randomised control trials for surgical innovations so rare, and, more importantly, what can be done to narrow this evidence base gap? They concluded that despite their challenges, surgical RCTs should still be the gold standard for researching new surgical innovations—and provided a path to get there [11, 12].

One pertinent barrier to surgical RCTs is the question of timing. Adopting a new technique is quickly followed by a learning curve as the user, often idiosyncratically, becomes more confident and efficient. Similarly, an early prototype will go through rapid development and iterative refinement. However, if we wait until a technique is near-perfect and clearly better than the gold standard before testing it, we may be doing wrong—or harm—to the patients who are subject to the old inferior method.

Barriers are raised by the intrinsic nature of surgery too: successful surgery relies upon inseparable components: preoperative care, the operating room environment, the surgical team (doctors, nurses, technicians, and more), and the post-operative environment. Standardising these and eliminating confounding factors are immensely challenging. Blinding can also be impossible or impracticable depending on the intervention—a patient cannot be blinded for WGL for instance.

We can look at the existing literature to see further weaknesses of a traditional approach. In a 2022 meta-analysis of 24 RCTs, ten studies investigated ROLL, six investigated RSL, and three investigated ultrasound-guided localisations. Five other

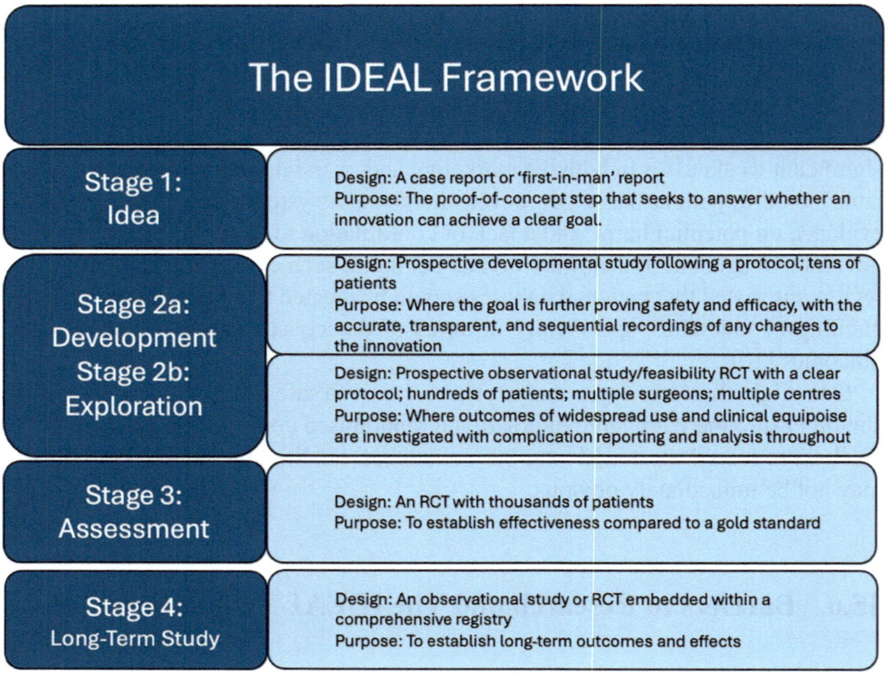

Fig. 15.1 The IDEAL framework. (Adapted from McCulloch et al. [11])

techniques were only investigated once [13]. Every paper used WGL as the control, with the largest of these papers (n = 659) being a 5-year long multicentre (n = 8) Australasian/Oceanic paper that investigated RSL [14]. However, of the 19 papers investigating those named devices, 8 had 100 patients or less. While this provides some evidence as regards device outcomes, when studies lack in size, a definitive statement on superiority cannot be made, and so the traditional approach to research (multiple centres publishing their data for separate studies) can take several years and still have some pitfalls.

Given these challenges, the IDEAL collaborative recognised the role that non-randomised trials must play, though they should still be prospective and protocol-driven (wherein a plan is published ahead of the study to ensure they stick to their stated methodology, thereby reducing any bias). As techniques develop and differences between the intervention and comparator become less, RCTs will then have an important role in differentiating between devices.

Hence, the collaborative put forward the IDEAL framework for surgical innovation (Fig. 15.1).

It addresses some of the reasons why the evidence-base gap exists when comparing surgical innovations with medicines and provides a practicable and realistic set of standards that teams behind surgical innovations should strive towards—an example being that innovators should not imply that the final iteration of their device was always used in early-stage research.

15.7 Shared Learning

The IDEAL framework emphasises transparent and accurate recording of changes to an innovation as well as any complications. As experience using an innovation grows, the users will become more efficient, and reporting their findings can help others through the learning curve. Similarly, for complications, the reporting can alert other clinicians and mitigate patient harm. In traditional approaches to research, multiple centres often carry out their own studies without communicating, thus even with diligent recording, their findings—and therefore learning points—may not be available until after publication. This could lead to patient harm through complications not being reported quickly enough, or, the learning curve may be prolonged with patients not benefiting from a more refined technique informed by shared learning. Indeed, in the Draft Guidelines for Adverse Event Reporting and Learning Systems, the World Health Organisation stated, 'too often neither health-care providers nor health-care organizations advise others when a mishap occurs, nor do they share what they learned...as a consequence, the same mistakes occur repeatedly' [15].

Thus 'shared learning'—the communication of errors and lessons learned—should be a key principle in researching new innovations. In the same document, the WHO discusses barriers to shared learning, such as different countries (and even different regions or hospitals in the same country) using different terms to describe or report errors, posing a barrier to understanding when sharing results. An international collaborative approach can mitigate this. Instead of multiple centres across the world following their own protocols and terminology, multiple centres could work internationally in one study, following a single protocol. Accompanied by a central data system, the study leads can analyse data from all sites and disseminate shared learning through regular updates to all participating centres on safety, improvements, and complications.

However, though shared learning has intuitive benefits and is advised by the WHO, there is no gold standard for incorporating it into a study, nor has its effect and impact been analysed. iBRA-NET have attempted to put into practice the principles of IDEAL and of shared learning through their platform study.

15.8 A Modern Audit: The iBRA-Platform Study

iBRA-NET followed their national questionnaires with a national audit—a prospective platform study aligned with the 2a/2b level of IDEAL, comparing devices against WGL. By using a standardised protocol, this enables new devices to be quickly adopted into the study as a new arm within a 6-month period, meaning that research can potentially keep up with changes in practice [16]. They incorporated shared learning by asking surgeons to report any issues pre-, intra-, and post-operatively, and addressed the impact of the learning curve by requiring involved surgeons to have performed a minimum number of cases with any investigated techniques [17].

Over the 6-year period of study, it has enabled nearly 6000 localisation device outcomes to be assessed, with 1000 cases approximately of each device. These studies rely on goodwill and are not fully prospective data collection, hence do not provide the robustness of data collection in a fully prospective RCT.

Nevertheless, their results comparing magnetic seeds and WGL have been published and suggest non-inferiority of magnetic seeds as regards resection of the index lesion. Moreover, they also found the logistical benefit of magnetic seed cases starting earlier in the day [16].

This study functioned not only as the largest study comparing WGL and magnetic seed localisation at the time, but also as a proof of concept for the platform study as a robust method to evaluate devices in a short period of time.

The shared learning element of this study was analysed and published separately. They used a mixed methodology—not only by asking surgeons to report any issues as above, but also by inviting clinicians to focus groups. They found both methods complemented each other, with focus groups often eliciting more responses per respondent, but with the reporting system being a lot more efficient [18].

15.9 Modern RCTs

Though the large multicentre platform study above has its strengths, one must not discount the value of randomised control trials even when working with smaller sample sizes. MAGTOTAL is a recently published RCT (2023), carried out not just to compare Magseed® and WGL alone, but in combination with superparamagnetic iron oxide (SPIO) for sentinel lymph node detection (SNLD), i.e. a 'totally magnetic technique' versus mixed techniques for the breast and axilla [19]. This was prompted by a concern that using a paramagnetic tumour marker and SPIO simultaneously could produce interfering signals, leading to increased resection size. With 426 patients, MAGTOTAL demonstrated equivalence in resection volumes, and even found that the totally magnetic approach had a shorter operative time and increased satisfaction amongst clinicians and theatre coordinators.

Another RCT published recently is that by [14]. Their work compared RSL to WGL, and like MAGTOTAL, sought to provide clarity on unanswered questions. In this instance, whether there is a difference between RSL and WGL with respect to reoperation rate or free margin status. With 659 patients, they found a significant reduction in reoperation rates using RSL compared to WGL (13.9% vs. 18.9%)—the first RCT to do so [14].

Both RCTs demonstrate that while we may not be in the position to hold the large thousands-of-patient-RCT mentioned in the latter stages of the IDEAL framework, smaller RCTs can still be used as a vehicle for problem-solving issues and questions that arise as a result of the changing landscape of innovations. MAGTOTAL in particular is an example wherein a new innovation can influence practice change for other procedures.

15.10 Future Avenues in Research

In the papers cited thus far that investigate the efficacy of new devices, the general trend is that they are non-inferior compared to WGL. Some papers have suggested a non-statistically significant benefit in newer technologies, but in general, more information through further studies is needed. The iBRA-NET platform study has showcased the benefit of large studies: instead of having multiple centres or health systems run their own trials and not communicating, resulting in a staggered reporting of results, a single large multicentre (and ideally international) study that utilises shared learning can bring all centres up to speed, using the same terminology, and publish results with adequately powered methodology.

The MELODY study (Methods for Localisation of Different types of breast lesions) is a multinational prospective non-interventional (i.e. participating centres do not need to change their practice) cohort study, spearheaded by the European Breast Cancer Research Association of Surgical Trialists (EUBREAST) and the iBRA-NET group. The study is an IDEAL stage 2b/3 observational study: aiming to truly assess effectiveness of new interventions when compared to the gold standard of WGL [7].

Their primary endpoints are as follows: (1) intended target lesion and/or marker removal (irrespective of histopathological margin status) and (2) negative resection margin rates at first surgery. With a target—guided by power calculations—of 7416 patients, they will be able to answer questions on efficacy. Their secondary endpoints are the gaps in the literature that are only starting to be explored in depth, such as, among others, patient-reported outcomes, radiologist and surgeon satisfaction, economic evaluation of the technique, and rates of second surgery and secondary mastectomy. Enrolment began in January 2023, and as of their latest newsletter (May 2025), they have recruited over 5000 patients, across 186 study sites in 21 countries (and all 6 inhabited continents). Melody aims to compare modern devices with further control groups, such as intraoperative ultrasound, and to assess the qualitative benefit of the devices to patients [7].

Indeed, the patient perspective is often overlooked. A 2024 paper investigating research gaps in breast cancer sought to compare the priorities of patients, members of the public, clinicians, and scientists as regards avenues for research [20]. Among 22 chosen topics were 'safety for new equipment' (defined as 'ensure checking of new treatments, materials and equipment to make sure they are safe, cost-effective and used in the best situation') 'better clinical trials' ('for example, find out more quickly if new treatments work and if patients think the side effects are worth the benefits'), and 'better surgery' ('improve surgery so that patients need less operations, have improved outcomes, with less side effects; work out which patients could have less surgery or no surgery at all').

Of these, 'better surgery' ranked 6th amongst patients and the public, with 'better clinical trials' at 10th and 12th, and 'safety for new equipment' at 21st and 22nd, respectively. The overall top three were 'better prevention', 'cancer blood tests', and 'target prevention.'

Bringing patients into the fold through paying special attention to patient-reported outcomes and making them active participants in research may raise the betterment of equipment as a priority for all stakeholders. This in turn may clarify that improving 'new equipment' goes hand-in-hand with 'better surgery'. It is vital that as research advances along the IDEAL framework, it brings patients with it.

15.11 Future Avenues in Technology

The breast cancer localisation techniques discussed thus far provide a point of reference for the surgeon and give information on how to get there. It would be fair to describe these widely used techniques as two-dimensional, as they more commonly rely upon ultrasound or mammography for marking. The device then gives the operator a point of reference relative to the lesion, rather than a true three-dimensional volumetric map. The surgeon can also attempt to fill in the gaps intraoperatively with palpation (assuming the tumour is palpable), referring to preoperative imaging, and specimen imaging intraoperatively.

15.11.1 Breast Cancer Locator™

Current localisation techniques localise a single point (the device) during excision surgery. Breast Cancer Locator™ (CairnSurgical, New Hampshire, The United States of America) aims to visualise the tumour bed and the volume for excision rather than a single point. It requires patients to have a prone and supine MRI mapping of the tumour bed [21].

The device is a patient-specific bra-like plastic form that is designed using the supine MRI. It is printed out, delivered to the surgeon, and placed temporarily on the breast after anaesthetic induction, with a cutout for the nipple allowing correct orientation. Further small holes allow the surgeon to mark the cancer's borders on the skin, with larger holes allowing for the insertion of wires at the centre and periphery of the cancer with a 1 cm margin. The BCL™ can then be removed and surgery can proceed to cut around the wires that mark a clear margin around the tumour bed [21].

The BCL™ is coupled with a visualizer: a virtual 3D view of the cancer that the surgeon can refer to with pertinent measurements such as the dimensions of the cancer and its distance to the skin and chest wall. The optimal specimen volume is also provided. A pilot study first carried out on palpable cancers [21] has informed a recently published paper using BCL™ on non-palpable cancers in 33 patients, with promising results [22]. An international randomised study of the device has now fully recruited with results awaited to see if MRI guidance can reduce re-excision rate [23].

15.11.2 EnVisio™

A different recent device is perhaps more similar to its antecedents. The EnVisio™ Surgical Navigation System (Elucent, Minnesota, The United States of America) utilises SmartClips™: wireless soft tissue markers that are inserted any time before surgery. Each clip has a unique signal that relays information to a pad placed under the patient. This pad generates electromagnetic waves to track the smart clips relative to the position of a transducer that is attached to the surgeon's electrocautery instrument. This is also relayed to a wire navigation screen thus producing an integrated system wherein the surgeon can see on the screen the distance (in millimetres), depth, and direction between the instrument and the individual SmartClips™ (with their own unique colour on screen) [24]. A pilot study on the EnVisio™ Surgical Navigation system at a single site with 22 patients has again shown promise, with no re-excisions or close margins reported [24].

15.11.3 NaviKnife

Finally, the NaviKnife (Queen's University, Ontario, Canada—supported by the Canadian Institutes of Health Research) is another device seeking to give surgeons 3D information on the tumour and its ideal margins. It is derived from WGL: a needle is inserted into or near a cancer under ultrasound guidance intraoperatively and hooked wires are deployed to prevent slippage of the needle. A tracker on the base of the needle ensures the tumour position is always known. A navigation system uses the tumour position information alongside information from the ultrasound machine and position trackers on the electrocautery instrument and a reference point [25]. This information is fed into a mounted display that shows a 3D image of the tumour with respect to the electrocautery device. The green 3D tumour model turns red when the surgeon enters the tumour—giving real-time feedback on when a surgeon needs to withdraw to maintain the oncological margin. This feasibility study of 40 patients again demonstrated positive results with ease of use and a reduction in resection size being highlighted [26].

15.12 Chapter Summary

WGL has been the gold-standard as a localisation technique and maintains its position as an effective and cheap solution. However, there now exist a variety of devices that clinicians can choose from that provide a single point of reference within the breast tissue and enable the device placement to be uncoupled from the date of surgery, providing logistical advantages. Prospective post-marketing surveillance has provided good data on efficacy and logistical benefits but have not directly compared new technologies with each other.

The reasons that RCTs are challenging as regards surgical innovations have been clearly laid out by the IDEAL collaborative, who have set out a clear framework to approach researching new devices, with the ultimate goal of producing high-quality RCTs.

Recognising these challenges and evidence gaps, clinicians should be, and are, working together on the national and international level to participate in large-scale audits (iBRA-NET, UK) and trials (MELODY, Europe). These examples have already proven to be very efficient in recruiting clinicians and patients, further overcoming some of the shortfalls of traditional research by incorporating shared learning and following standardised protocols. This helps to ensure adequate device surveillance wherein any problems with—or improvements to—techniques can be shared quickly, addressing the issue of the learning curve that arises with adopting a novel method as well as helping to maintain safety for patients.

There is still a role for RCTs, an example being MAGTOTAL, which has shown that innovation breeds further innovation by providing evidence for a 'totally magnetic' technique. RCTs ultimately are the best way of collecting prospective data sets and allowing direct robust comparison between devices. Prospective audits enable us to provide relatively high-quality data to power the subsequent studies.

The development of new devices requires strong collaboration between clinicians and commercial partners, not only for the development of new techniques, but also to devise a research development strategy. This strategy aims to combine the needs of patients and clinicians for strong efficacy data and the commercial needs of manufacturers to demonstrate the benefits of their potential new product.

Finally, in the same way that the past decade has seen the move from WGL to modern devices, innovation will continue in the coming years. Devices are being developed that aim to provide three-dimensional real-time feedback to surgeons.

15.13 Tips and Pitfalls

Tip: Despite its flaws, wire-guided localisation remains the gold standard for breast cancer localisation, with the highest level of evidence (Cochrane review) affirming this.

Tip: Collaboration between industry and clinicians is key to the development of new devices and to ensure research and development is at the heart of the commercial strategy.

Tip: Collaboration is key for future research—multicentre studies overall accelerate recruitment, reduce bias, and help standardise technique and terminology.

Tip: There is no gold standard for incorporating shared learning into a study, but mixed-method approaches (e.g. structured reporting plus focus groups) can provide both quantitative trends and qualitative insights.

Tip: Shared learning does not happen automatically; it needs structure, accountability, and leadership within collaborative networks.

Tip: Modestly sized RCTs can answer focused, practical questions and should be used to clarify specific uncertainties for devices.

Pitfall: Avoid conflating 'preference for change' with proven superiority—many reported advantages are logistical, not oncological.

Pitfall: A randomised control trial remains the best way to prove the efficacy of any new technique compared to the gold standard, but one must consider the time and cost it takes to produce results for surgical interventions.

Pitfall: Consider how studies handle shared learning and adverse event reporting—by leaving their analysis until the end they may not be addressing the learning curve and preventing patient harm.

Pitfalls: Patients and the public do not perceive the safety of a new equipment as high a priority as other research targets—consider whether a study is involving these stakeholders and addressing their priorities.

References

1. Dua SM, Gray RJ, Keshtgar M. Strategies for localisation of impalpable breast lesions. Breast. 2011;20(3):246–53.
2. Tabár L, Dean PB, Chen TH, Yen AM, Chen SL, Fann JC, Chiu SY, Ku MM, Wu WY, Hsu CY, Chen YC. The incidence of fatal breast cancer measures the increased effectiveness of therapy in women participating in mammography screening. Cancer. 2019;125(4):515–23.
3. Chan BK, Wiseberg-Firtell JA, Jois RH, Jensen K, Audisio RA. Localization techniques for guided surgical excision of non-palpable breast lesions. Cochrane Database Syst Rev. 2015;2015(12):CD009206.
4. Schermers B, van Riet YE, Schipper RJ, Vrancken Peeters MJ, Voogd AC, Nieuwenhuijzen GA, Ten Haken B, Ruers TJ. Nationwide registry study on trends in localization techniques and reoperation rates in non-palpable ductal carcinoma in situ and invasive breast cancer. Br J Surg. 2022;109(1):53–60.
5. Somasundaram SK, Potter S, Elgammal S, Maxwell AJ, Sami AS, Down SK, Dave RV, Harvey J. Impalpable breast lesion localisation, a logistical challenge: results of the UK iBRA-NET national practice questionnaire. Breast Cancer Res Treat. 2021;185(1):13–20.
6. Mavor F, Somasundaram SK, Carmichael AR, Elgammal S, Foster R, Lowes S, Masannat Y, Milligan R, Morgan JL, St John ER, Vidya R. Adoption of nonwire localisation devices in UK breast units: an iBRA-NET survey to assess changes in practice. Ann R Coll Surg Engl. 2025. https://doi.org/10.1308/rcsann.2024.0106.

7. Banys-Paluchowski M, Kühn T, Masannat Y, Rubio I, de Boniface J, Ditsch N, Karadeniz Cakmak G, Karakatsanis A, Dave R, Hahn M, Potter S. Localization techniques for non-palpable breast lesions: current status, knowledge gaps, and rationale for the MELODY study (EUBREAST-4/iBRA-NET, NCT 05559411). Cancer. 2023;15(4):1173.
8. Morgan JL, Bromley HL, Dave RV, Masannat Y, Masudi T, Mylvaganam S, Elgammal S, Barnes N, Down S, Holcombe C, Potter S. Results of shared learning of a new magnetic seed localisation device–a UK iBRA-NET breast cancer localisation study. Eur J Surg Oncol. 2022;48(12):2408–13.
9. Seifalian A, Basma Z, Digesu A, Khullar V. Polypropylene pelvic mesh: what went wrong and what will be of the future? Biomedicines. 2023;11(3):741.
10. Haskell H. Cumberlege review exposes stubborn and dangerous flaws in healthcare. BMJ. 2020;370:m3099.
11. McCulloch P, Altman DG, Campbell WB, Flum DR, Glasziou P, Marshall JC, Nicholl J. No surgical innovation without evaluation: the IDEAL recommendations. Lancet. 2009;374(9695):1105–12.
12. Ergina PL, Cook JA, Blazeby JM, Boutron I, Clavien PA, Reeves BC, Seiler CM. Challenges in evaluating surgical innovation. Lancet. 2009;374(9695):1097–104.
13. Davey MG, O'Donnell JP, Boland MR, Ryan ÉJ, Walsh SR, Kerin MJ, Lowery AJ. Optimal localization strategies for non-palpable breast cancers–a network meta-analysis of randomized controlled trials. Breast. 2022;62:103–13.
14. Taylor DB, Bourke AG, Westcott EJ, Marinovich ML, Chong CY, Liang R, Hughes RL, Elder E, Saunders CM. Surgical outcomes after radioactive 125I seed versus hookwire localization of non-palpable breast cancer: a multicentre randomized clinical trial. Br J Surg. 2021;108(1):40–8.
15. World Alliance for Patient Safety; World Health Organization. WHO draft guidelines for adverse event reporting and learning systems: from information to action. Geneva: World Health Organization; 2005. WHO Reference Number: WHO/EIP/SPO/QPS/05.3. Available from: https://www.who.int/publications/i/item/WHO-EIP-SPO-QPS-05.3.
16. Dave RV, Barrett E, Morgan J, Chandarana M, Elgammal S, Barnes N, Sami A, Masudi T, Down S, Holcombe C, Potter S. Wire-and magnetic-seed-guided localization of impalpable breast lesions: iBRA-NET localisation study. Br J Surg. 2022;109(3):274–82.
17. Bromley HL, Dave R, Holcombe C, Potter S, Maxwell AJ, Kirwan C, Mylvaganam S, Elgammal S, Morgan J, Down S, Masudi T. A novel mixed-methods platform study protocol for investigating new surgical devices, with embedded shared learning: iBRA-NET breast lesion localisation study. Int J Surg Protoc. 2021;25(1):26–33.
18. Morgan JL, Harvey J, Lowes S, Milligan R, Krizak S, Masannat Y, Carmichael A, Elgammal S, Youssef M, Petralia G, Dave RV. Results of shared learning of a new radiofrequency identification localization device—a UK iBRA-NET breast cancer localisation study. Clin Radiol. 2024;79(11):e1288–95.
19. Pantiora E, Jazrawi A, Hersi AF, Abdsaleh S, Ahlstedt H, Molnar E, Wärnberg F, Eriksson S, Karakatsanis A. Magnetic seed vs guidewire breast cancer localization with magnetic lymph node detection: a randomized clinical trial. JAMA Surg. 2024;159(3):239–46.
20. Wilson RL, Boundouki G, Jackson RJ, Dave RV, Harvey JR, Wray J, Ballance L, Henderson JR, Duxbury P, Ibrahim I, Appanah V. Breast cancer research gaps: a questionnaire-based study to determine overall priorities and compare the priorities of patients, the public, clinicians and scientists. BMJ Open. 2024;14(8):e084573.
21. Barth RJ Jr, Krishnaswamy V, Paulsen KD, Rooney TB, Wells WA, Rizzo E, Angeles CV, Marotti JD, Zuurbier RA, Black CC. A patient-specific 3D-printed form accurately transfers supine MRI-derived tumor localization information to guide breast-conserving surgery. Ann Surg Oncol. 2017;24(10):2950–6.

22. Thill M, Ghilli M, Roncella M, Kelling K, Fansa H, Golatta M, Heil J, Haasteren V, Freitag A, Togawa R, Sagona A. A multi-institutional study to evaluate the effectiveness and safety of a supine MRI-based guidance system, the breast cancer LocatorTM, for breast conserving surgery in patients with nonpalpable breast cancer. Ann Surg Oncol. 2025;6:1–8.
23. ClinicalTrials.gov [Internet]. NCT04397185: randomized prospective trial of Breast Cancer Locator guided vs. wire-localized partial mastectomy for breast cancer. United States. [2020] [cited 2025 Oct 1]. Available from: https://clinicaltrials.gov/study/NCT04397185.
24. Carlson KA, Checka C, Hunt KK, Jung J, Bridges C, Singh P, Refinetti A, Moseley T, Perez F, Mayo C, Tamirisa N. Evaluation of a surgical navigation system for localization and excision of nonpalpable lesions in breast and axillary surgery. Breast J. 2023;2023(1):9993852.
25. Ungi T, Gauvin G, Lasso A, Yeo CT, Pezeshki P, Vaughan T, Carter K, Rudan J, Engel CJ, Fichtinger G. Navigated breast tumor excision using electromagnetically tracked ultrasound and surgical instruments. IEEE Trans Biomed Eng. 2015;63(3):600–6.
26. Gauvin G, Yeo CT, Ungi T, Merchant S, Lasso A, Jabs D, Vaughan T, Rudan JF, Walker R, Fichtinger G, Engel CJ. Real-time electromagnetic navigation for breast-conserving surgery using NaviKnife technology: a matched case-control study. Breast J. 2020;26(3):399–405.

Chapter 16
The Future of Breast and Axilla Localisation

Raghavan Vidya and Nisha Sharma

Contents

16.1 Introduction

Globally, breast cancer remains the most common cancer, with early detection and precision surgical treatment being vital to improving survival and quality of life. Central to this surgical strategy is the accurate localisation of impalpable breast and axillary disease. As breast oncological surgery is shifting towards minimally invasive, conservative approach, the demand for safe, accurate, and patient-centred localisation techniques have grown.

R. Vidya (✉)
Department of Breast Surgery, The Royal Wolverhampton NHS Trust, Wolverhampton, UK
e-mail: Raghavan.Vidya@nhs.net

N. Sharma
Department of Breast Radiology, St. James's University Hospital, Leeds, UK
e-mail: nisha.sharma2@nhs.net

R. Vidya, N. Sharma (eds.), *Breast and Axilla Localisation Techniques*,
https://doi.org/10.1007/978-3-032-17995-1_16

While conventional methods such as wire-guided localisation have laid the foundation for lesion localisation, they have drawbacks including workflow inflexibility, dislocation, and patient discomfort. Hence, new methods of localisation have emerged including radiation free, wireless alternatives with improved patient-centred care.

In the future, a new wave of innovations is poised to revolutionise localisation entirely, leveraging real-time imaging, machine learning, nanotechnology, and augmented reality to enable more accurate, less invasive, and more adaptive surgical interventions [1, 2].

16.2 Emerging Technologies

The present localisation technologies including mechanical and radioactive systems would be replaced by digital and biological innovation. These systems are less invasive and offer higher integration with diagnostic imaging and intraoperative navigation.

16.2.1 Image-Guided and Fluorescence-Guided Surgery

Indocyanine Green (ICG) fluorescence imaging represents a particularly promising innovation for localisation. It provides real-time, high-contrast visualisation, aiding in the precise localisation of breast lesions and axillary targets. ICG fluorescence is a radiation-free localisation technique providing dynamic, intraoperative feedback to the surgeon [3, 4]. Optical Coherence Tomography (OCT) provides microscopic, high-resolution cross-sectional imaging of tissue microstructure. This enables precise delineation of tumour margins and aids accurate intraoperative decision-making in breast-conserving surgery [5]. Similarly, Near-Infrared Fluorescence (NIRF) imaging systems use a combination of real-time fluorescence imaging with molecular specificity. This enables the potential to improve margin assessment, optimise resection accuracy, and enhance cosmetic outcomes [6, 7].

Together, these image-guided and fluorescence-based technologies mark a transition towards precision-guided breast and axillary surgery. As imaging resolution, intraoperative integration, and molecular targeting continue to advance, these techniques are likely to play an increasingly central role in the future of breast and axilla localisation.

16.2.2 Nanotechnology and Theranostic Agents

Nanotechnology is offering new horizons for dual-function agents that provide both localisation and treatment, referred to as theranostics. Theranostic agents can be engineered to target tumour-specific receptors or microenvironments. For instance, iron oxide nanoparticles coated with antibodies can be visualised via MRI while simultaneously delivering cytotoxic agents directly to tumour tissue. Gold nanoparticles, owing to their photothermal properties, can support both localisation and ablation during surgery [8, 9].

The combination of diagnostic and therapeutic functionality is being explored in ongoing trials and may offer unprecedented precision in both detecting and treating breast and axillary lesions. Such novel techniques promise to decrease the need for repeated interventions and may contribute to tumour eradication during a single surgical encounter [10].

16.2.3 Artificial Intelligence and Machine Learning

Artificial intelligence (AI) is revolutionising breast imaging interpretation, and AI algorithms can automatically detect impalpable lesions, classify tumour types, and predict the possibility of axillary nodal metastasis based on imaging and histopathological features. Deep learning models have demonstrated performance that can match or exceed human capability, particularly in detecting subtle abnormalities [11, 12].

In the future, integration of AI in the operating theatre with intraoperative imaging systems, including recognition of anatomical landmarks, will guide localisation of tumours both in the breast and axilla while providing information on tumour margins. This technology may be particularly valuable in dense breast tissue. Furthermore, AI can assist in post-operative assessments, helping predict recurrence risk or the need for adjuvant therapy based on surgical outcomes and tumour characteristics [13, 14].

16.2.4 Augmented Reality and 3D Visualisation

Augmented reality (AR) is transforming surgical navigation by overlaying critical preoperative imaging data directly onto the patient in real time. 3D visualisation supports enhanced preoperative planning. The use of head-mounted displays or projection-based systems permits the surgeon to visualise tissue and locate structures including lesions or lymph nodes non-invasively [15, 16].

Patient-specific models generated from imaging scans provide tangible representations of tumour location and surrounding anatomy. These models have proved useful in both educational environments and multidisciplinary tumour boards, leading to improved surgical consensus and execution [17].

16.2.5 Smart Implants and Biosensors

Smart implants appear to be at the forefront of emerging real-time monitoring with localisation. Biosensors embedded in biocompatible implants can detect microenvironmental changes such as pH, temperature, or oxygen saturation, which can wirelessly transmit data, enabling continuous intraoperative or postoperative monitoring [18, 19]. The real-time detection provides dynamic updates on tumour status during surgery or follow-up care. While still largely experimental, these devices could represent the next leap in combining diagnostics, monitoring, and therapy in a seamless manner. The integration of emerging novel technologies provides a platform towards non-invasive, intelligent, and hyper-personalised localisation systems, which will also support and transform surgical planning, execution, and follow-up.

16.2.6 Personalised Localisation Pathways

The progressive evolution of precision medicine will lead to localisation protocols tailored to an individual's tumour biology, clinical risk profiles, and radiogenomic signatures. AI-based intelligent decision-support systems could recommend optimal localisation techniques based on real-time integration of imaging, pathology, and molecular data. For instance, patients undergoing neoadjuvant therapy or with triple-negative breast cancer may benefit from more precise localisation approaches given their higher likelihood of multifocal disease [20, 21]. In the future, multidisciplinary tumour boards may adopt digital twins—virtual models of individual patients that simulate surgical outcomes and help to guide decisions. This would enable personalised planning adopting AI-predicted response models, enabling dynamic, flexible, adaptable preparatory tool for treating individual patients.

16.2.7 Integration with Smart Operating Rooms

Future theatres will be built as intelligent environments, where devices and systems interact seamlessly. AI-driven platforms and robotic-assisted surgery will integrate intelligence-driven localisation and imaging data in real time. This would enable precise patient-centred mapping, intraoperative margin assessment, and targeted node mapping with fluorescence overlays [22, 23]. Voice-commanded navigation, gesture-control interfaces, and intraoperative analytics dashboards could become part of routine practice, allowing the surgeon to operate within a highly responsive, data-rich ecosystem. This would minimise cognitive load while improving surgical accuracy and safety.

16.2.8 Non-invasive and Real-Time Localisation

New technologies and research are now focused on novel non-contact localisation techniques, eliminating the need for any form of physical marker placement. Emerging imaging modalities including photoacoustic imaging, hyperspectral imaging, and high-resolution elastography can detect tumour boundaries based on tissue optical and acoustic properties [24].

Real-time feedback from techniques such as contrast-enhanced ultrasound or dynamic optical imaging, when coupled with machine learning interpretation, can lead to the development of autonomous or semi-autonomous surgical localisation systems. These systems would be capable of adjusting a surgeon's technique in response to intraoperative changes, offering a powerful avenue for precision medicine.

16.2.9 Ethical Considerations and Data Privacy

Ethical considerations are paramount with the progressive development and advancements in localisation technologies. The combination of AI and digital imaging generates enormous data, which mandates careful monitoring with robust frameworks needed for security and ownership while addressing ethical dilemmas and biases. Clearly informed consent processes would need to mirror the evolving landscape and promote patient-centred care [25, 26].

16.2.10 Health Equity and Access to Innovation

Advancement in localisation technologies must be balanced against the potential to exacerbate healthcare disparities. Expensive tools such as robotic systems, augmented reality platforms, and AI systems may not be universally accessible, particularly in under-resourced health systems. It can pave the way leading to a digital divide between high- and low-income countries and resulting in wider inequities in cancer outcomes. Global collaborations with low-cost, open-access technologies can provide the solution to mitigate this risk. Furthermore, clinical trials need to ensure diverse involvement to make innovations generalisable across populations and healthcare settings [23].

16.3 Conclusion

The evolution from wire-localised to wireless technologies is a major step forward in managing non-palpable breast and axillary lesions. Advances in technology have led to precision surgery, greater flexibility, and improved patient-centred care. The future depends on combining artificial intelligence, engineering, and biology with data science, paving the pathway to novel innovations and personalised care.

References

1. Masud M, Rahman A, Chowdhury S, Patel V. AI in breast cancer localisation: current evidence and future prospects. J Surg Innov. 2023;30(2):130–41. https://doi.org/10.1177/15533506221150495.
2. Kuemmel S, Krug D, Holtschmidt J, Kühn T. Emerging tools for axillary lymph node localisation. Eur J Surg Oncol. 2020;46(8):1445–51. https://doi.org/10.1016/j.ejso.2020.03.016.
3. Ogasawara Y, Ikeda T, Nakamura M, Sato K. Near-infrared fluorescence imaging with indocyanine green for sentinel node detection in breast cancer. Breast Cancer Res Treat. 2021;187(2):345–53. https://doi.org/10.1007/s10549-021-06180-2.
4. Bloomquist EV, As'adi N, Garcia M, Li J. Fluorescence-guided surgery in breast oncology: a systematic review. Ann Surg Oncol. 2019;26(1):325–34. https://doi.org/10.1245/s10434-018-07089-3.
5. Kang JW, Park SY, Choi JH, Kim SH. Optical molecular imaging in breast cancer: current state and future directions. Cancers (Basel). 2020;12(6):1608. https://doi.org/10.3390/cancers12061608.
6. Yang Y, Zhang Q, Chen L, Liu X. Nanoparticles in surgical oncology: applications for localisation and drug delivery. Cancer Nanotechnol. 2022;13(1):16. https://doi.org/10.1186/s12645-022-00109-7.
7. Sun T, Zhang Y, Wang H, Li J. Smart theranostic nanoplatforms for cancer diagnosis and therapy. ACS Nano. 2021;15(1):50–70. https://doi.org/10.1021/acsnano.0c08174.
8. Riley RS, Day ES, Zeman KL, West JL. Nanotechnology for cancer diagnosis and therapy: recent advances. ACS Nano. 2019;13(3):2831–50. https://doi.org/10.1021/acsnano.8b08756.
9. McKinney SM, Sieniek M, Godbole V, Liu Y. International evaluation of an AI system for breast cancer screening. Nature. 2020;577(7788):89–94. https://doi.org/10.1038/s41586-019-1799-6.
10. Kontos D, Bakic PR, McCarthy AM, Conant EF. Artificial intelligence in breast imaging: a radiologist's perspective. Acad Radiol. 2021;28(2):259–69. https://doi.org/10.1016/j.acra.2020.10.002.
11. Ahmed M, Rossi P, Patel K, Thomas S. Augmented reality in surgical oncology: a new frontier. J Surg Technol. 2021;24(2):157–69. https://doi.org/10.1177/1553350620958611.
12. Fotouhi J, Armand M, Navab N, Sauer F. Navigated augmented reality in breast surgery: a feasibility study. PLoS One. 2019;14(10):e0223164. https://doi.org/10.1371/journal.pone.0223164.
13. Cho HH, Kim MJ, Park JH, Lee SY. 3D printing in breast cancer surgery: potential and current limitations. Breast. 2022;65:24–30. https://doi.org/10.1016/j.breast.2022.06.002.
14. Park S, Lee J, Kim D, Cho K. Implantable biosensors for real-time cancer monitoring. Adv Healthc Mater. 2020;9(22):e2001157. https://doi.org/10.1002/adhm.202001157.
15. Dong Y, Wang J, Chen X, Huang P. Smart implants in oncologic surgery: an overview. Sensors (Basel). 2021;21(11):3788. https://doi.org/10.3390/s21113788.

16. Houssami N, Cuzick J, Dixon JM, Lord SJ. Predicting lymph node metastasis in breast cancer: molecular subtypes and clinical variables. Breast Cancer Res. 2018;20(1):140. https://doi.org/10.1186/s13058-018-1065-x.
17. Duffy MJ, Crown J, Mullooly M, Nicolini A. Personalised medicine and tumour markers: current concepts and future perspectives. Crit Rev Clin Lab Sci. 2021;58(4):283–94. https://doi.org/10.1080/10408363.2020.1834277.
18. Hashimoto DA, Rosman G, Rus D, Meireles OR. Artificial intelligence in surgery: promises and perils. Ann Surg. 2020;271(4):610–5. https://doi.org/10.1097/SLA.0000000000002693.
19. Müller PC, Wengenmayer T, Clavien PA, Käser SA. The smart operating room: surgical data science and digital surgery. Ann Surg Oncol. 2021;28(10):5543–53. https://doi.org/10.1245/s10434-021-09852-z.
20. Houssami N, Cuzick J, Dixon JM, Lord SJ. Predicting lymph node metastasis in breast cancer. Breast Cancer Res. 2018;20(1):140.
21. Duffy MJ, Crown J, Mullooly M, Nicolini A. Personalised medicine and tumour markers. Crit Rev Clin Lab Sci. 2021;58(4):283–94.
22. Hashimoto DA, Rosman G, Rus D, Meireles OR. Artificial intelligence in surgery. Ann Surg. 2020;271(4):610–5.
23. Müller PC, Wengenmayer T, Clavien PA, Käser SA. The smart operating room. Ann Surg Oncol. 2021;28(10):5543–53.
24. Kang JW, Park SY, Choi JH, Kim SH. Optical molecular imaging in breast cancer. Cancers (Basel). 2020;12(6):1608.
25. Hashimoto DA, Rosman G, Rus D, Meireles OR. AI in surgery: promises and perils. Ann Surg. 2020;271(4):610–5.
26. Müller PC, Wengenmayer T, Clavien PA, Käser SA. Surgical data science and digital surgery. Ann Surg Oncol. 2021;28(10):5543–53.

Batch number: 10726060

Printed by Printforce, the Netherlands